A COMPREHENSIVE REVIEW OF URTICARIA AND ANGIOEDEMA

Edited by **Selda Pelin Kartal** and **Zekayi Kutlubay**

A Comprehensive Review of Urticaria and Angioedema
http://dx.doi.org/10.5772/65526
Edited by Selda Pelin Kartal and Zekayi Kutlubay

Contributors
Jesús Jurado-Palomo, Alexandru Daniel Vlagea, Teresa Caballero, Irina Bobolea, Ragıp Ertaş, Asli Gelincik, Semra Demir, Selda Pelin Kartal, Isil Bulur, Hilal Gokalp, Sevgi Akarsu, Ecem Canturk, Müzeyyen Gönül, Havva Hilal Ayvaz, Erol Koc, Asli Gunaydin Tatliparmak, Berna Aksoy, Burhan Engin, M Çiğdem Oba, Server Serdaroglu, murat borlu, Salih Levent Cinar, Demet Kartal, Emel Calikoglu, Asli Feride Kaptanoglu, Didem Mullaaziz

Published by InTech
Janeza Trdine 9, 51000 Rijeka, Croatia

Publishing Process Manager Maja Bozicevic
Technical Editor SPi Global
Cover InTech Design team

First published May, 2017
Printed in Croatia
Legal deposit, Croatia: National and University Library in Zagreb

Additional hard copies can be obtained from orders@intechopen.com

A Comprehensive Review of Urticaria and Angioedema, Edited by Selda Pelin Kartal and Zekayi Kutlubay
p. cm.
Print ISBN 978-953-51-3167-0
Online ISBN 978-953-51-3168-7

Meet the editors

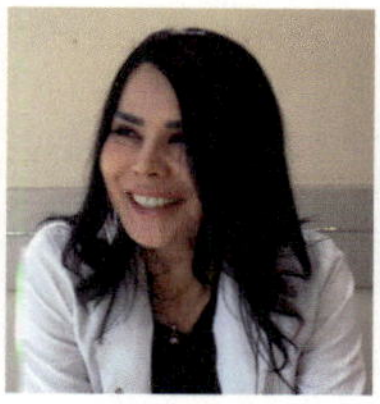

Assoc. Prof. Dr. Selda Pelin Kartal graduated from Hacettepe University School of Medicine. Currently, she is an Associate Professor in the Department of Dermatology at University of Health Sciences, Dışkapı Yıldırım Beyazıt Training and Research Hospital in Ankara, Turkey. She has co-authored over 100 published articles and supervised several master's and postdoctoral students. Her actual interests are focused on acne, psoriasis, urticaria, autoimmune bullous diseases, Behçet's disease and cosmetic dermatology.

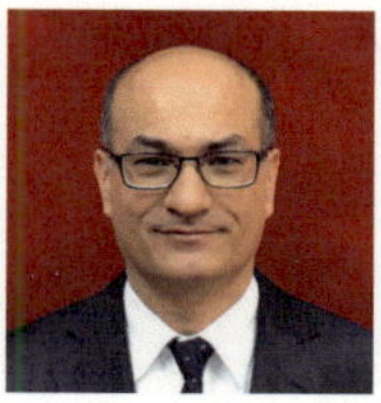

Zekayi Kutlubay, MD, is a chief physician of Istanbul University Cerrahpasa Medical Faculty Hospital. He is also an Associate Professor in the Department of Dermatology at Istanbul University Cerrahpasa Medical Faculty in Turkey. He has co-authored over 50 publications and supervised several master's, doctoral, and postdoctoral students. His actual research interests are focused on psoriasis, pediatric dermatology, autoimmune bullous diseases, urticaria and allergic diseases, Behçet's disease, vasculitis, lasers, cosmetic dermatology, facial rejuvenation, hair diseases, mesotherapy, botulinum toxin, and fillers.

Contents

Preface

The aim of this book is to give readers a broad review of urticaria and angioedema, which may affect people from birth to death, and their treatment options. The book contains the latest advances and scientific knowledge from the leading experts.

The book consists of 15 chapters in which urticaria classification, urticaria etiopathogenesis, urticaria clinics, urticarial syndromes, angioedemas, diagnosis, pathogenesis and pathophysiology of urticaria, and treatment options are discussed. This book also emphasizes on the various laboratory tests necessary for urticarias. One chapter of the book is devoted to comorbidities in chronic spontaneous urticaria. Another chapter is related with pathophysiology and treatment of hereditary angioedema.

We are thankful to our families for understanding our missed family time and grateful to all the contributors and leading experts for their valuable chapters, which provide an in-depth view of all aspects of the content.

We express our heartfelt gratitude to magnificent Ataturk who said "Our true mentor in life is science" and inspired us the importance of working on positive science.

Assoc. Prof. Dr. Selda Pelin Kartal
University of Health Sciences,
Department of Dermatology,
Dışkapı Yıldırım Beyazıt Training and Research Hospital in Ankara,
Turkey

Assoc. Prof. Dr. Zekayi Kutlubay
Istanbul Cerrahpasa University,
Department of Dermatology,
Turkey

Section 1

Introduction

Chapter 1

Introductory Chapter: Urticaria

Selda Pelin Kartal, Uğur Çelik and Zekayi Kutlubay

Additional information is available at the end of the chapter

http://dx.doi.org/10.5772/intechopen.68997

1. Introduction

Urticaria, also known as hives, is a common pruritic skin disease which is characterized by erythematous and edematous papules and plaques. These lesions have a transient nature which means a single-lesion heals within 24 h but new lesions may occur recurrently. The disease may be idiopathic or inducible and it is called chronic when intermittent attacks last for more than 6 weeks [1].

The lifetime prevalence of urticaria is 10–20%, while this rate is approximately 2% in its chronic form [1, 2]. Urticaria can occur at any age but the chronic urticaria form is more common in adults. The disease can affect both genders but female predominance is evident [2].

Cutaneous mast cells and mediators that are released as a result of mast cell degranulation are located at the center of urticaria pathogenesis [3]. Triggering factors may cause mast cell degranulation via different mechanisms such as direct activation or IgE-mediated allergic activation. The common outcomes are the release of mediators such as histamine and their clinical effects. Beside pruritus, these vasoactive mediators are responsible for vasodilation and subsequent erythema and edema [3, 4]. Activation of mast cells in superficial dermis causes urticarial papules and plaques while angioedema occurs as a result of mast cell involvement in deeper tissues [5].

There are many triggering factors for urticaria but determining a specific cause is not always possible. This quest is more complicated in some cases, especially in chronic ones. In addition to classification as acute or chronic, the disease may also be defined with etiologic factors, such as physically induced, autoimmune, or idiopathic urticarial [6]. Drugs, viral, bacterial or parasitic infections, insect bites, foods, physical factors, autoimmune diseases, and emotional stress are leading causes in etiology [6, 7].

It is known that infections may cause urticaria but the mechanism is unclear [8]. It is also difficult to determine if the trigger was an infection or a drug used for the treatment of infection. Nonsteroidal anti-inflammatory drugs and antibiotics, especially beta lactams, constitute a significant proportion of drug etiology. These drugs mainly cause urticarial reaction via

IgE-mediated immunologic pathways [9]. In addition, some drugs such as vancomycin, narcotic analgesics, barbiturates, neuromuscular blockers, and radiocontrast agents may cause urticarial eruption via direct mast cell degranulation [9, 10]. Nonsteroidal anti-inflammatory drugs may also trigger urticaria by interfering with arachidonic acid metabolism via cyclo-oxygenase 1 enzyme inhibition. This blockage leads to increased synthesis of cysteinyl leukotrienes. This form of urticarial reaction is called pseudoallergy [10].

Physically induced urticarias are thought to occur as a result of increased mast cell sensitivity to environmental stimuli. Physical factors that may trigger urticaria include ultraviolet light, pressure, vibration, exercise, water contact, cold or heat exposures, and increased body temperature [11].

Systemic diseases can also be the underlying cause of urticaria. Therefore, the presence of any accompanying systemic symptoms is significant. Autoimmune and rheumatologic diseases constitute the majority of this group [12]. Systemic diseases include cutaneous vasculitis, systemic lupus erythematosus, celiac disease, diabetes mellitus, Sjögren's syndrome, rheumatoid arthritis, autoimmune thyroid disease, and mastocytosis [1, 12]. Malignancies may also trigger urticaria and the disease tends to be persistent in this case [13].

Elementary lesion of urticarial eruption is papule or plaque with erythema and edema. Circumscribed, pink-to-red lesions elevated from the skin vary in size and shape. These plaques which may tend to merge with central pallor can affect any region of the body [14]. Pruritus is the main annoying symptom which mostly interferes with daily activities of the patients [15]. Although a single urticarial lesion is transient, repetitive character of the eruption is a significant problem. Lesions persisting beyond 24 h with residual petechia or hyperpigmentation, especially if accompanied by systemic symptoms such as fever and arthralgia, may suggest urticarial vasculitis in differential diagnosis and warrant skin biopsy [16].

Angioedema may accompany urticaria if the mast cells in the deeper dermis and subcutaneous tissue were involved in reactions. When this occurs, the lips and eyelids are the regions mainly affected [1]. Urticaria may also be a component of severe systemic allergic reactions, anaphylaxis, and so patients should always be examined for accompanying signs and symptoms such as flushing, swollen lips and tongue, difficulty in breathing, hoarse voice, hypotension, dizziness, hypotonia, syncope, nausea, vomiting, abdominal pain, and incontinence [17].

Diagnosis of urticaria is mostly based on anamnesis and physical examination. Due to the transient nature of the rash, there may be no lesions during a doctor visit. In this case, the clinical history of intensely pruritic lesions that heal within a few hours may be the only clue for urticaria diagnosis. In uncertain cases, asking patients to take a photo when they have a rash is a helpful method. It may be advisable to mark a single lesion and note the time it appeared and disappeared to determine the duration. Observation of characteristic erythematous and edematous papules and plaques supports the diagnosis. Association with angioedema and/or anaphylaxis should always be kept in mind and questioned [1, 2].

Skin biopsy is not indicated for the diagnosis of urticaria unless there is suspicion of urticarial vasculitis or mastocytosis. If vasculitis is suspected, an additional skin sample should be taken for immunofluorescence examination. Histopathological findings of urticaria include interstitial edema and perivascular mixed cellular infiltrate. T lymphocytes are predominant cells in this infiltrate but eosinophils, neutrophils, and basophils may also exist in a lesser extent [18]. Leukocytoclasis and fibrinoid necrosis of vessel walls are signs in favor of vasculitis [16].

Once the diagnosis is confirmed, it becomes important to find out triggering factors, if possible. Detailed anamnesis is important to determine any triggering medication, infection, or physical stimuli such as scratching, sunlight, pressure, heat or cold contact, exercise, and water. Challenge tests may be performed for the diagnosis of physical urticaria but caution should be exercised during the procedure because serious systemic allergic reactions can develop.

Autologous serum skin tests may be used to differentiate autoimmune urticaria, but patients should cease antihistamines at least 3 days prior to the procedure. In this subtype of urticaria, intradermal injection of patient's own serum results in an urticarial reaction within 30 min [19].

It is not indicated to use laboratory tests for patients with acute urticaria unless they have signs and symptoms suggesting an underlying systemic disease [1]. In chronic cases, initial laboratory examinations may include complete blood count, fasting blood glucose, erythrocyte sedimentation rate, C-reactive protein, kidney and liver function tests, urinalysis, and total serum Immunoglobulin-E levels. Additional tests such as antinuclear antibody, rheumatoid factor, complement C_3 and C_4 levels, thyroid hormones and autoantibodies, serology of Hepatitis viruses, *Helicobacter pylori* antigen, and fecal parasite examination can be performed if an infectious disease or an autoimmune disease is suspected [1, 12].

After diagnosis, determining the severity of the disease becomes important to evaluate the treatment response objectively. There are some scoring systems used for this purpose, one of which is the urticaria activity score (UAS). It is a widely used scoring system questioning the intensity of pruritus and the number of wheals in a day. Higher scores mean a more severe disease [20].

2. Conclusion

Generally, the disease is self-limited and it shows regression in a few weeks for most cases. Some patients may have persistent symptoms for months or years and the disease is considered chronic beyond 6 weeks.

If possible, the prevention of trigger is the first step of treatment. Treatment aim is to control symptoms with minimal side effects. H_1 antihistamines are the drugs most commonly used for this purpose. Second-generation H_1 antihistamines, such as cetirizine and loratadine, are used as first-line treatment options. These newer, non-sedative antihistamines are more preferred than first-generation ones such as hydroxyzine and diphenhydramine. First-generation antihistamines may have also the disadvantage of anticholinergic side effects in addition to their sedative effects. In unresponsive cases, dose increment up to fourfold of standard therapeutic doses is recommended by the latest guidelines [1, 21]. Increasing the dose of a particular antihistamine is thought to be superior to the combined use of multiple antihistamines at standard doses [21]. H_2 antihistamines may be used in combination with H_1 antihistamines.

Short-term systemic glucocorticoid therapy may be administered in addition to antihistamines for acute urticarial attacks, particularly when accompanied by angioedema [1]. Long-term usage of systemic glucocorticoids is not recommended because of potential side effects.

Antileukotrienes, such as montelukast and zafirlukast, are generally added to antihistamines as second-line treatment options in chronic cases refractory to high-dose antihistamines. Immunosuppressive agents, especially cyclosporine, are efficient to treat chronic urticaria but potential side effects must always be kept in mind. Dapsone, hydroxychloroquine, sulfasalazine, and mycophenolate are other less recommended drugs for the treatment of urticarial [1, 21]. Omalizumab, which is a safer alternative to those mentioned above, has recently come to the forefront in the treatment of chronic urticaria. It is an anti-IgE monoclonal antibody which has a good efficacy and safety profile [22, 23]. It also has the ease of use with monthly subcutaneous injections.

Since chronic urticaria treatment may become complicated, treatment switch, or combination is not surprising for most cases.

Author details

Selda Pelin Kartal[1], Uğur Çelik[2] and Zekayi Kutlubay[3]*

*Address all correspondence to: zekayikutlubay@hotmail.com

1 University of Health Sciences, Dışkapı Yıldırım Beyazıt Training and Research Hospital in Ankara, Turkey

2 Department of Dermatology, Şişli Hamidiye Etfal Research and Training Hospital, Istanbul, Turkey

3 Department of Dermatology, Cerrahpaşa Medical Faculty, Istanbul University, Istanbul, Turkey

References

[1] Zuberbier T, Aberer W, Asero R, et al. The EAACI/GA2LEN/EDF/WAO Guideline for the definition, classification, diagnosis, and management of urticaria: The 2013 revision and update. Allergy. 2014;**69**:868–887.

[2] Zuberbier T, Balke M, Worm M, Edenharter G, Maurer M. Epidemiology of urticaria: A representative cross-sectional population survey. Clinical and Experimental Dermatology. 2010;**35**:869–873.

[3] Tharp MD. Chronic urticaria: Pathophysiology and treatment approaches. Journal of Allergy and Clinical Immunology. 1996;**98**:325–330.

[4] Jain S. Pathogenesis of chronic urticaria: An overview. Dermatology Research and Practice. 2014;**2014**:674709.

[5] Faisant C, Boccon-Gibod I, Mansard C, et al. Idiopathic histaminergic angioedema without wheals: A case series of 31 patients. Clinical & Experimental Immunology. 2016;**185**:81–85.

[6] Saini SS. Chronic spontaneous urticaria: Etiology and pathogenesis. Immunology and Allergy Clinics of North America. 2014;**34**:33–52.

[7] Schocket AL. Chronic urticaria: Pathophysiology and etiology, or what and why. Allergy and Asthma Proceedings. 2006;**27**:90–95.

[8] Sackesen C, Sekerel BE, Orhan F, Kocabas CN, Tuncer A, Adalioglu G. The etiology of different forms of urticaria in childhood. Pediatric Dermatology. 2004;**21**:102–108.

[9] Mathelier-Fusade P. Drug-induced urticarias. Clinical Reviews in Allergy & Immunology. 2006;**30**:19–23.

[10] Farnam K, Chang C, Teuber S, Gershwin ME. Nonallergic drug hypersensitivity reactions. International Archives of Allergy and Immunology. 2012;**159**:327–345.

[11] Abajian M, Młynek A, Maurer M. Physical urticaria. Current Allergy and Asthma Reports. 2012;**12**:281–287.

[12] Confino-Cohen R, Chodick G, Shalev V, Leshno M, Kimhi O, Goldberg A. Chronic urticaria and autoimmunity: Associations found in a large population study. Journal of Allergy and Clinical Immunology. 2012;**129**:1307–1313.

[13] Zhang Y, Morita E, Matsuo H, Ueda D, Dekio S. Urticarial erythema associated with IgA myeloma. Journal of Dermatology. 2004;**31**:661–665.

[14] Poonawalla T, Kelly B. Urticaria: A review. American Journal of Clinical Dermatology. 2009;**10**:9–21.

[15] Choi WS, Lim ES, Ban GY, et al. Disease-specific impairment of the quality of life in adult patients with chronic spontaneous urticaria. Korean Journal of Internal Medicine. 2016 Jun 1. doi: 10.3904/kjim.2015.195. [Epub ahead of print].

[16] Chang S, Carr W. Urticarial vasculitis. Allergy and Asthma Proceedings. 2007;**28**:97–100.

[17] Simons FE. Anaphylaxis. Journal of Allergy and Clinical Immunology. 2010;**125**:161–181.

[18] Kaplan AP. Chronic urticaria: Pathogenesis and treatment. Journal of Allergy and Clinical Immunology. 2004;**114**:465–474.

[19] Kumar YH, Bhaskar S, Shankar K. Comparative study of positive versus negative autologous serum skin test in chronic spontaneous urticaria and its treatment outcome. North American Journal of Medical Sciences. 2016;**8**:25–30.

[20] Młynek A, Zalewska-Janowska A, Martus P, Staubach P, Zuberbier T, Maurer M. How to assess disease activity in patients with chronic urticaria? Allergy. 2008;**63**:777–780.

[21] Powell RJ, Leech SC, Till S, Huber PA, Nasser SM, Clark AT, British Society for Allergy and Clinical Immunology. BSACI guideline for the management of chronic urticaria and angioedema. Clinical & Experimental Allergy. 2015;**45**:547–565.

[22] Maurer M, Rosén K, Hsieh HJ, et al. Omalizumab for the treatment of chronic idiopathic or spontaneous urticaria. New England Journal of Medicine. 2013;**368**:924–935.

[23] Saini SS, Bindslev-Jensen C, Maurer M, et al. Efficacy and safety of omalizumab in patients with chronic idiopathic/spontaneous urticaria who remain symptomatic on H1 antihistamines: A randomized, placebo-controlled study. Journal of Investigative Dermatology. 2015;**135**:925.

Section 2

Urticaria and Angioedema

Chapter 2

Urticaria and Angioedema

Burhan Engin, Muazzez Çiğdem Oba and
Server Serdaroğlu

Additional information is available at the end of the chapter

http://dx.doi.org/10.5772/67772

Abstract

Urticaria is a common mast cell–mediated dermatosis presenting with pruritic erythematous superficial plaques also known as hives or wheals. Angioedema is an acute condition manifesting as localized edema affecting the skin and mucous membranes. In contrast with urticaria, itching is often absent, the skin appears normal and the edema occurs in deeper dermal and subcutaneous tissues in angioedema. Spontaneous urticaria can either be acute lasting less than 6 weeks or chronic with a duration of more than 6 weeks. In acute urticaria cases, an underlying cause, mostly medications, foods and infections, may be found in approximately 50% of patients. However, spontaneous urticaria is generally idiopathic. First-line treatment option for both acute and chronic urticaria is non-sedating H_1 antihistamines. Patients with recalcitrant disease are candidates for therapy with corticosteroids, immunosuppressives or omalizumab treatment. There are two different mechanisms causing angioedema. The first is mast cell mediated and is considered to be part of the spectrum of spontaneous or inducible urticarias. Patients present with angioedema alone or angioedema combined with urticaria. The second is bradykinin-induced angioedema, as observed in the hereditary angioedema and angiotensin-converting enzyme (ACE) inhibitor–induced angioedema.

Keywords: angioedema, spontaneous urticaria

1. Introduction

Urticaria is a common mast cell–mediated dermatosis presenting with pruritic erythematous superficial plaques also known as hives or wheals. There may be associated swelling in deep dermis or subcutaneous tissue leading to angioedema [1]. Angioedema is rather painful than pruritic and takes longer time to resolve in contrast to the wheals which usually disappear within 24 hours [2, 3]. The disease has considerable impact on patients' quality of life with dissatisfaction in private life and work being frequent [4]. Non-sedating H_1 antihistamines are the first line therapy for both acute and chronic urticaria. Apart from angioedema which is part of the spectrum of urticaria, there is bradykinin-induced angioedema, such as that observed in the hereditary angioedema characterized by angioedema without wheals. Management of isolated angioedema differs from that of urticaria involving both preventive measures and treatment of acute attacks [5].

2. Classification

The current classification of urticaria is based upon the clinical course of the disease. Subtypes include spontaneous urticaria, physical urticarias and other urticaria types [2]. Spontaneous urticaria can either be acute lasting less than 6 weeks or chronic with a duration of more than 6 weeks. This arbitrary division for chronicity has been made as the etiologies and thus the clinical evaluation of acute and chronic urticaria vary considerably [3]. The physical and other urticaria types are elicited by external stimuli, such as heat, cold, pressure, vibration, friction, sunlight, water, etc. [6]. These two subtypes of urticaria are beyond the scope of this chapter.

3. Epidemiology

An episode of urticaria can occur in 15–25% of individuals at some point in their lifetime. Approximately 40% of patients with urticaria have wheals associated with angioedema and 1–13% of patients present with isolated angioedema [3, 7]. Socioeconomic status, ethnicity and education do not have any clear influence on the prevalence of the disease [3].

At first all cases of urticaria are acute; 30% of them progress to become chronic [7]. Acute episodic form of urticaria commonly presents in infancy and childhood, particularly in atopic subjects [1, 8]. Chronic urticaria peaks in adulthood between 20 and 40 years of age affecting women two times more frequently than men [1, 3, 4]. About 0.5–1% of population has chronic spontaneous urticaria at a specific point in time [3].

4. Etiology and pathogenesis

Drugs, foods, viral and parasitic infections, insect stings and contact allergens are present among the most common causes of acute urticaria [8]. Drugs most commonly implicated in acute urticaria are antibiotics (penicillins and sulfonamides), nonsteroidal anti-inflammatory drugs, acetylsalicylic acid, opiates and narcotics. Foods, such as milk, eggs, nuts, fish and shellfish are common offenders, as well as food additives, such as tartrazine dyes, benzoic acid derivatives like sodium benzoate. Approximately 50% of cases of acute urticaria are idiopathic [5, 9].

The relationship between stress and chronic spontaneous urticaria is not fully understood. There are reports showing stressful life events, such as loss of close family member, financial problems, major personal illness preceded onset or exacerbation of the disease in a considerable subset of patients with chronic spontaneous urticaria [10, 11]. Although many patients report stress to exacerbate their disease, there is a lack of well-controlled studies on this subject [3].

In 35–40% of patients with chronic urticaria, circulating immunoglobulin G (IgG) autoantibodies against alpha subunit of the IgE receptors are found and in 5–10% of chronic urticaria patients, there is IgG antibody to IgE. This subtype of chronic urticaria is designated as chronic autoimmune urticaria [12]. The remainder of the patients with chronic urticaria is classified under the name of chronic idiopathic urticaria. In this form of urticaria, the mechanism for stimulation of mast cells is unknown [5].

Pathophysiological mechanisms leading to formation of urticaria and angioedema can be immune-mediated, complement-mediated, non-immune–mediated and autoimmune-mediated [13]. As in most cases of acute urticaria, immune-mediated urticaria is an IgE-mediated hypersensitivity reaction. This allergic reaction is commonly triggered in response to drugs, foods and insect bites [7, 13]. Complement activation leading to release of C3a, C4a and C5a can stimulate mast cells. Non-immune–mediated urticaria involves direct activation of mast cells by non-IgE mechanisms examples of which are physical stimuli, radiocontrast dyes, drugs, such as opiates and vancomycin. Autoimmune urticaria involves autoantibodies causing mast cell degranulation [12, 13]. As noted all mechanisms lead to activation of mast cells causing liberation of histamine, leukotriene C4 and prostaglandin D2. These vasoactive mediators cause vasodilatation and extravasation of plasma from postcapillary venules. In 4–5 hours, an inflammatory cytokine response including tumor necrosis factor, interleukin 4 and interleukin 5 recruits a perivascular inflammatory infiltrate. The result is the formation a pruritic urticarial plaque or angioedema [7].

5. Clinical features

Urticarial wheals consist of circumscribed erythematous plaques of various sizes with central swelling, with or without a surrounding flare (**Figure 1**). There is accompanying intense pruritus or occasional burning sensations. Lesions typically have round to oval shape but occasionally irregular, serpiginous or gyrate configurations may occur. Wheals are blanchable by diascopy. Individual lesions usually disappear within 1–24 hours without scarring but some lesions may take up to 48 hours to resolve [14–16]. Patients often report a poorly localized pruritus starting before the appearance of wheals [7]. Pruritus may impair sleep, private life and work leading to a diminished quality of life [4].

Angioedema is a descriptive term for abrupt onset of swellings of the deep dermis and subcutaneous tissue. In contrast to edema, angioedema is asymmetrical and can occur on nondependent sites. Most common sites of involvement are the lips (**Figure 2**), tongue, eyelids and genitalia although any part of the body can be involved. Due to the tissue distention, the lesions are usually painful rather than pruritic. Swellings of angioedema can be pink or skin-colored [9, 17, 18]. Involvement of the mucous membranes is a common feature. Stridor, abdominal pain, rarely intestinal obstruction may result from edema of respiratory or gastrointestinal tract. Lesions may take up to 72 hours to resolve [9, 18].

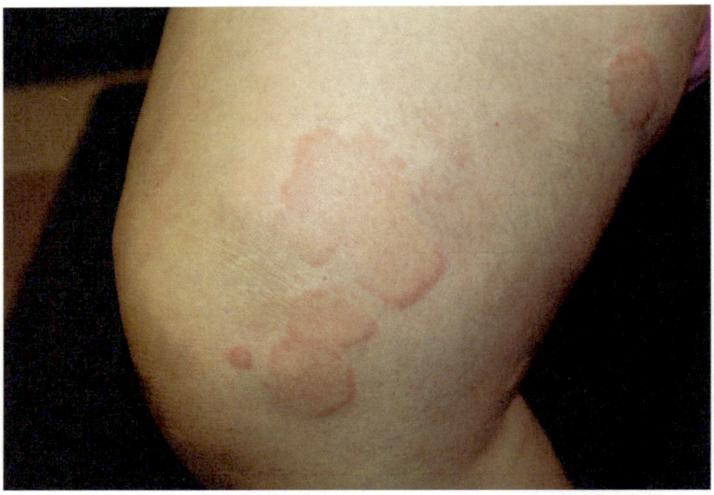

Figure 1. Typical urticarial plaques are observed on the leg of the patient.

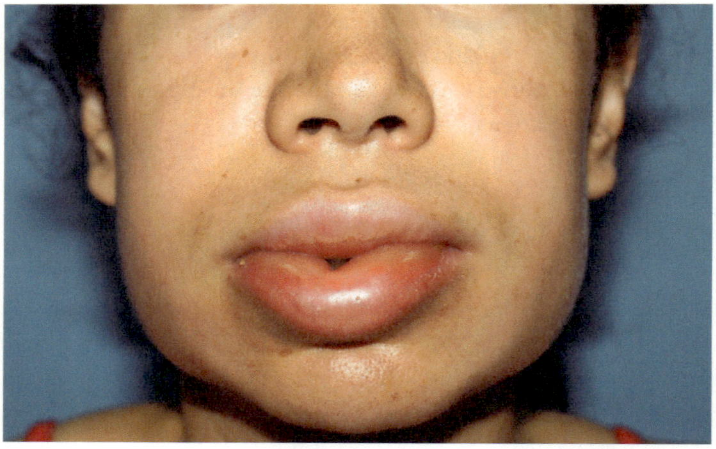

Figure 2. Angioedema involving the lips.

6. Prognosis

Cases of acute urticaria have a benign course with most patients being managed with conventional treatments [8].

Studies concerning duration of chronic spontaneous urticaria have yielded varying results. However, it is clear that many patients are affected for more than one year and an important proportion of patients have a long-term course of the disease exceeding 5 years [3].

In chronic spontaneous urticaria, there are four factors that potentially predict long disease duration, namely disease severity, presence of angioedema, autoreactivity and combination with physical urticaria. Patients with moderate to severe disease tend to have a more persistent disease as compared to patients with mild disease. Presence of angioedema with or without wheals in patients with chronic spontaneous urticaria predicts a longer course [3]. Autoreactivity, which is defined by a positive autologous serum skin test, reflects the finding of autoantibodies against IgE receptor or IgE. These patients have more severe disease with a longer duration and require higher doses of antihistamines to control disease activity than patients with negative autologous serum skin test [19]. Patients suffering from both chronic spontaneous urticaria and physical urticaria are likely to have longer disease duration in comparison with patients with chronic spontaneous urticaria alone [3].

7. Associated diseases

An increased prevalence of concomitant allergic diseases including rhinitis, asthma and atopic dermatitis is observed in cases of acute urticaria [8].

Chronic autoimmune urticaria is associated with antithyroid antibodies namely anti-microsomal and anti-thyroglobulin antibodies, observed in 27% of cases [12]. In patients with chronic urticaria, other autoimmune conditions such as vitiligo, type I diabetes mellitus, systemic lupus erythematosus and rheumatoid arthritis are more prevalent than in general population [5, 16].

Patients with chronic spontaneous urticaria often have concomitant physical urticaria that present with wheals lasting 2 hours or less [6].

Role of *Helicobacter pylori* infection in etiology of chronic autoimmune urticaria is still controversial [5]. However, it has been shown that *H. pylori* infection may contribute to the exacerbation of urticaria and that 2 weeks long triple therapy for eradication of the bacteria led to improvement of symptoms. As most patients infected with *H. pylori* are asymptomatic, screening of chronic urticaria patients for the presence of *H. pylori* infection by a non-invasive test, such as urea breath test or fecal antigen test is recommended [20].

8. Diagnosis

A through history is the most important tool in the diagnosis of urticaria. Duration, timing and localization of lesions, history of a recent viral infection, recent insect bite, medications, suspected foods, associated systemic symptoms, such as fever and arthralgia, and response to previous treatments should be questioned [5, 13]. In majority of cases of acute urticaria, history taking and physical examination is sufficient for the diagnosis. Further investigations are generally not required in patients with acute urticaria except those with a clinical history or physical examination suggesting an underlying cause, such as upper respiratory tract infection, food- or drug-induced urticaria [8]. Skin prick tests and serum-specific IgE tests can be used to confirm allergic reaction to foods, latex and certain antibiotics [5].

In chronic urticaria, complete blood count, liver enzymes, urinalysis and thyroid function tests can be checked; however, these laboratory tests are of minor significance, if there is not a suspected underlying etiology for persistent urticarial lesions [13, 21].

Skin testing to aeroallergens can be of value only if the patient has concomitant allergic rhinitis and/or asthma. If the patient reports a specific food to be strongly related with the attacks, a serologic test to the specific food can be performed. Serologic testing would be more reliable than skin testing as an interpretation of wheal and flare response would be misleading in patients under recurrent bouts of urticaria [16].

Autologous serum skin test is a practical clinical test to detect circulating functional autoantibodies in patients with chronic urticaria. The test is performed by intradermal injection of patient's own serum obtained while the patient is symptomatic and injection of 0.9% saline on volar aspect of the forearm. It is of importance to stop antihistamines 2 days before application. A positive autologous serum skin test is defined as a red serum-induced wheal having a diameter greater than 1.5 mm than the saline-induced wheal at 30 min. The test is performed when an immunomodulatory treatment is planned for patients with severe chronic urticaria. However, this is a controversial issue as the presence or absence of autoantibodies does not predict efficacy to most therapies [5, 16]. Basophil histamine release assays, western blot analysis or ELISA are also used to detect autoantibodies. However, these tests are sophisticated tests not readily available to most clinicians [22].

Urticaria activity score (UAS) is commonly used to assess disease activity and treatment response in patients with chronic urticaria. UAS is calculated based on the daily number of wheals (1–3 points) and the intensity of pruritus (0–3 points) and ranges from 0 to 6 [23]. UAS7 is calculated by summing UAS recorded by the patient on 7 consecutive days. A UAS7 score of less than 7 indicates control of disease, whereas a score exceeding 28 indicates poorly controlled symptoms [24].

9. Histopathology

Skin biopsies of acute lesions demonstrate a minimal inflammatory infiltrate along with dilatation of small vessels, flattened rete pegs and swollen collagen fibers. Histology of chronic urticaria lesions reveals a perivascular cuffing by predominantly T lymphocytes and also monocytes, neutrophils, eosinophils and basophils [25].

Observation of fragmentation of neutrophils, red cell extravasation and swelling of endothelial cells in persistent lesions points to the diagnosis of leukocytoclastic vasculitis [13].

http://dx.doi.org/10.5772/67772

10. Differential diagnosis

Urticarial rash may be seen in the course of many diseases (**Table 1**). Urticaria and angioedema can be manifestations of underlying systemic diseases, such as collagenopathies, endocrinopathies, tumors and hemolytic diseases [1].

Urticarial vasculitis is a rare condition mainly affecting adult females in 4th decade of life. It may manifest with urticarial plaques, which generally persist for 48–72 hours. Pain and tenderness is a common complaint. The wheals may resolve leaving residual purpuric or hyperpigmented discoloration of the skin. Underlying pathogenesis is a type III hypersensitivity reaction mediated by immune complexes. It is mostly idiopathic, however cases associated with connective tissue diseases (systemic lupus erythematosus), infections (hepatitis B and hepatitis C), medications (diltiazem, fluoxetine, potassium iodide, etc.) and malignancies have been reported. In histopathology, leukocytoclastic vasculitis is seen with signs of vessel damage, such as leukocytoclasis and fibrinoid deposits around venules. In contrast to urticaria, immunofluorescence of the skin shows deposits of immunoglobulins and complement [26, 27].

Systemic mastocytosis is a rare disorder in which atypical mast cells proliferate in the liver, spleen, lymph nodes, bone marrow and other organs. Involvement of the skin manifests as wheals and itching [5].

Urticarial lesions that persist beyond 24 hours should warrant alternative diagnosis, such as erythema multiforme minor, morbilliform drug eruption, dermatitis herpetiformis and bullous pemphigoid [9]. Erythema multiforme minor is an acute condition that differs from urticaria with its persistent targetoid lesions, and is typically less pruritic than urticaria [13].

Urticarial rash in a young child accompanied by fever, edema of hands and feet and arthralgias should prompt a diagnosis of serum sickness-like reaction. In this condition, urticarial plaques usually have an associated ecchymotic pattern. Serum sickness-like reaction is a hypersensitivity reaction that is often due to medications or infections. It develops 1–3 weeks

Urticarial vasculitis
Systemic mastocytosis
Erythema multiforme minor
Morbilliform drug eruption
Dermatitis herpetiformis
Bullous pemphigoid
Serum sickness-like reaction
Urticaria multiforme
Cryopyrin-associated periodic syndromes

Table 1. Differential diagnosis of urticaria.

after the initial antigen exposure and has a self-limited course. Urticaria multiforme is also a hypersensitivity reaction marked with annular urticarial plaques and bruise-like areas similar to that seen in serum sickness-like reaction. The triggering factor is often a viral infection; urticarial lesions are preceded by 1–3 days of fever [28].

Cryopyrin-associated periodic syndromes are autoinflammatory diseases including familial cold autoinflammatory syndrome, Muckle-Wells syndrome and the neonatal onset multisystem inflammatory disease. They present often early in infancy with a variable severity of clinical manifestations. Main symptoms are fever, arthralgias and skin involvement with urticaria-like nonpruritic lesions. Histopathologically, the perivascular infiltration is composed of polymorphonuclear cells in contrast with classical urticaria [29].

11. Management

Management of acute urticaria should initially focus on avoidance of any triggering factors, such as foods, drugs, insect venoms and latex. First-line treatment agents are antihistamines, corticosteroids and immunomodulatory agents are reserved for patients resistant to antihistamines [5].

11.1. Antihistamines

For the first-line management of acute or chronic urticaria, second-generation H_1 antihistamines are used. Fexofenadine, desloratadine, loratadine, cetirizine and levocetirizine are the most commonly prescribed agents [5, 10]. Symptomatic relief with suppression of the pruritus and reduction of the number and size of wheals is the main goal of treatment. Loratadine and cetirizine can be used starting from 6 months of age and are also safe during pregnancy [9, 10]. Efficacy of antihistamines is often patient specific and none are consistently superior [16].

Antihistamines target H_1 receptors located on endothelial cells and sensory nerves. First-generation antihistamines (hydroxyzine, diphenhydramine and chlorpheniramine) can penetrate central nervous system and thus have sedating effects lasting longer than 12 hours. However relief of pruritus is much short-lived and lasts only up to 6 hours. Older first-generation antihistamines are not recommended for the management of chronic urticaria in the European Guidelines because they place patients at risk for serious side-effects and drug interactions. In contrast to first-generation antihistamines, the second-generation antihistamines are devoid of sedating and anticholinergic effects [30]. Similar to first-generation H_1 antihistamines, the use of H_2 receptor blockers (cimetidine and ranitidine) are not recommended in European Guidelines.

Updosing of antihistamines is safe in therapy resistant patients. Fourfold higher doses of licensed doses of antihistamines should be used before considering other treatments [30]. However, according to US guidelines treatment by updosing second-generation H_1 antihistamines can substituted with an add-on treatment with other second-generation H_1 antihistamines, H_2 antagonists, leukotriene receptor antagonists or first-generation H_1 antihistamines as alternative second step treatment options [31].

11.2. Corticosteroids

Corticosteroids can be used in the management of antihistamine-resistant cases of acute urticaria and exacerbations of chronic spontaneous urticaria. Long-term therapy with corticosteroids is strictly dismissed because of the risk of side effects and development of tolerance. Oral corticosteroids such as 7 days of prednisone up to 40 mg/day are often used to alleviate symptoms unresponsive to antihistamines in chronic urticaria [5]. Likewise, addition of a brief course of prednisone to antihistamines in acute urticaria significantly improves symptom control [32].

11.3. Leukotriene receptor antagonists

Leukotriene receptor antagonists, such as montelukast and zafirlukast, may have a role in the management of chronic urticaria. According to European Guidelines, leukotriene receptor antagonists may be considered in patients who do not respond to updosing of H_1 antihistamines, although evidence is low as compared to cyclosporine or omalizumab [30, 33].

11.4. Immunosuppressives

Cyclosporine has been shown to be effective in the treatment of recalcitrant cases of chronic spontaneous urticaria in combination with second-generation antihistamines especially cetirizine. Its mechanism of action depends on the inhibition of anti-IgE–induced histamine release from basophils and skin mast cells. Cyclosporine at 3–5 mg/kg/day is administered with monitorization of diastolic blood pressure and levels of serum creatinine, serum potassium, serum bilirubin and liver enzymes at each visit [34, 35]. Common adverse effects of cyclosporine therapy include hypertension, fatigue, gastrointestinal problems and headache [33].

Immunosuppressive therapy with mycophenolate, tacrolimus and methotrexate can also be considered in recalcitrant cases [31].

11.5. Omalizumab

Omalizumab is a recombinant humanized monoclonal anti-immunoglobulin E antibody that prevents binding of IgE to the high-affinity IgE receptor and thus prevents urticaria and angioedema. This new biologic treatment, applied by monthly subcutaneous injections in a standardized protocol, provides a rapid and effective control of treatment-refractory urticaria patients. Omalizumab is generally well-tolerated and safe. Major risks of omalizumab treatment include anaphylaxis, increased risk of cardiac and neurovascular events, and a controversial increased risk of lymphoma [16, 36, 37].

11.6. Phototherapy

Efficacy of phototherapy, both narrowband UVB and PUVA, has been shown in several studies. Phototherapy is not recommended in urticaria guidelines; still it appears to be a safe and effective therapeutic modality for patients with refractory chronic urticaria [38–40].

12. Angioedema without wheals

As described previously in this chapter, angioedema is defined as swellings of the deep dermis and subcutaneous tissue. Clinically, there is non-pitting asymmetrically distributed edema usually involving the face. Angioedema typically resolves spontaneously in less than 72 hours [41].

Clinically a variety of conditions may cause swellings that resemble angioedema. Acute contact dermatitis develops after exposure to a foreign substance. When acute contact dermatitis involves the face, it is frequently misdiagnosed as angioedema. Abrupt onset of angioedema associated with diffuse maculopapular rash, fever, eosinophilia and lymphadenopathy is seen in drug rash with eosinophilia and systemic symptoms (DRESS) Syndrome. Periorbital edema of dermatomyositis may mimic angioedema [41]. Other diseases to consider in differential diagnosis of angioedema are superior vena cava syndrome, myxedema of hypothyroidism, photodermatitis, Crohn's disease of the mouth and lips, facial cellulitis and Melkersson-Rosenthal syndrome [18, 41].

Angioedema without wheals can be classified as hereditary angioedema, acquired angioedema, drug-induced angioedema and idiopathic angioedema [42].

12.1. Hereditary angioedema

12.1.1. Epidemiology

Hereditary angioedema is rare genetic disease with a prevalence of about 1:10,000–1:50,000. The inheritance is autosomal dominant. In 20% of cases, a positive family history of the disease cannot be obtained because these cases occur due to spontaneous mutations [42].

12.1.2. Etiology and pathogenesis

Two types of the disease have been defined, both concerning the inhibitor of the first component of human complement (C1). Type I accounts for 80–85% of cases and is characterized by low C1 inhibitor levels and function. Type II comprises the remaining 15–20% of cases and it is associated with normal levels of poorly functioning C1 inhibitor. Both types of hereditary angioedema result in low levels of C4; during acute attacks C2 levels may also decrease [42].

The recently described hereditary angioedema type III is not associated with C1 inhibitor deficiency or dysfunction. The etiology of this very rare type of hereditary angioedema is not fully understood. It mostly affects women. Estrogens and mutations in factor XII are thought be involved in pathogenesis [43, 44].

C1 inhibitor is the major regulator of complement and contact system activation. With the decreased activity of C1 inhibitor, unopposed activation of contact system leads to generation of bradykinin. Bradykinin induces relaxation in vascular smooth muscle and increases vascular permeability causing angioedema [42, 44].

Trauma, stress, infection, menstruation, oral contraceptives, hormonal replacement therapy and angiotensin-converting enzyme (ACE) inhibitors can trigger the attacks. However an underlying trigger cannot be found in most of the cases [42, 44].

12.1.3. *Clinical features*

Clinically angioedema mostly involves the face, tongue and lips, abdomen, larynx, extremities and genitalia [42]. Any part of the body can be affected including chest, joints, muscles, etc. Abdominal colicky pain, nausea and vomiting are manifestations of gastrointestinal involvement. Edema of the upper airway tract can be life threatening [42, 43]. The onset of disease is usually in childhood mostly between 8 and 12 years. Episodic swellings last 1–5 days before subsiding. A serpiginous rash called erythema marginatum, fatigue and muscle aches are prodromal symptoms reported by 50% of patients with hereditary angioedema [44].

12.1.4. *Prophylaxis and treatment*

Management of hereditary angioedema can be classified under three different categories, which are treatment of the attacks, short-term or procedural prophylaxis and long-term prophylaxis [43].

Management of acute attacks can be accomplished by replacement of C1 inhibitor or alternatively by using icatibant or ecallantide. Plasma-derived or recombinant C1 inhibitors are available for intravenous replacement of C1 inhibitor. Icatibant is bradykinin B2 receptor antagonist. Human C1 inhibitors and icatibant are approved for self-administration. These agents are most effective when given as early as possible during the attacks. Ecallantide works by reversible inhibition of kallikrein and is approved by FDA for use in patients older than 12 years of age. Application by a healthcare professional is imperative because of a high risk of developing anaphylactic reaction [43].

As noted above trauma is among the well-known triggers of an angioedema attack. Thus a short-term prophylaxis is indicated before interventions in the upper aerodigestive tract, such as intubation, bronchoscopy or esophagogastroduodenoscopy. For this purpose C1 inhibitors are the first-choice agents. Androgens, which have been the mainstay of management of patients with hereditary angioedema in the past, are no longer considered as first-line options because of associated side effects and are only used when C1 inhibitor therapy is not available. Weight gain, hepatotoxicity, virilism and hypertension are among the various side effects of androgen therapy [43, 44].

Long-term prophylaxis can be initiated if treatment of acute attacks does not result in adequate symptom control. C1 inhibitor concentrates are recommended as first-line agents. Androgens and tranexamic acid are less favored because of high risk of adverse effects and low treatment efficacy, respectively [43].

12.2. Acquired angioedema

12.2.1. Etiology and pathogenesis

Acquired angioedema is an autoimmune disease characterized by autoantibodies against C1 inhibitor [44]. A lymphoproliferative disorder such as non-Hodgin lymphoma or monoclonal gammopathy or an autoimmune disease is found in many of the cases. These associations suggest that pathological B cell clones may be responsible for acquired angioedema [45].

Acquired angioedema is divided into two types. Type I acquired angioedema is due to massive consumption of C1 inhibitor, presumably by tumor-related immune complexes. Type II acquired angioedema occurs due to the production of anti-C1 inhibitor autoantibodies [25].

12.2.2. Clinical features

Clinical features of acquired angioedema are similar to those seen in hereditary angioedema. Abdominal involvement is less frequent [44]. Absence of family history and late onset of symptoms at 4th decade are distinguishing features [42]. Laboratory evaluation of patients with acquired angioedema reveals low C4 levels and decreased C1 inhibitor activity similar to hereditary angioedema; but also decreased levels of C1q [44].

12.2.3. Treatment

Treatment of acquired angioedema mostly depends on treatment of the underlying disease [42]. Although response rates are low, treatments used for hereditary angioedema are frequently applied. Acute attacks can be managed by administration of C1 inhibitor concentrate or alternatively by using icatibant or ecallantide. High-dose corticosteroid therapy is used in order to reduce production of autoantibodies but it is frequently ineffective and has many adverse effects. Rituximab has also been shown to be effective in decreasing autoantibody production against C1 inhibitor. Although several reports of patients successfully treated with rituximab exist, the responses can be inconsistent [44, 46].

12.3. Drug-induced angioedema

Drug-induced angioedema is most typically associated with the use of angiotensin-converting enzyme (ACE) inhibitors. Angiotensin receptor blockers, nonsteroidal anti-inflammatory drugs, fibrinolytics and oral contraceptives can also induce isolated angioedema [18].

http://dx.doi.org/10.5772/67772

Angioedema due to angiotensin-converting enzyme inhibitors occurs in 0.1–6% of patients under treatment with ACE inhibitors. It tends to develop more commonly in women, smokers and in patients of African American descent [47]. ACE inhibitor angioedema mostly develops at the first month of treatment but may also occur years after starting the medication [42].

As the underlying mechanism involves elevated levels of bradykinin, antihistamines and corticosteroids are not helpful in the management of drug-induced angioedema. Although not FDA-approved for this indication, bradykinin receptor antagonist icatibant and kallikrein inhibitors are effective treatment agents [42, 48].

12.4. Idiopathic angioedema

The term idiopathic angioedema is used when there is no identifiable cause for the recurrent angioedema attacks without wheals. Idiopathic angioedema is a diagnosis of exclusion. C1 inhibitor deficiency, factor XII mutation, treatment with ACE inhibitors must be ruled out [49]. The condition is mostly well-controlled with prophylactic antihistamines [5].

Author details

Burhan Engin*, Muazzez Çiğdem Oba and Server Serdaroğlu

*Address all correspondence to: burhanengin2000@yahoo.com

Dermatology Department, Cerrahpaşa Medical Faculty, Istanbul University, Istanbul, Turkey

References

[1] Novembre E, Cianferoni A, Mori F, et al. Urticaria and urticaria related skin condition/disease in children. Eur Ann Allergy Clin Immunol 2008; **40**:5–13.

[2] Zuberbier T. Classification of urticaria. Indian J Dermatol 2013; **58**:208–210.

[3] Maurer M, Weller K, Bindslev-Jensen C, et al. Unmet clinical needs in chronic spontaneous urticaria. A GA²LEN task force report. Allergy. 2011; **66**:317–330.

[4] Baiardini I, Giardini A, Pasquali M, et al. Quality of life and patients' satisfaction in chronic urticaria and respiratory allergy. Allergy 2003; **58**:621–623.

[5] Kanani A, Schellenberg R, Warrington R. Urticaria and angioedema. Allergy Asthma Clin Immunol 2011;**7**:9.

[6] Magerl M, Borzova E, Giménez-Arnau A, et al. The definition and diagnostic testing of physical and cholinergic urticarias—EAACI/GA2LEN/EDF/UNEV consensus panel recommendations. Allergy. 2009; **64**:1715–1721.

[7] Amar SM, Dreskin SC. Urticaria. Prim Care 2008; **35**:141–157.

[8] Sánchez-Borges M, Capriles-Hulett A, Caballero-Fonseca F. Demographic and clinical profiles in patients with acute urticaria. Allergol Immunopathol 2015; **43**:409–415.

[9] Krishnaswamy G, Youngberg G. Acute and chronic urticaria. Challenges and considerations for primary care physicians. Postgrad Med. 2001; **109**:107–108, 111–114, 119–123.

[10] Malhotra SK, Mehta V. Role of stressful life events in induction or exacerbation of psoriasis and chronic urticaria. Indian J Dermatol Venereol Leprol 2008; **74**:594–599.

[11] Yang HY, Sun CC, Wu YC, Wang JD. Stress, insomnia, and chronic idiopathic urticaria–a case-control study. J Formos Med Assoc 2005; **104**:254–263.

[12] Kaplan AP. Chronic urticaria: pathogenesis and treatment. J Allergy Clin Immunol 2004; **114**:465–474.

[13] Baxi S, Dinakar C. Urticaria and angioedema. Immunol Allergy Clin North Am 2005; **25**:353–367.

[14] Frigas E, Park MA. Acute urticaria and angioedema: diagnostic and treatment considerations. Am J Clin Dermatol 2009; **10**:239–250.

[15] Dibbern DA Jr, Dreskin SC. Urticaria and angioedema: an overview. Immunol Allergy Clin North Am 2004; **24**:141–162.

[16] Fine LM, Bernstein JA. Guideline of chronic urticaria beyond. Allergy Asthma Immunol Res 2016; **8**:396–403.

[17] Greaves MW. Urticaria. Clin Allergy Immunol 2002; **16**:381–400.

[18] Kaplan AP, Greaves MW. Angioedema. J Am Acad Dermatol 2005; **53**:373–388.

[19] Poonawalla T, Kelly B. Urticaria: a review. Am J Clin Dermatol 2009; **10**:9–21.

[20] Abdou AG, Elshayeb EI, Farag AG, Elnaidany NF. *Helicobacter pylori* infection in patients with chronic urticaria: correlation with pathologic findings in gastric biopsies. Int J Dermatol 2009; **48**:464–469.

[21] Kozel MM, Bossuyt PM, Mekkes JR, Bos JD. Laboratory tests and identified diagnoses in patients with physical and chronic urticaria and angioedema: a systematic review. J Am Acad Dermatol 2003; **48**:409–416.

[22] Sabroe RA, Grattan CE, Francis DM, Barr RM, Kobza Black A, Greaves MW. The autologous serum skin test: a screening test for autoantibodies in chronic idiopathic urticaria. Br J Dermatol 1999; **140**:446–452.

[23] Młynek A, Zalewska-Janowska A, Martus P, Staubach P, Zuberbier T, Maurer M. How to assess disease activity in patients with chronic urticaria? Allergy 2008; **63**:777–780.

[24] Moolani Y, Lynde C, Sussman G. Advances in understanding and managing chronic urticaria. F1000Res. 2016; **5**:177.

[25] Huston DP, Bressler RB. Urticaria and angioedema. Med Clin North Am 1992; **76**:805–840.

[26] Davis MD, Brewer JD. Urticarial vasculitis and hypocomplementemic urticarial vasculitis syndrome. Immunol Allergy Clin North Am 2004; **24**:183–213.

[27] Black AK. Urticarial vasculitis. Clin Dermatol 1999; **17**:565–569.

[28] Mathur AN, Mathes EF. Urticaria mimickers in children. Dermatol Ther 2013; **26**:467–475.

[29] Neven B, Prieur AM, Quartier dit Maire P. Cryopyrinopathies: update on pathogenesis and treatment. Nat Clin Pract Rheumatol. 2008; **4**:481–489.

[30] Zuberbier T, Asero R, Bindslev-Jensen C, et al. EAACI/GA(2)LEN/EDF/WAO guideline: management of urticaria. Allergy. 2009; **64**:1427–1443.

[31] Bernstein JA, Lang DM, Khan DA, et al. The diagnosis and management of acute and chronic urticaria: 2014 update. J Allergy Clin Immunol 2014; **133**:1270–1277.

[32] Pollack CV Jr, Romano TJ. Outpatient management of acute urticaria: the role of prednisone. Ann Emerg Med 1995; **26**:547–551.

[33] Staubach P, Zuberbier T, Vestergaard C, Siebenhaar F, Toubi E, Sussman G. Controversies and challenges in the management of chronic urticaria. J Eur Acad Dermatol Venereol 2016; **30**:16–24.

[34] Vena GA, Cassano N, Colombo D, Peruzzi E, Pigatto P, Neo-I-30 Study Group. Cyclosporine in chronic idiopathic urticaria: a double-blind, randomized, placebo-controlled trial. J Am Acad Dermatol. 2006; **55**:705–709.

[35] Grattan CE, O'Donnell BF, Francis DM, et al. Randomized double-blind study of cyclosporin in chronic 'idiopathic' urticaria. Br J Dermatol 2000; **143**:365–372.

[36] Metz M, Ohanyan T, Church MK, Maurer M. Omalizumab is an effective and rapidly acting therapy in difficult-to-treat chronic urticaria: a retrospective clinical analysis. J Dermatol Sci 2014; **73**:57–62.

[37] Viswanathan RK, Moss MH, Mathur SK. Retrospective analysis of the efficacy of omalizumab in chronic refractory urticaria. Allergy Asthma Proc 2013; **34**:446–452.

[38] Berroeta L, Clark C, Ibbotson SH, Ferguson J, Dawe RS. Narrow-band (TL-01) ultraviolet B phototherapy for chronic urticaria. Clin Exp Dermatol 2004; **29**:97–98.

[39] Engin B, Ozdemir M, Balevi A, Mevlitoglu I. Treatment of chronic urticaria with narrowband ultraviolet B phototherapy: a randomized controlled trial. Acta Derm Venereol 2008; **88**:247–251.

[40] Bishnoi A, Parsad D, Vinay K, Kumaran MS. Phototherapy using narrowband ultraviolet B and psoralen plus ultraviolet A is beneficial in steroid-dependent antihistamine-refractory chronic urticaria: a randomized, prospective observer-blinded comparative study. Br J Dermatol 2017; **176**:62–70.

[41] Andersen MF, Longhurst HJ, Rasmussen ER, Bygum A. How not to be misled by disorders mimicking angioedema: a review of pseudoangioedema. Int Arch Allergy Immunol 2016;**169**:163–170.

[42] Banerji A, Sheffer AL. The spectrum of chronic angioedema. Allergy Asthma Proc 2009; **30**:11–16.

[43] Greve J, Strassen U, Gorczyza M, et al. Prophylaxis in hereditary angioedema (HAE) with C1 inhibitor deficiency. J Dtsch Dermatol Ges 2016; **14**:266–275.

[44] Zeerleder S, Levi M. Hereditary and acquired C1-inhibitor-dependent angioedema: from pathophysiology to treatment. Ann Med 2016; **48**:256–267.

[45] Castelli R, Deliliers DL, Zingale LC, Pogliani EM, Cicardi M. Lymphoproliferative disease and acquired C1 inhibitor deficiency. Haematologica 2007; **92**:716–718.

[46] Branellec A, Bouillet L, Javaud N, et al. Acquired C1-inhibitor deficiency: 7 patients treated with rituximab. J Clin Immunol. 2012; **32**:936–941.

[47] Byrd JB, Adam A, Brown NJ. Angiotensin-converting enzyme inhibitor-associated angioedema. Immunol Allergy Clin North Am 2006; **26**:725–737.

[48] Bas M. The angiotensin-converting-enzyme-induced angioedema. Immunol Allergy Clin North Am 2017; **37**:183–200.

[49] Cicardi M, Suffritti C, Perego F, Caccia S. Novelties in the diagnosis and treatment of angioedema. J Investig Allergol Clin Immunol 2016; **26**:212–221.

Chapter 3

Chronic Inducible Urticaria Part I

Murat Borlu, Salih Levent Cinar and Demet Kartal

Additional information is available at the end of the chapter

http://dx.doi.org/10.5772/68069

Abstract

Urticaria is a common mast cell-driven disease which is characterized by red, itchy swellings. Urticaria, that persists more than 6 weeks in a repetitive manner (each lesion disappearing in <24 h), is called chronic urticaria. Chronic urticaria can be either spontaneous without the need of a trigger, or inducible in which with a known trigger the lesions can be provoked. Chronic inducible urticarias include the physical urticarias and some other forms such as cholinergic urticaria.

Keywords: urticaria, chronic urticaria, inducible urticaria, cholinergic urticaria, contact urticaria

1. Introduction

Urticaria, also known as hives, is a common, mast cell-driven, itchy condition which is characterized by red/pink, swollen whealing of the skin [1]. The lesions can vary from a few millimeters to tens of centimeters. Chronic urticaria is defined when the transient lesions that disappear in <24 h and last more than 6 weeks in repetitive manner [2]. Most of the chronic urticaria cases are idiopathic [3]. Chronic spontaneous urticaria is the spontaneous appearance of wheals, angioedema or both due to known or unknown causes for a period longer than 6 weeks. In case of a known trigger that causes whealing, angioedema or both at every exposure, chronic inducible urticaria term is used. Chronic inducible urticarias consist of physical urticarias (PUs) and cholinergic urticaria (CU) [1, 3, 4]. **Figure 1** demonstrates the classification of urticaria according to EAACI/GA^{2}LEN/WAO 2013 guideline.

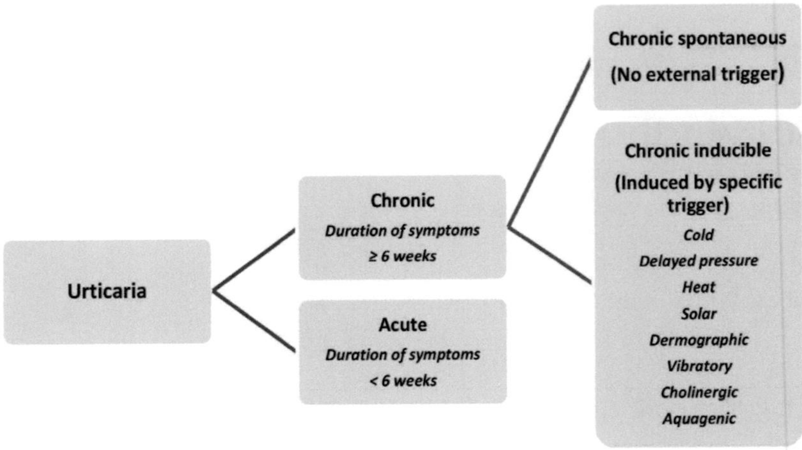

Figure 1. Classification of urticaria, according to EAACI/GA2LEN/WAO 2013 guideline.

Physical urticaria (PU) is a subgroup of acquired, chronic inducible urticaria which is associated with a known physical trigger [5]. In PU, the symptoms are induced by exogenous physical triggers such as friction, pressure, vibration, cold, heat or solar radiation. All the PUs may manifest with both wheals and angioedema at the sites of the triggers with the exceptions that urticaria factitia (symptomatic dermographism) presents with wheals only and pressure urticaria presents with angioedema only [6, 7]. **Table 1** summarizes the types and subtypes of chronic inducible urticaria and the triggering agents.

Cholinergic urticaria is another subtype of inducible urticaria. Because of the fact that the symptoms are not triggered by exogenous physical exposure, cholinergic urticaria is not considered as PU. Rather, it is induced by an increase in the body core temperature [8].

Almost 0.5% of the population suffers from chronic inducible urticaria that makes nearly 15–25% of all chronic urticarias [7]. All forms of urticaria do not only cause impaired quality of

Type	Subtypes	Trigger
Physical urticarias	Cold urticaria	Cold contact (air, water and solid)
	Delayed pressure urticaria	Vertical pressure
	Heat urticaria	Hot contact (air, water and solid)
	Solar urticaria	UV or visible light
	Symptomatic dermographism	Mechanical stroking
	Vibratory urticaria	Vibration
Other inducible urticarias	Aquagenic urticaria	Water at any temperature
	Contact urticaria	(Non)immunological contactant
	Cholinergic urticaria	Increment of body temperature
	Exercise-induced anaphylaxis	Physical exercise

Table 1. Classification of chronic inducible urticaria.

life but also affect performance at social life, school and work [9]. PU is classified depending on the type of the physical trigger. They are diagnosed by using different provocation tests inducing wheals and sometimes angioedema [3]. It is important to make provocation tests after taking the patient's history in order to get a proper diagnosis. One must be very careful during the provocation tests as systemic symptoms including shock can develop along the course [10]. In chronic inducible urticaria, the threshold of the causative trigger must be established to assess the severity of the condition. These threshold levels also allow us to evaluate the activity of the diseases and the response to the therapy [11]. PU generally accompanies other forms of chronic urticaria such as spontaneous urticaria and/or other inducible urticaria types. Therefore, every patient with one of the PUs must be tested with all physical triggers that seem to be relevant from the medical history [12]. The result of the provocation test changes according to the medical status of the patient. That's why the test should be done prior to the treatment if possible. Testing should be performed on skin areas which have not been complicated with wheals recently. Because affected skin areas exhibit a refractory period after urticarial reactions. In case of a negative result despite a strong suspicion, the testing can be repeated several times. In cholinergic urticaria, the patient must be asymptomatic for 48 h before testing [6].

2. Cholinergic urticaria (CU)

Cholinergic urticaria, simply, is a type of chronic urticaria which is triggered by elevated body temperature. Physical exercise, strong emotions, hot or spicy food and hot showers seem to be the most common causes [13]. CU accounts for 5% of all chronic urticaria cases [7]. Generalized flushing, itching and wheals surrounded by macular erythema make the clinical picture in CU. The lesions spread from the trunk and neck to the extremities. Some of the CU cases are complicated with systemic symptoms such as hypotension, angioedema and bronchospasm [14]. CU due to exercise starts 5–10 min after the beginning of the exercise and maximizes after 12–25 min [15].

The pathophysiology in CU is thought to be related to the elevation of histamine in the serum. Adachi et al. proposed that CU occurs after a type 1 allergic reaction to the patient's own sweat. They reported that the patients underwent autologous sweat testing and demonstrated an immediate skin reaction [8].

In case of a suspicion, confirmatory testing should be conducted. Appearance of whealing after the intradermal injection of 0.01 mg methacholine in 0.1 ml saline is diagnostic. Assuming that only one-third of the patients demonstrate positive testing CU cannot be ruled out with a negative provocation test [9]. Specific provocative challenges such as exercise, hot showers or spicy food trials can also be tried. The best way to provoke is to increase the individual's body temperature by submerging the patient in a hot water bath at 40°C. Developing of generalized hives confirms the diagnosis [6]. Unfortunately, this testing can have interference with aquagenic urticaria (AU) or heat urticaria.

Best treatment of CU is the avoidance of the offending stimulus in cases where possible. First-line medical therapy is the oral antihistamines. Hydroxyzine is believed to be more effective than the others [16]. Oral anticholinergics have been tried with failure mostly. Use of pre-exercise propranolol 80 mg daily has been found effective in controlling the symptoms of CU [17]. These data have not been supported by further studies because of the fact that beta-blockers, themselves, cause allergic reactions.

The prognosis of CU is mostly pleasing. About 70% of the patients heal within 10 years of the diagnosis. Sibbald et al. estimated the duration of CU to be 3–16 years with an average of 7.5 years [2].

Cholinergic urticaria must be distinguished from exercise-induced anaphylaxis (EIA). The main symptoms of EIA include laryngospasm, bronchospasm, vascular collapse, fatique, vocal changes, gastrointestinal upset, flushing and hives [18]. In contrast to CU, the urticarial plaques are larger, up to 10–15 mm. All types of exercise including walking can be the trigger. In EIA, although the anaphylaxis symptoms are at the forefront, only a few cases of death have been reported [19].

EIA is treated like any other forms of anaphylaxis. Epinephrine is the life-saving treatment. Diphenhydramine 25–50 mg is helpful. Systemic steroids are used to prevent delayed biphasic reactions [20]. Any individual with the diagnosis of EIA should carry an epinephrine auto-injector [21]. Cetirizine and montelukast combination also has been reported to be useful in preventing symptoms of EIA [22].

CU can be differentiated from EIA with the size of the whealings. Also, in CU, the hives are in the front, whereas the edema and the anaphylaxis are in the front in case of EIA. In addition, passive warming test in a bath and methacholine injection tests are positive in CU [23].

3. Aquagenic urticaria (AU)

Aquagenic urticaria (AU) is a rare form PU which is characterized by wheals following cutaneous exposure to water, including tears and sweat. Mostly, 1–3 mm follicular wheals and 1–3 cm erythematous flares surrounding them are present. The lesions develop 20–30 min after exposure to water. Lesions usually resolve in 30–60 min after the cessation of contact to water [4]. Most of the patients are peri-pubertal females. Trunk and proximal arms are the most commonly affected sites, sparing palms and soles [5]. Wheezing and dyspnea can accompany the lesions. When there is such a systemic symptom, large lesions rather than 1–3 mm punctate lesions are present [24].

Most of the AU cases are sporadic. However, there are some reports of familial cases. No specific gene locus has been identified so far [5]. There are few cases showing the association of AU and HIV infection and papillary thyroid gland carcinoma [25, 26].

The pathogenesis of AU is not clear yet. In 1981, Tkach hypothesized that sudden changes in osmotic pressure around hair follicles, leading to passive diffusion of water caused whealing [27]. A recent proposal involves existence of water-soluble antigens in the epidermis which later migrate to dermis and cause histamine release [10]. The lack of a proper etiologic mechanism makes AU difficult to treat.

Water challenge test is necessary for the proper diagnosis. For this, water at room temperature is applied to a cloth, and this cloth is applied to patient's skin for 20 min. In case of an urticarial lesion, the provocation test is considered as positive. Water should be at room temperature. Because, if the temperature is higher or lower, the test could give arise to other forms of PU (cold or heat urticaria) [28]. Bayle et al. reported a case with AU, dermatographism and cholinergic urticaria at the same time [29]. It is possible to induce AU, heat urticaria, cold urticaria and cholinergic urticaria with applying water at different temperatures [30]. So, one should be very careful to differentiate among these conditions.

Management of AU is difficult. Avoidance is almost impossible. The first-line therapy is H1 antihistamines [11]. Long acting newer antihistamines with fewer side effects are usually preferred. H2 receptors are thought to be not operating in the pathogenesis of PU. Yet there is a case report that claims that H2 antihistamines reduce wheal response [31].

Topical barrier therapies show promising results in AU. They are also safer. Application of oil-in-water emulsions before bathing can reduce wheals. Such physical barriers must be used in the pediatric patients before everything else to prevent the potential side effects of the antihistamines [29].

Phototherapy, both PUVA and narrow-band UVB, has been reported to be effective in AU treatment. Possible action of mechanism is the reduction of mast cell activity and thickening of the skin, mostly epidermis, leading to decreased water penetration [32].

Stanozolol which is used in the treatment of hereditary angioedema was shown to be effective in one male patient at a dose of 10 mg daily [25].

4. Contact urticaria

Contact urticaria is the transient whealing and flare of the skin after contact with certain agents. The lesions appear within 60 min of contact and mostly resolve in 2–24 h [33]. Contact urticaria can be both immunological (IgE mediated) or non-immunological. Mostly, non-immunological mechanisms are seen. It can be provoked in all persons without the need of prior sensitization [34].

The lesions in contact urticaria appear as a result of the release of vasoactive amines such as histamine, leukotrienes, substance P and prostaglandins, independent from immunological processes. The lesions are localized to the contact area causing no systemic symptoms. The causative contact agents can be insects, metals, alcohol, balsam of Peru, sodium benzoate, sorbic acid, fruits, vegetables, jellyfish, sea anemones and corals [33–35].

Contact urticaria is rarely due to immunological causes, that is, allergic. In this case, it is caused by antigen-antibody type 1 IgE-mediated hypersensitivity reaction. The contact antigen penetrates the skin and binds with specific IgE antibodies on dermal mast cells. Histamine and some other mediators such as kinin and prostaglandins are released. As a result, erythema and hives are observed [35]. Sometimes systemic symptoms (rhinitis, conjunctivitis and asthma) can accompany the cutaneous manifestations [36]. The triggering agent in contact urticaria can be rubber latex, antibiotics (cephalosporins and streptomycin), foods (potato, fish and apple), cosmetics (hair bleaching products and paraphenylenediamine) and chemicals (isocyanates, chlorhexidine and aluminum) [35].

The mainstay of the therapy is mainly avoidance in contact urticaria [7]. Barrier creams are being used recently with good results [37]. H1 antihistamines make the first line therapy. In case of failure, dose increment, leukotriene antagonists, cyclosporine, omalizumab can be used with variable success rates [34, 35, 37].

5. Conclusion

As a result, we should keep in mind that chronic urticaria is hard to manage. The treatment should be individualized most of the time because of the fact that one patient can respond well to a specific treatment but another patient cannot. Another fact, to remember, is to differentiate cholinergic urticaria from exercise-induced anaphylaxis. Because they are similar entities, but they have different therapy options and courses.

Author details

Murat Borlu, Salih Levent Cinar* and Demet Kartal

*Address all correspondence to: sleventcinar@yahoo.com

Erciyes University Faculty of Medicine, Kayseri, Turkey

References

[1] Zuberbier T, Maurer M. Urticaria: current opinions about etiology, diagnosis and therapy. *Acta Derm Venereol*. 2007;87(3):196–205. doi:10.2340/00015555-0240

[2] Sibbald RG, Cheema AS, Lozinski A, Tarlo S. Chronic urticaria. Evaluation of the role of physical, immunologic, and other contributory factors. *Int J Dermatol*. 1991;30(6):381–386. doi:10.1111/j.1365-4362.1991.tb03891.x

[3] Zuberbier T, Bindslev-Jensen C, Canonica W, et al. EAACI/GA²LEN/EDF guideline: definition, classification and diagnosis of urticaria. *Allergy*. 2006;61(3):316–320. doi:10.1111/j.1398-9995.2005.00964.x

[4] Shelley WB, Rawnsley HM. Aquagenic urticaria. Contact sensitivity reaction to water. *JAMA*. 1964;189:895–898. doi:10.1001/jama.1964.03070120017003

[5] Kai AC, Flohr C. Aquagenic urticaria in twins. *World Allergy Organ J*. 2013;6(1):2. doi:10.1186/1939-4551-6-2

[6] Magerl M, Borzova E, Giménez-Arnau A, et al. The definition and diagnostic testing of physical and cholinergic urticarias – EAACI/GA [2] LEN/EDF/UNEV consensus panel recommendations. *Allergy*. 2009;64(12):1715–1721. doi:10.1111/j.1398-9995.2009.02177.x

[7] Dice JP. Physical urticaria. *Immunol Allergy Clin North Am*. 2004;24(2):225–46, vi. doi:10.1016/j.iac.2004.01.005

[8] Adachi J, Aoki T, Yamatodani A. Demonstration of sweat allergy in cholinergic urticaria. *J Dermatol Sci*. 1994;7(2):142–149. http://www.ncbi.nlm.nih.gov/pubmed/7520273. Accessed February 13, 2017.

[9] Jaqua NT, Peterson MR, Davis KL. Exercise-induced anaphylaxis: a case report and review of the diagnosis and treatment of a rare but potentially life-threatening syndrome. *Case Rep Med*. 2013;2013:1–4. doi:10.1155/2013/610726

[10] Rothbaum R, McGee J. Aquagenic urticaria: diagnostic and management challenges. *J Asthma Allergy*. 2016;9:209–213. doi:10.2147/JAA.S91505

[11] Zuberbier T, Aberer W, Asero R, et al. The EAACI/GA [2] LEN/EDF/WAO guideline for the definition, classification, diagnosis, and management of urticaria: the 2013 revision and update. *Allergy*. 2014;69(7):868–887. doi:10.1111/all.12313

[12] WANDERER A. Cold temperature challenges for acquired cold urticaria. *J Allergy Clin Immunol*. 2005;115(5):1096–1096. doi:10.1016/j.jaci.2005.01.013

[13] Ammann P, Surber E, Bertel O. Beta blocker therapy in cholinergic urticaria. *Am J Med*. 1999;107(2):191. http://www.ncbi.nlm.nih.gov/pubmed/10460061. Accessed February 13, 2017.

[14] Cuervo-Pardo L, Gonzalez-Estrada A, Lang DM. Diagnostic utility of challenge procedures for physical urticaria/angioedema syndromes. *Curr Opin Allergy Clin Immunol*. 2016;16(5):511–515. doi:10.1097/ACI.0000000000000298

[15] Hirschmann JV, Lawlor F, English JS, Louback JB, Winkelmann RK, Greaves MW. Cholinergic urticaria. A clinical and histologic study. *Arch Dermatol*. 1987;123(4):462–467. doi:10.1001/archderm.1987.01660280064024

[16] Ortonne J-P. Urticaria and its subtypes: the role of second-generation antihistamines. *Eur J Intern Med*. 2012;23(1):26–30. doi:10.1016/j.ejim.2011.09.008

[17] Trevisonno J, Balram B, Netchiporouk E, Ben-Shoshan M. Physical urticaria: review on classification, triggers and management with special focus on prevalence including a meta-analysis. *Postgrad Med*. 2015;127(6):565–570. doi:10.1080/00325481.2015.1045817

[18] Tokura Y. New Etiology in Cholinergic Urticaria. Cur Probl Dermatol. 2016;51:94-100. doi: 10.1159/000446787

[19] Sweeney TM, Dexter WW. Cholinergic urticaria in a jogger: ruling out exercise-induced anaphylaxis. *Phys Sportsmed*. 2003;31(6):32–36. doi:10.3810/psm.2003.06.399

[20] Silpa-archa N, Kulthanan K, Pinkaew S. Physical urticaria: prevalence, type and natural course in a tropical country. *J Eur Acad Dermatology Venereol*. 2011;25(10):1194–1199. doi:10.1111/j.1468-3083.2010.03951.x

[21] Lebrun CM. Care of the high school athlete: prevention and treatment of medical emergencies. *Instr Course Lect*. 2006;55:687–702. http://www.ncbi.nlm.nih.gov/pubmed/16958502. Accessed February 13, 2017.

[22] Peroni DG, Piacentini GL, Piazza M, Cametti E, Boner AL. Combined cetirizine-montelukast preventive treatment for food-dependent exercise-induced anaphylaxis. *Ann Allergy, Asthma Immunol*. 2010;104(3):272–273. doi:10.1016/j.anai.2009.12.002

[23] Montgomery SL. Cholinergic urticaria and exercise-induced anaphylaxis. *Curr Sports Med Rep*. 2015;14(1):61–63. doi:10.1249/JSR.0000000000000111

[24] Gimenez-Arnau A, Serra-Baldrich E, Camarasa JG. Chronic aquagenic urticaria. *Acta Derm Venereol*. 1992;72(5):389. http://www.ncbi.nlm.nih.gov/pubmed/1361294. Accessed February 12, 2017.

[25] Fearfield LA, Gazzard B, Bunker CB. Aquagenic urticaria and human immunodeficiency virus infection: treatment with stanozolol. *Br J Dermatol*. 1997;137(4):620–622. doi:10.1111/j.1365-2133.1997.tb03798.x

[26] Ozkaya E, Elinç-Aslan MS, Yazici S. Aquagenic urticaria and syncope associated with occult papillary thyroid carcinoma and improvement after total thyroidectomy. *Arch Dermatol*. 2011;147(12):1461–1462. doi:10.1001/archderm.147.12.1461

[27] Tkach JR. Aquagenic urticaria. *Cutis*. 1981;28(4):454, 463. http://www.ncbi.nlm.nih.gov/pubmed/7307567. Accessed February 12, 2017.

[28] McGee JS, Kirkorian AY, Pappert AS, Milgraum SS. An adolescent boy with urticaria to water: review of current treatments for aquagenic urticaria. *Pediatr Dermatol*. 2014;31(1):116–117. doi:10.1111/j.1525-1470.2012.01801.x

[29] Bayle P, Gadroy A, Messer L, Bazex J. Localized aquagenic urticaria: efficacy of a barrier cream. *Contact Dermatitis*. 2003;49(3):160–161. doi:10.1111/j.0105-1873.2003.0185c.x

[30] Torchia D, Francalanci S, Bellandi S, Fabbri P. Multiple physical urticarias. *Postgrad Med J*. 2008;84(987):e1–e2. doi:10.1136/pgmj.2007.062760

[31] Sharpe GR, Shuster S. In dermographic urticaria H2 receptor antagonists have a small but therapeutically irrelevant additional effect compared with H1 antagonists alone. *Br J Dermatol*. 1993;129(5):575–579. doi:10.1111/j.1365-2133.1993.tb00487.x

[32] Martínez-Escribano JA, Quecedo E, De la Cuadra J, Frías J, Sánchez-Pedreño P, Aliaga A. Treatment of aquagenic urticaria with PUVA and astemizole. *J Am Acad Dermatol*. 1997;36(1):118–119. http://www.ncbi.nlm.nih.gov/pubmed/8996279. Accessed February 13, 2017.

[33] Wakelin SH. Contact urticaria. *Clin Exp Dermatol.* 2001;26(2):132–136. doi:10.1046/j.1365-2230.2001.00780.x

[34] Bensefa-Colas L, Telle-Lamberton M, Faye S, et al. Occupational contact urticaria: lessons from the French National Network for Occupational Disease Vigilance and Prevention (RNV3P). *Br J Dermatol.* 2015;173(6):1453–1461. doi:10.1111/bjd.14050

[35] Chowdhury MMU. Occupational contact urticaria: a diagnosis not to be missed. *Br J Dermatol.* 2015;173(6):1364–1365. doi:10.1111/bjd.14250

[36] von Krogh G, Maibach HI. The contact urticaria syndrome–an updated review. *J Am Acad Dermatol.* 1981;5(3):328–342. http://www.ncbi.nlm.nih.gov/pubmed/6455450. Accessed February 13, 2017.

[37] Adisesh A, Robinson E, Nicholson PJ, Sen D, Wilkinson M, Standards of Care Working Group. U.K. standards of care for occupational contact dermatitis and occupational contact urticaria. *Br J Dermatol.* 2013;168(6):1167–1175. doi:10.1111/bjd.12256

Chapter 4

Chronic Inducible Urticaria: Part II

Murat Borlu, Salih Levent Cinar and Demet Kartal

Additional information is available at the end of the chapter

http://dx.doi.org/10.5772/intechopen.68754

Abstract

Physical urticaria (PU) is a subgroup of acquired, chronic inducible urticaria which is associated with a known physical trigger. In PU, the symptoms are induced by exogenous physical triggers, such as friction, pressure, vibration, cold, heat, or solar radiation. All the PUs may manifest with both wheals and angioedema at the sites of the triggers with the exceptions that urticaria factitia (UF) (symptomatic dermatographism) presents with wheals only and pressure urticaria presents with angioedema only. More than one form of physically induced urticarias can be present in one patient.

Keywords: physical urticaria, dermatographism, cold urticaria, heat urticaria, solar urticaria

1. Introduction: physical urticarias

Physically induced urticarias are symptomatic dermatographism, cold contact urticaria, heat contact urticaria, solar urticaria, delayed pressure urticaria, and vibratory urticaria. More than one of these can be present in a single patient making it difficult to manage. A known and repeatable physical trigger is the causative agent in these entities.

2. Urticaria factitia (dermatographism)

Urticaria factitia (UF) is also known as dermographic urticaria and symptomatic dermatographism. UF is the most common type of physical urticaria (PU) [1]. It must be differentiated from simple dermatographism in which whealing without itching is seen after moderate stroking of the skin [2]. White dermatographism which is seen in atopic patients is not related to UF [3]. UF is commonly seen in young adults and the mean duration of the disease was reported 3–9 years in different studies. The etiology of UF is still unknown [4]. Infections (hepatitis, upper respiratory tract infections), medications (progesterone, statins), and diabetes mellitus have been accused, but still, there is less evidence [5]. The pathogenic mechanism is believed to be the release of histamine following a mechano-immunological trigger [6].

In UF, itchy, white/pink/red wheals are observed after friction, scratching, rubbing, or tight clothing. Wheals appear in a few minutes following the trigger and may last a few hours. UF should come to mind in such cases, and the diagnosis should be made after positive skin provocation test [7].

The provocation in UF can be done by scratching or rubbing the skin with a blunt object (e.g., closed ballpoint pen tip or wooden tongue depressor). The flexor aspect of the forearm is the most suitable site for the provocation. Five to ten minutes of waiting time is mostly enough to conclude [8]. Recent guidelines suggest threshold testing with more advanced devices called the dermographometer. With this device, predefined and reproducible pressures can be applied to the testing area. The minimal force which is necessary to induce whealing can be determined with dermographometer and the disease activity in time (i.e., the patient's response to therapy) can be easily monitored. A positive response is noted when the patient shows a wheal response and complain pruritus [9].

Treatment of UF is mostly symptomatic. Avoidance is the best strategy. It is possible to prevent or minimize whealing by some precautions. Decreasing mechanical irritation in daily life is the essential of the therapy [10]. For symptomatic cases, new generation, nonsedating antihistamines are suggested as first-line treatment. In case of failure, the dose can be increased to fourfold. Type of the antihistamine can be changed, leukotriene antagonists and/or H2 antihistamines can be added [11]. Next two drugs in the treatment course are cyclosporine A and omalizumab [10, 12].

3. Delayed pressure urticaria (DPU)

Delayed pressure urticaria (DPU) manifests with pink/red whealing or angioedema of the skin at sites of sustained pressure, such as tight clothing, walking, or sitting down. It is called delayed because hours (6–8 h) are necessary for it to manifest [9, 13]. The patients suffer from severe pain and burning sensation in contrast to other PUs. Fatigue and arthralgia can accompany. The quality of life is much more affected in DPU patients when compared with other forms of PU. Sometimes, the lesions can last up to 72 h [14].

The diversity of symptoms suggests that other mediators such as cytokines and interleukins play a role in addition to histamine in the pathogenesis of DPU. There is evidence that IL-1, IL-3, IL-6, and tumor necrosis factor alpha (TNF-α) play a role in the etiopathogenesis [12]. More recently, neuropeptides, such as substance P and calcitonin gene-related peptide, have also shown to be taking a part in the formation of DPU [15].

http://dx.doi.org/10.5772/intechopen.68754

After taking proper history of the patient, if there is a suspicion of DPU, skin provocation test should be performed. Either weighted rods (7 kg weight with a 3 cm wide strap over the shoulder) or dermographometer can be used for this purpose. Weighted rods should be applied for 15 min and the dermographometer for 70 sec. If a red-colored edema appears after 6 h of the trigger, the test result is accepted as positive [16].

The etiology of DPU is not clear, so symptomatic treatment and avoidance are the mainstay of the therapy. Angioedema can be made less frequent or less severe with H1 antihistamines [3]. Most of the time, additional efforts are necessary to control the attacks. Leukotriene antagonists, dapsone, sulfasalazine, or combinations of these have been reported to be successfully used in the literature. Systemic steroids can be used in flare-ups. Recent studies show the benefit of omalizumab, but further controlled studies are necessary [17]. Anecdotal reports have shown the efficacy of intravenous immunoglobulins, tranexamic acid, and chloroquine [18, 19]. More recently, good results with gluten-free diet have been reported [14]. Cassano et al. reported remission of DPU after eradication of Blastocystis hominis surprisingly [13].

4. Heat contact urticaria (HCU)

Heat contact urticaria (HCU) is a rare type of PU in which wheals appear after contact to objects with temperature higher than the skin temperature itself [20]. The lesions emerge within a few minutes after the trigger and last for a few hours. Most of the patients are 20–45-year-old females. Most of the patients with HU have additional systemic symptoms such as weakness, headache, flushing, diarrhea, shortness of breath, and, even sometimes, syncope [21–23]. Some familial cases with autosomal dominant inheritance have been shown [2]. Most of the time, the trigger is a warm bath. Hot air, heating pads, open fire, heated stove, hair dryers, and indirect sunlight can also cause HU [24].

In case of a suspicion, container filled with hot water should be applied for about 5 min to the skin, or the patient should be asked to shower with hot water at a temperature of 45°C. If the testing area shows a palpable and clearly visible wheal and flare, it is accepted as a positive test. In most of the cases, a burning sensation can accompany the itching. In patients with a positive test result, stimulation time and temperature threshold levels should be measured [25].

Generalized HU must be differentiated from cholinergic urticaria. In HU, the whealing and flares are limited to the contact areas. The lesions are mostly in similar size and morphology. On the contrary, cholinergic urticaria is caused by an increase in the body core temperature and the lesions are small pinpoint hives with flushing [26].

In HCU, the principal of the treatment is to avoid heat if possible. Sometimes, heat desensitization can be effective. For symptomatic cases, H1 antihistamines are the first-line treatment, and in case of failure, the dose can be increased up to fourfold [26]. Omalizumab, montelukast, and cyclosporine are the third-line treatments [27]. Systemic steroids, colchicine, and disodium cromoglycate can be used in resistant cases [8].

5. Cold contact urticaria (CCU)

Cold contact urticaria (CCU) is characterized by the appearance of wheals and angioedema after exposure to cold. Lesions occur a few minutes following the cold contact. Lesions usually do not spread beyond the contact area [28]. This form of PU can be fatal in some cases. After extensive cold contact, severe angioedema or shock can be seen, mostly following swimming in cold water [29]. CCU is mostly seen in young adults and can continue for 5–8 years [2].

There are some rare variants of CCU. In some cases, CCU lesions develop 24–48 h after cold exposure. In this case, it is called *delayed CCU*. In *cold- dependent dermatographism,* the lesions are seen in cold-exposed and mechanically stimulated areas. *Cold- induced cholinergic urticaria* is the case that happens after physical exercise in cold air [30]. Familial cold auto-inflammatory syndrome (FCAS) is a rare autosomal dominant condition in which wheals appear within 2 h of systemic cold exposure. The lesions in this syndrome cannot be brought out by localized cold exposure. In FCAS, CIAS1/NLRP3 mutation leads to the activation of NLRP3 inflammasome complex, and finally, interleukin-1β is released from the mast cells. That is why FCAS responds dramatically to interleukin-1 antagonists [31].

CCU lesions and symptoms arise as a result of the release of some mediators such as histamine, prostaglandin D2, platelet-activating factor, and leukotrienes. Yet, it is not known why cold exposure causes the release of these mediators [32]. Half of the CCU patients are positive for antibodies against immunoglobulin E (IgE). IgE binding of some possible, unproven cold-depended skin antigens can be the reason of mast cell degradation [33]. It is also shown that CCU patients have circulating histamine-releasing factors and positive autologous serum skin test (ASST) [34].

Suspecting CCU or angioedema, one should perform cold stimulation test since fatality has been reported in several cases. In this test, the volar aspect of the forearm is exposed to ice cube in a thin plastic bag for 5 min. Ten minutes after the removal of the bag, the response should be assessed. If a well-demarcated, palpable wheal with a pruritic and burning sensation is present, the test is considered as positive. Ice cube should be in a thin bag in order to avoid any confusion with aquagenic urticaria [35]. Further critical temperature threshold tests with sophisticated devices can enable the patients to avoid situations that cause whealing [28]. More accurate testing is possible with computer-aided thermoelectric Peltier device. This device can also be used for the evaluation of the success of the treatments. In most of the studies, the critical temperature threshold is about 15–20°C [36]. The avoidance of below threshold temperatures is hard to manage in daily life. Even so, the patients should be warned to avoid contact with subthreshold temperatures.

The essential of the treatment of CCU is to avoid cold exposure. Non-sedating H1 antihistamines are accepted as the first-line therapy by the current European Academy of Allergy and Clinical Immunology (EAACI)/Global Allergy and Asthma European Network (GA^{2}LEN)/European Dermatology Forum (EDF)/World Allergy Organization (WAO) guidelines [5]. Usually high doses of H1 antihistamines are necessary to control CCU. Siebenhaar et al. claimed that high dose of desloratadine is better in controlling CCU when compared with the standard dose [37]. Likewise, Magerl et al. reported that H1 antihistamine up-dosing increases the success rate in the treatment of CCU [38].

In case of failure of therapy with H1 antihistamines, there is lack of well-studied alternative treatment options. Boyce JA reported successful treatment of cold-induced urticaria/anaphylaxis with omalizumab (anti-IgE) [39]. In 2011, Gualdi et al. claimed that a patient who had CCU healed with the use of etanercept for the treatment of co-existing psoriasis vulgaris. It was the first case report regarding the efficacy of etanercept in CCU [40]. Interleukin-1 receptor antagonist (anakinra) was shown to be effective in controlling severe idiopathic cold urticaria [41]. But more controlled studies are necessary to show the effects of omalizumab, etanercept, and anakinra in CCU.

Cold tolerance induction and maintenance therapy can also be tried with precaution due to the risk of anaphylaxis. In this procedure, the patient starts daily showers, first with water temperatures above the threshold and in time, the temperature of the water is decreased gradually. Acquired tolerance is maintained with daily cold showers for a long time [42].

6. Vibratory urticaria (VU)

Vibratory urticaria (VU) is a rare form of PU in which whealing and pruritus of the skin is observed after vibration at the contact area [43]. For proper diagnosis, provocation testing can be done by using a laboratory vortex mixer at a frequency of 1000 r.p.m. Test is considered positive with swelling 10 min after provocation [4]. Nonsedating H1 antihistamines are the first-line therapy [9].

7. Solar urticaria (SU)

Solar urticaria (SU) is characterized by wheals and sometimes angioedema after visible or ultraviolet (UV) light exposure [44]. Young adults are more commonly affected with a female predominance. The lesions which develop within 10 min of solar exposure are limited to the exposed areas. There are some variants of SU. Monfrecola et al. reported a case of solar urticaria with delayed onset [45]. Torinuki reported two cases with solar urticaria manifesting pruritic erythema but no whealing [46].

It is thought that some unknown photo-allergens that are produced in the skin after sun exposure cross-react with IgE on mast cells, and as a result, histamine and other inflammatory mediators are released. Norris et al. and Esdaile et al. claimed that bruised skin is more prone to the formation of SU. They tried to explain this by the migration of photo-allergens into the skin through damaged vessels [47, 48].

In a chronic urticaria patient, after history taking, if there is a suspicion of SU, we should perform provocation test. For this purpose, solar simulators can be used. Provocation should be performed on body areas which are usually not exposed to sunlight, such as the buttocks, and

UVA, UVB, and visible light should be used separately. In a positive test result which means flare and whealing within 10 min of the exposure, threshold testing should also be done using increasing radiation doses [8].

It is difficult to manage SU. Avoidance of the sunlight exposure is almost impossible. According to the guidelines, H1 antihistamines are the first-line treatment options. But only one-third of the patients respond well to the antihistamines. Repeated sunlight exposure can induce tolerance [45]. For this purpose, PUVA and narrow-band UVB can be used. Güzelbey et al. reported successful treatment of SU with anti-immunoglobulin E therapy [49]. There are few other studies in the literature showing the efficacy or inefficacy of omalizumab [50, 51].

Hughes et al. and Correia et al. reported that SU can be successfully treated with intravenous immunoglobulin [52, 53]. On the contrary, Llamas-Velasco et al. claimed that intravenous immunoglobulin was ineffective in the treatment of SU [54]. In 2011, Haylett et al. revealed that systemic photoprotection was possible with alpha-melanocyte-stimulating hormone (afamelanotide). Its mechanism of action is to increase melanization of the skin. With this effect, it protects the skin from the penetration of UV and visible wavelengths [55].

8. Conclusion

Physically induced urticarias are hard to manage. Avoidance is the best treatment option, but it is impossible most of the time. We should be alert that more than one form can be together in a patient. Although antihistamines are the first-line therapy, usually other options are required to manage.

Author details

Murat Borlu, Salih Levent Cinar* and Demet Kartal

*Address all correspondence to: sleventcinar@yahoo.com

Faculty of Medicine, Erciyes University, Kayseri, Turkey

References

[1] Abajian M, Młynek A, Maurer M. Physical urticaria. Current Allergy and Asthma Reports. 2012 Aug;**12**(4):281-287. DOI: 10.1007/s11882-012-0269-0

[2] Dice JP. Physical urticaria. Immunology and Allergy Clinics of North America. 2004 May;**24**(2):225-246. DOI: 10.1016/j.iac.2004.01.005

[3] Black AK, Lawlor F, Greaves MW. Consensus meeting on the definition of physical urticarias and urticarial vasculitis. Clinical and Experimental Dermatology. 1996 Nov;**21**(6):424-426. DOI: 10.1111/j.1365-2230.1996.tb00146.x

[4] Zuberbier T, Aberer W, Asero R, et al. The EAACI/GA(2) LEN/EDF/WAO guideline for the definition, classification, diagnosis, and management of urticaria: The 2013 revision and update. Allergy. 2014 Jul;**69**(7):868-887. DOI: 10.1111/all.12313

[5] Zuberbier T, Bindslev-Jensen C, Canonica W, et al. EAACI/GA2LEN/EDF guideline: Management of urticaria. Allergy. 2006 Mar;**61**(3):321-331. DOI: 10.111/j.1398-9995.2005.00964.x

[6] Breathnach SM, Allen R, Ward AM, et al. Symptomatic dermatographism: Natural history, clinical features laboratory investigations and response to therapy. Clinical and Experimental Dermatology. 1983 Sep;**8**(5):463-476. DOI: 10.1111/j.1365-2230.1983.tb01814.x

[7] Kontou-Fili K, Borici-Mazi R, Kapp A, et al. Physical urticaria: Classification and diagnostic guidelines. An EAACI position paper. Allergy. 1997 May;**52**(5):504-513. DOI: 10.1111/j.1398-9995.1997.tb02593.x

[8] Magerl M, Borzova E, Giménez-Arnau A, et al. The definition and diagnostic testing of physical and cholinergic urticarias—EAACI/GA2LEN/EDF/UNEV consensus panel recommendations. Allergy. 2009 Dec;**64**(12):1715-1721. DOI: 10.1111/j.1398-9995.2009.02177.x

[9] Magerl M, Schmolke J, Metz M, et al. Prevention of signs and symptoms of dermographic urticaria by single-dose ebastine 20 mg. Clinical and Experimental Dermatology. 2009 Jul;**34**(5):e137-e140. DOI: 10.1111/j.1365-2230.2008.03097.x

[10] Mecoli CA, Morgan AJ, Schwartz RA. Symptomatic dermatographism: Current concepts in clinical practice with an emphasis on the pediatric population. Cutis. 2011 May;**87**(5):221-225

[11] Sastre J. Ebastine in allergic rhinitis and chronic idiopathic urticaria. Allergy. 2008 Dec;**63**(Suppl 89):1-20. DOI: 10.1111/j.1398-9995.2008.01897.x

[12] Metz M, Altrichter S, Ardelean E, et al. Anti-immunoglobulin E treatment of patients with recalcitrant physical urticaria. International Archives of Allergy and Immunology. 2011;**154**(2):177-180. DOI: 10.1159/000320233

[13] Cassano N, Scoppio BM, Loviglio MC, et al. Remission of delayed pressure urticaria after eradication of Blastocystis hominis. Acta Dermato-Venereologica. 2005;**85**(4):357-358. DOI: 10.1080/00015550510026695

[14] Lawlor F, Black AK. Delayed pressure urticaria. Immunology and Allergy Clinics of North America. 2004 May;**24**(2):247-258. DOI: 10.1016/j.iac.2004.01.006

[15] Trevisonno J, Balram B, Netchiporouk E, et al. Physical urticaria: Review on classification, triggers and management with special focus on prevalence including a meta-analysis. Postgraduate Medical. 2015 Aug;**127**(6):565-570. DOI: 10.1080/00325481.2015.1045817

[16] Cuervo-Pardo L, Gonzalez-Estrada A, Lang DM. Diagnostic utility of challenge procedures for physical urticaria/angioedema syndromes: A systematic review. Current Opinion in Allergy and Clinical Immunology. 2016 Oct;**16**(5):511-515. DOI: 10.1097/ACI.0000000000000298

[17] Tonacci A, Billeci L, Pioggia G, et al. Omalizumab for the treatment of chronic idiopathic urticaria: Systematic review of the literature. Pharmacotherapy. 2017;37(4): 464-480. DOI:10.1002/phar.1915

[18] Kulthanan K, Thumpimukvatana N. Positive impact of chloroquine on delayed pressure urticaria. Journal of Drugs in Dermatology. 2007 Apr;**6**(4):445-446

[19] Shedden C, Highet AS. Delayed pressure urticaria controlled by tranexamic acid. Clinical and Experimental Dermatology. 2006 Mar;**31**(2):295-296. DOI: 10.1111/j.1365-2230.2005.02014.x

[20] Chang A, Zic JA. Localized heat urticaria. Journal of the American Academy of Dermatology. 1999 Aug;**41**(2 Pt 2):354-356. DOI: 10.1016/S0190-9622(99)70387-7

[21] Grant JA, Findlay SR, Thueson DO, et al. Local heat urticaria/angioedema: Evidence for histamine release without complement activation. Journal of Allergy and Clinical Immunology. 1981 Jan;**67**(1):75-77. DOI: 10.1016/0091-6749(81)90049-X

[22] Irwin RB, Lieberman P, Friedman MM, et al. Mediator release in local heat urticaria: Protection with combined H1 and H2 antagonists. Journal of Allergy and Clinical Immunology. 1985 Jul;**76**(1):35-39. DOI: 10.1016/0091-6749(85)90801-2

[23] Johansson EA, Reunala T, Koskimies S, et al. Localized heat urticaria associated with a decrease in serum complement factor B (C3 proactivator). British Journal of Dermatology. 1984 Feb;**110**(2):227-231. DOI: 10.1111/j.1365-2133.1984.tb07472.x

[24] Baba T, Nomura K, Hanada K, et al. Immediate-type heat urticaria: Report of a case and study of plasma histamine release. British Journal of Dermatology. 1998 Feb;**138**(2):326-328. DOI: 10.1046/j.1365-2133.1998.02084.x

[25] Pezzolo E, Peroni A, Schena D, et al. Preheated autologous serum skin test in localized heat urticaria. Clinical and Experimental Dermatology. 2014 Dec;**39**(8):921-923. DOI: 10.1111/ced.12447

[26] Pezzolo E, Peroni A, Gisondi P, et al. Heat urticaria: A revision of published cases with an update on classification and management. British Journal of Dermatology. 2016 Sep;**175**(3):473-478. DOI: 10.1111/bjd.14543

[27] Bullerkotte U, Wieczorek D, Kapp A, et al. Effective treatment of refractory severe heat urticaria with omalizumab. Allergy. 2010 Jul;**65**(7):931-932. DOI: 10.1111/j.1398-9995.2009.02268.x

[28] Wanderer AA. Cold temperature challenges for acquired cold urticaria. Journal of Allergy and Clinical Immunology. 2005 May;**115**(5):1096. DOI: 10.1016/j.jaci.2005.01.013

[29] Alangari AA, Twarog FJ, Shih MC, et al. Clinical features and anaphylaxis in children with cold urticaria. Pediatrics. 2004 Apr;**113**(4):e313-e317. DOI: 10.1542/peds.113.4.e313

[30] Katsarou-Katsari A, Makris M, Lagogianni E, et al. Clinical features and natural history of acquired cold urticaria in a tertiary referral hospital: A 10-year prospective study. Journal

of the European Academy of Dermatology and Venereology. 2008 Dec;**22**(12):1405-1411. DOI: 10.1111/j.1468-3083.2008.02840.x

[31] Nakamura Y, Kambe N, Saito M, et al. Mast cells mediate neutrophil recruitment and vascular leakage through the NLRP3 inflammasome in histamine-independent urticaria. Journal of Experimental Medicine. 2009 May;**206**(5):1037-1046. DOI: 10.1084/jem.20082179

[32] Wasserman SI, Ginsberg MH. Release of platelet factor 4 into the blood after cold challenge of patients with cold urticaria. Journal of Allergy and Clinical Immunology. 1984 Sep;**74**(3 Pt 1):275-279

[33] Gruber BL, Baeza ML, Marchese MJ, et al. Prevalence and functional role of anti-IgE autoantibodies in urticarial syndromes. Journal of Investigative Dermatology. 1988 Feb;**90**(2):213-217. DOI: 10.1111/1523-1747.ep12462239

[34] Asero R, Tedeschi A, Lorini M. Histamine release in idiopathic cold urticaria. Allergy. 2002 Dec;57(12):1211-1212. DOI: 10.1034/j.1398-9995.2002.23893_3.x

[35] Gimenez-Arnau A, Serra-Baldrich E, Camarasa JG. Chronic aquagenic urticaria. Acta Dermato-Venereologica. 1992 Sep;**72**(5):389

[36] Siebenhaar F, Staubach P, Metz M, et al. Peltier effect-based temperature challenge: an improved method for diagnosing cold urticaria. Journal of Allergy and Clinical Immunology. 2004 Nov;**114**(5):1224-1225. DOI: 10.1016/j.jaci.2004.07.018

[37] Siebenhaar F, Degener F, Zuberbier T, et al. High-dose desloratadine decreases wheal volume and improves cold provocation thresholds compared with standard-dose treatment in patients with acquired cold urticaria: A randomized, placebo-controlled, crossover study. Journal of Allergy and Clinical Immunology. 2009 Mar;**123**(3):672-679. DOI: 10.1016/j.jaci.2008.12.008

[38] Magerl M, Schmolke J, Siebenhaar F, et al. Acquired cold urticaria symptoms can be safely prevented by ebastine. Allergy. 2007 Dec;**62**(12):1465-1468. DOI: 10.1111/j.1398-9995.2007.01500.x

[39] Boyce JA. Successful treatment of cold-induced urticaria/anaphylaxis with anti-IgE. Journal of Allergy and Clinical Immunology. 2006 Jun;**117**(6):1415-1418. DOI: 10.1016/j.jaci.2006.04.003

[40] Gualdi G, Monari P, Rossi MT, et al. Successful treatment of systemic cold contact urticaria with etanercept in a patient with psoriasis. British Journal of Dermatology. 2012 Jun;**166**(6):1373-1374. DOI: 10.1111/j.1365-2133.2011.10797.x

[41] Bodar EJ, Simon A, de Visser M, et al. Complete remission of severe idiopathic cold urticaria on interleukin-1 receptor antagonist (anakinra). Netherlands Journal of Medicine. 2009 Oct;**67**(9):302-305

[42] von Mackensen YA, Sticherling M. Cold urticaria: Tolerance induction with cold baths. British Journal of Dermatology. 2007 Oct;**157**(4):835-836. Epub 2007 Aug 17. DOI: 10.1111/j.1365-2133.2007.08109.x

[43] Sarmast SA, Fang F, Zic J. Vibratory angioedema in a trumpet professor. Cutis. 2014 Feb;93(2):E10-E11

[44] Chong WS, Khoo SW. Solar urticaria in Singapore: An uncommon photodermatosis seen in a tertiary dermatology center over a 10-year period. Photodermatology, Photoimmunology and Photomedicine. 2004 Apr;20(2):101-104. DOI: 10.1111/j.1600-0781.2004.00083.x

[45] Monfrecola G, Nappa P, Pini D. Solar urticaria with delayed onset: A case report. Photodermatology. 1988 Apr;**5>**(2):103-104

[46] Torinuki W. Two patients with solar urticaria manifesting pruritic erythema. Journal of Dermatology. 1992 Oct;**19**(10):635-637. DOI: 10.1111/j.1346-8138.1992.tb03745.x

[47] Norris PG, Hawk JL. Bruising and susceptibility to solar urticaria. British Journal of Dermatology. 1991 Apr;**124**(4):393. DOI: 10.1111/j.1365-2133.1991.tb00607.x

[48] Esdaile B, Grabczynska S, George S. Solar urticaria confined to areas of bruising. Photodermatology, Photoimmunology and Photomedicine. 2010 Aug;**26**(4):211-212. DOI: 10.1111/j.1600-0781.2010.00515.x

[49] Güzelbey O, Ardelean E, Magerl M, et al. Successful treatment of solar urticaria with anti-immunoglobulin E therapy. Allergy. 2008 Nov;**63**(11):1563-1565. DOI: 10.1111/j.1398-9995.2008.01879.x

[50] Goetze S, Elsner P. Solar urticaria. Journal der Deutschen Dermatologischen Gesellschaft. 2015 Dec;**3**(12):1250-1253. DOI: 10.1111/ddg.12809

[51] Müller S, Schempp CM, Jakob T. Failure of omalizumab in the treatment of solar urticaria. Journal of the European Academy of Dermatology and Venereology. 2016 Mar;**30**(3):524-525. DOI: 10.1111/jdv.12922

[52] Hughes R, Cusack C, Murphy GM, et al. Solar urticaria successfully treated with intravenous immunoglobulin. Clinical and Experimental Dermatology. 2009 Dec;**34**(8):e660-e662. DOI: 10.1111/j.1365-2230.2009.03374.x

[53] Correia I, Silva J, Filipe P, et al. Solar urticaria treated successfully with intravenous high-dose immunoglobulin: A case report. Photodermatology, Photoimmunology and Photomedicine. 2008 Dec;**24**(6):330-331. DOI: 10.1111/j.1600-0781.2008.00386.x

[54] Llamas-Velasco M, Argila DD, Eguren C, et al. Solar urticaria unresponsive to intravenous immunoglobulins. Photodermatology, Photoimmunology and Photomedicine. 2011 Feb;**27**(1):53-54. DOI: 10.1111/j.1600-0781.2010.00553.x

[55] Haylett AK, Nie Z, Brownrigg M, et al. Systemic photoprotection in solar urticaria with α-melanocyte-stimulating hormone analogue [Nle4-D-Phe7]-α-MSH. British Journal of Dermatology. 2011 Feb;**164**(2):407-414. DOI: 10.1111/j.1365-2133.2010.10104.x

Chapter 5

Contact Urticaria

Isil Bulur and Hilal Gokalp

Additional information is available at the end of the chapter

http://dx.doi.org/10.5772/67994

Abstract

The term "contact urticaria" was first used by Fisher in 1973 as a pruritic wheal and flare reaction appearing within minutes after the contact of the skin with the substance causing the reaction. The incidence is not clearly known due to misdiagnosis. The causative agents can be plants, food substances, drugs, cosmetic products, chemicals and animal products. Contact urticaria is classified according to the underlying mechanism as non-immunologic (irritant), immunologic (allergic) and mixed (undetermined). It is usually local but can rarely cause systemic symptoms and sometimes result in anaphylaxis. Diagnostic tests include the prick test, open test and RAST test. The main treatment step is avoiding the causative agent.

Keywords: urticaria, contact, sensitization, immunologic, irritant, occupational

1. Introduction

The term "contact urticaria" was first described by Fisher in 1973 as a pruritic wheal and flare reaction occurring within minutes after contact with the suspected contact substance [1]. Contact urticaria is accepted as one of the chronic inducible urticaria disorders and is seen in 1–2% of chronic urticaria patients [2, 3]. Although the disorder is thought to be common, its clear incidence is not known due to underreporting and underdiagnosis [4–6]. It is often seen on the face, hands and arms and is characterized by itching, redness and swelling [7]. A wide variety of allergens including animal products, plants, food, chemicals, cosmetics, flavoring, medications, enzymes and metals are responsible for contact urticaria development (**Table 1**).

Contact urticaria is classified according to the underlying mechanism as non-immunologic/irritant, immunologic/allergic urticaria and those with mixed/undetermined pathomechanism [4]. Non-immunologic contact urticaria (NICU) is often characterized by localized reactions regressing within a short time. Immunologic contact urticaria (ICU) occurs as a type 1

- Animal-animal derivated products (blood, urine, saliva, seminal fluid, hair), meat, milk, cheese, eggs, honey silk, wool
- Cosmetic components: hair care products (ammonium persulphate, henna, parafenilendiamin), emulsifiers, fragnances, allantoin, aloe gel
- Dyes: an azo, anthraquinone or phthalocyanine derivative
- Enzymes
- Foods: furits, vegetables, meat, fish, spice, plants, grains
- Food additives:flavoring, fragnansec, taste enhancer
- Metals: aluminum, chromium cobalt, copper, gold, nickel, zinc
- Natural rubber latex
- Plants: weed, wood, ornamental
- Preservatives and disenfectants: sodium benzoate, benzoic acid, benzyl alcohol, sorbic acid, formaldehyde, parabens, povidone-iodine, chloramine, chlorhexidine

Table 1. Contact allergens causing contact urticaria [5, 6].

hypersensitivity reaction in previously sensitized individuals and there may be involvement in the respiratory and gastrointestinal system in addition to the skin, resulting in anaphylactic reaction [7]. Contact urticarial syndrome (CUS) is characterized by systemic findings occurring within minutes after contact with the contact allergen, and it was first identified in 1975 by Maibach and Johnson [8, 9].

Contact urticaria usually causes a localized and transient reaction and the diagnosis is therefore often missed. However one must consider that it leads to a marked decrease in the patient's quality of life. It is therefore essential to diagnose the condition and determine the suspect agent.

This chapter reviews the definition of contact urticaria together with the causative agents, diagnostic tests and ways to avoid the disorder together with a survey of the literature.

2. Classification of contact urticaria

2.1. Non-immunologic contact urticaria

Non-immunologic contact urticaria occurs with the first contact of the person to the substance causing reaction. It is the most common type of contact urticaria. NICU is thought to occur with the stimulation of vasogenic mediators without involvement of immunological processes [4]. In addition to nonspecific histamine secretion, leukotriene, prostaglandin, substance A and eicosanoids are also responsible for this reaction [4, 10].

"Stinging nettle (Urtica dioica)" is best known among the agents that lead to NICU. Preservatives, fragrances, foodstuffs, cosmetics, toiletries, topical medications, chemicals and insecticides can

http://dx.doi.org/10.5772/67994

also cause NICU (**Table 2**). The severity and duration of the reaction in NICU vary according to the size of the contact area and the substance. It is characterized by localized redness, swelling, itching and burning. The lesion tends to regress within hours [4]. NICU is mostly seen on the face, antecubital fossa, upper back, upper arm, volar forearm and lower back.

2.2. Immunologic contact urticaria

Immunologic contact urticaria is a type 1 hypersensitivity reaction after contact of the allergen to the skin and mucosa. It often occurs with IgE sensitization but IgG and IgM can also be responsible for complement activation [10]. The penetration of the allergen to the epidermis results in IgE binding to the mast cells and the secretion of vasoactive substances such as histamine, prostaglandin, leukotriene and quinine [6]. While proteins with a molecular weight over 10,000 lead to sensitization directly, chemicals with a low molecular weight (below 1000) act like a hapten and bind to carrier proteins such as albumin to cause ICU [6, 10].

Atopic individuals are more prone to ICU development [10–12]. The identification and diagnosis of the disorder therefore become difficult especially in individuals with eczema. One of the significant characteristics of the disease is that it is not only related to the skin but can be generalized with respiratory and gastrointestinal system involvement and anaphylactic shock, leading to systemic findings [4]. Protein (animal proteins, plants) and non-protein (chemicals, drugs and metals) materials can cause ICU (**Table 3**).

Natural rubber latex is the most common allergen held responsible for ICU [4]. Latex is a fluid obtained from the body of the tropical rubber tree (*Hevea brasiliensis*) and is a natural rubber resource. Latex proteins are allergenic and preserve their antigenic characteristics in the final product. Gloves, catheters, tourniquets, stethoscopes, masks, electrode tips, balloons, condoms, pacifiers, stretch clothes, shoe soles and underwater goggles contain latex [13]. Health workers, cleaning workers and hairdressers are often at risk. However, natural latex rubber is common in daily life and the general population is also at risk in terms of ICU development [13–15]. Cross-reaction with latex has been identified with fruits (avocado, banana, apple and kiwi), vegetables (paprika, carrot, celery, potato and tomato), plants and pollens [4, 16–21]. It must also remember that the raw food protein can show allergenic reaction, but the reaction disappears when these cooked. This applies to raw fish, garlic and herbs in particular [22].

2.2.1. Contact urticaria syndrome

The term "contact urticaria syndrome" was first used in 1975 by Maibach and Johnson to identify the systemic reaction developing after contact with a substance [8]. CUS is more common in ICU, but can also develop in NICU [23]. It is characterized by a heterogeneous clinical picture including systemic findings occurring immediately following a contact urticaria reaction. The systemic involvement consists of four stages identified by von Krogh and Maibach [9] (**Table 4**). Localized urticaria is seen at stage 1 and generalized urticaria at stage 2. Stage 3 is characterized by bronchial asthma, rhinoconjunctivitis, orolaryngeal syndrome and gastrointestinal dysfunction and

Immunological contact urticaria

- Acetylsalicylic acid
- Aminophenazone
- Bacitracin
- Benzophenone
- Benzoyl peroxide
- Benzylic alcohol
- Butylhydroxytoluene
- Cephalosporins
- Chloramine T
- Chlorhexidine
- Chlorpromazine
- Colophony
- Copper
- Di(2-ethylhexyl) phthalate (DOP)
- Diethyltoluamide I
- Diglycidyl ether of bisphenol A (DGEBA) epoxy resin
- Etofenamate
- Gentamycin
- Levomepromazine
- Lindane
- Methylhexahydrophthalic anhydride
- Methylmetacrylate
- Naphthylacetic acid
- Nickel
- Neomycin
- Nylon
- Oleic acid
- *O*-phenylphenate
- Penicillins
- Phenoxyethanol
- Phenylmercuric acetate
- Platinum salts
- Polyethylene
- Polyfunctional aziridine hardener

http://dx.doi.org/10.5772/67994

- Promethazine
- Propylene glycol
- Pyrazolone
- Rifamycin
- Wool alcohol
- Xylene

Non-immunological contact urticaria

- Acetic acid
- Amyl alcohol
- Balsam of Friar
- Benzaldehyde
- Benzoic acid
- Butyl alcohol
- Butyric acid
- Capsaicin
- Chlorocresol
- Chloroform
- Cinnamaldehyde
- Cinnamic acid
- Cobalt chloride
- Diethyl fumarate
- Ethyl alcohol
- Isopropyl alcohol
- Nicotinic acid
- Sodium benzoate
- Sorbic acid
- Tar

Immunological/non-immunological contact urticaria

- Benzocaine
- Balsam of Peru (*Myroxylon pereirae*)
- Formaldehyde
- Fragrances
- Iodine
- Menthol
- Persulfates

Table 2. Non protein molecules responsible for contact urticaria [10].

Animals and their derivates

- Aminiotic fluid
- Blood
- Calf
- Cow
- Caterpillar
- Dogs
- Guinea pig
- Horse
- Hair (human, mice, rat)
- Jellyfish
- Mites
- Pig
- Plasenta
- Rat
- Saliva
- Serum
- Silk
- Urine
- Worm

Plant and derviates

- Algae
- Aloe
- Birch
- Camolile
- Corn powder
- Elm tree
- Larch
- Lime
- Mulbery
- Poppy flowers
- Sunflower seeds
- Tobacco
- Tropical woods
- Tulips

Plant derivates

- Abietic acid
- Colophony
- Cornstrach
- Latex rubber
- Turpedine

Vegetables

- Asparagus
- Beans
- Cabbage
- Celery
- Fungi
- Garlic
- Lettuce
- Mushroom
- Mustard
- Onion
- Rice
- Soybean
- Tomato

Fruit

- Apple
- Apricot
- Banana
- Kiwi
- Lemon
- Lime
- Mango
- Orange
- Peach
- Peanut
- Plum
- Strawbery
- Watermelon

Meat: beef, calf, lamb, chicken, Turkey
Fish: cod, crab, frog, seafood, raw fish
Other animal product: cheese, egg, honey, milk

Table 3. Protein molecules responsible for contact urticaria [6].

stage 4 by anaphylaxis [9]. CUS is characterized by itching, burning and pain associated with an urticarial plaque in the localized form. The disease can result in nasal symptoms, conjunctivitis, bronchospasm, dyspepsia and anaphylactic shock following angioedema. Non-dermatologic symptoms can be seen in 15% of the patients [9].

2.3. Mixed/undetermined pathomechanism

The pathogenesis is not clear for some of the substance, while certain agents result in only immunologic or non-immunologic urticaria. Ammonium persulfate is an example of these substance that can cause contact urticaria with an undetermined pathomechanism [4, 9] (**Table 2**).

- Stage 1: Localized urticaria, dermatitis, nonspecific symptoms (itching, tingling, burning, etc.)
- Stage 2: Generalize urticaria
- Stage 3: Bronchial asthma, rhinoconjunctivitis, orolaryngeal symptom and gastointestinal dysfunction
- Stage 4: Anaphylactic and anaphylactoid reaction

Table 4. Contact urticaria syndrome staging [9].

3. Special types of contact urticaria

3.1. Occupational contact urticaria

Skin diseases are the second most common occupational diseases in Europe and occupational contact urticaria (OCU) makes up 1–8% of occupational skin disorders [12]. The most commonly affected professional groups are healthcare employees, food handlers, farmers and hairdressers [24, 25]. Immunologic and non-immunologic contact urticaria types can be seen in OCU. The risk of sensitization against all proteins is high in presence of atopy in OCU [10]. Besides, atopy is also important in OCU associated with NICU [10].

Natural rubber latex is the most commonly identified allergen and this allergy is seen in 1–3% in general population and 5–10% of healthcare workers in Europe [10]. *H. brasiliensis* proteins are the main responsible agents for natural rubber latex allergy [10]. A reaction against modified proteins (wheat, soy and Croetin Q) that are added to shampoo and especially ammonium persulfate is often observed in hairdressers [26, 27]. Reactions against saliva, amniotic fluid, urine and seminal fluid of animals have been defined in animal handlers, farmers and veterinarians. Dyes cause contact urticaria at significant levels in the cosmetic and industrial sectors [4, 6].

3.2. Oral allergy syndrome (food contact dermatitis)

"Oral allergy syndrome" is used to identify ICU developing in the mucosa [28]. It is characterized by mucosal edema, itching and a burning sensation after contact of the oral mucosa with respiratory allergens [29]. Cross-reactivity between homologous pollen and food allergens is accused in the etiology [29]. The term pollen-food allergy syndrome (PFAS) can therefore also be used [30].

Fruits and vegetables especially apples, carrots, tomatoes, pears, cherries, plums, celery, spices and hazelnuts are the agents that are often blamed for the oral allergy syndrome. The individuals who have oral allergy syndrome frequently suffer from atopy and pollen allergy, therefore a cross allergy against IgE antibodies has been observed [30].

3.3. Physical contact urticaria

Some physical urticaria cases occur following skin contact with hot, cold, light (UV: solar urticaria), water or as dermographism, pressure hives and vibratory angioedema. A physical agent does not cause a reaction alone but leads to the activation of a chemical product in some cases. It is possible to see this mechanism in induced contact urticaria. Benzophenones, chlorpromazine, methenamine hippurate and formaldehyde are included among the agents that can cause such a reaction [31–33].

3.4. Delayed and prolonged contact urticaria

Contact urticaria, protein contact dermatitis and allergic contact dermatitis can sometime coexist. The patients can primarily present with an urticarial lesion and the contact dermatitis and eczematous lesions can develop later [32, 34]. Elm, vaseline and castor oil are agents that often cause delayed and prolonged contact urticaria [10].

4. Diagnosis

The contact urticaria diagnosis is made with a detailed history and dermatologic examination. The detailed history should include the occupation, hobbies, additional systemic disorders and current medication of the patient, and when the lesion started, how long it lasted and the presence of accompanying symptoms (allergic rhinitis, conjunctivitis, gastrointestinal symptoms and angioedema) [7]. An open test, patch test, prick test, scratch test and intradermal test are the test mainly used for diagnosis.

The allergens are properly prepared and applied to the skin of the inner surface of the forearm or back in the open test. The test is conducted both with cooked and uncooked samples of the foods. The evaluation of the contact urticaria response should be performed 45-60 minutes after the contact of allergen with the skin [13]. This duration can be extended to 1 hour if NICU is suspected. A positive response in contact urticaria consists of edema and/or erythema [6].

The test substances for the rubbing test are prepared as in the open test and are applied by rubbing with a finger or cotton swab 15–20 times to increase the absorption. Dermographism should be tested before the rubbing procedure and the test should not be performed with latex gloves. The evaluation is performed 15–20 minutes after the test substances are removed [13].

The short-term patch test can be used to prevent the contact urticarial factors from spreading or drying. In the closed test method, the patch test sites are opened after 20 minutes and the urticarial reaction evaluated [13].

The prick test demonstrates the presence of specific tissue IgE against the allergen. It is used in the diagnosis of immunologic contact urticaria [13]. Commercial antigens in 2–3 ml bottles are used for the test. The test can be conducted on the skin of the inner surface of the forearm or the back. The evaluation is performed 15–20 minutes after the contact of the allergen with the skin. However, the test should be finalized early in case of severe reaction development. The most important point during the test is to use a separate lancet for each allergen and to apply the allergens 2 cm away from each other [13].

After a superficial scratch of 5–10 mm is formed with the lancet, the test substance is applied to the scratch and evaluation is performed 5–20 minutes later [13].

In the closed scratch test, the test substance is applied similarly and then covered. The evaluation of the test is performed 20 minutes later [13].

It is possible to use histamine hydrochloride as a positive control and aqueous sodium hydroxide as a negative control for the prick and scratch tests.

The radioallergosorbent test (RAST) measures specific IgE in the serum. It can be used for the diagnosis of ICU and CUS and also detect cross-allergenicity [16].

If a strong early reaction is suspected, the first step should be specific IgE measurement and it should be followed by non-invasive skin tests (open test-rubbing test and close test) and invasive skin tests (prick test, scratch test and closed scratch test) at the final stage [13]. Besides specific IgE measurement, open test should be used first when a direct puncture test is risky in latex allergy. It should not be forgotten that latex can cause cross-react with fruits, vegetables and seafood, plants and pollen while latex allergy is evaluated [18–21].

It is necessary to discontinue H1 antihistamines for 1 week, H2 antihistamines for 1 day, steroids (if used for longer than 1 week) for 1–3 weeks and phototherapy for a couple of weeks before skin tests [13, 35]. The possibility of an anaphylactic reaction should be considered during skin tests. All skin tests should therefore be conducted in the special clinic where the proper and necessary equipment are available.

5. Prevention and treatment

The first step in the treatment is to avoid and eliminate the allergen. Identification of the allergens is therefore the main step of the treatment [36].

The secretion of histamine and other mediators from mast cells should be prevented to decrease symptoms. The first treatment step consists of 2nd generation H1 antihistamines. The antihistamine dose can be increased if there is no benefit at first. In addition to oral antihistamines, systemic steroid treatment can also be used in severe cases. Conducting the treatment in units where resuscitation can be performed is appropriate for anaphylaxis and anaphylactic shock cases [6].

Author details

Isil Bulur[1]* and Hilal Gokalp[2]

*Address all correspondence to: isilbulur@yahoo.com

1 Department of Dermatology, Memorial Şişli Hospital, Istanbul, Turkey

2 Department of Dermatology, Koç University School of Medicine, Istanbul, Turkey

References

[1] Fisher AA. Contact Dermatitis, 2nd ed. Philadelphia: Lea & Febiger, 1973.

[2] Gomułka K, Panaszek B. Contact urticaria syndrome caused by haptens. Postepy Dermatol Alergol 2014;31:108–112. doi: 10.5114/pdia.2014.40915.

[3] Greaves MW. Pathology and classification of urticaria. Immunol Allergy Clin North Am 2014;34:1–9. doi: 10.1016/j.iac.2013.07.009.

[4] Wakelin SH. Contact urticaria. Clin Exp Dermatol 2001;26(2):132–136.

[5] Giménez-Arnau A. Contact urticaria and the environment. Rev Environ Health 2014;29:207–215. doi: 10.1515/reveh-2014-0042.

[6] Gimenez-Arnau A, Maurer M, De La Cuadra J, Maibach H. Immediate contact skin reactions, an update of contact urticaria, contact urticaria syndrome and protein contact dermatitis—"a never ending story". Eur J Dermatol 2010;20:552–562. doi: 10.1684/ejd.2010.1049.

[7] Bhatia R, Alikhan A, Maibach HI. Contact urticaria: present scenario. Indian J Dermatol 2009;54:264–268. doi: 10.4103/0019-5154.55639.

[8] Maibach HI, Johnson HL. Contact urticaria syndrome. Contact urticaria to diethyltoluamide (immediate-type hypersensitivity). Arch Dermatol 1975;111:726–730.

[9] von Krogh G, Maibach HI. The contact urticaria syndrome—an updated review. J Am Acad Dermatol 1981;5:328–342.

[10] Bourrain JL. Occupational contact urticaria. Clin Rev Allergy Immunol 2006;30:39–46. doi: 10.1385/CRIAI:30:1:039.

[11] Amin S, Tanglertsampan C, Maibach HI. Contact urticaria syndrome: 1997. Am J Contact Dermat 1997;8:15–19.

[12] Nicholson PJ, Llewellyn D, English JS. Guidelines development group. Evidence-based guidelines for the prevention, identification and management of occupational contact dermatitis and urticaria. Contact Dermatitis. 2010;63:177–186. doi: 10.1111/j.1600-0536.2010.01763.x.

[13] Lachepelle J-M, Maibach HI. The methodology of open (non-prick) testing, prick testing, and its variants. In Patch Testing and Prick Testing A Practical Guide, edited by Lachpella J-M, Maibach HI, 2nd ed. Berlin: Springer Verlag, 2009:141–152.

[14] Wu M, McIntosh J, Liu J. Current prevalence rate of latex allergy: why it remains a problem? J Occup Health 2016;58:138–144. doi: 10.1539/joh.15-0275-RA.

[15] Wagner S, Breiteneder H. Hevea brasiliensis latex allergens: current panel and clinical relevance. Int Arch Allergy Immunol 2005;136:90–97. doi: 10.1159/000082938.

[16] Wang CY, Maibach HI. Immunologic contact urticaria—the human touch. Cutan Ocul Toxicol 2013;32:154–160. doi: 10.3109/15569527.2012.727519.

[17] de Lagrán ZM, de Frutos FJ, de Arribas MG, Vanaclocha-Sebastián F. Contact urticaria to raw potato. Dermatol Online J 2009;15:14.

[18] Blanco C, Carrillo T, Castillo R, Quiralte J, Cuevas M. Latex allergy: clinical features and cross-reactivity with fruits. Ann Allergy 1994;73:309–314.

[19] Wagner S, Breiteneder H. The latex-fruit syndrome. Biochem Soc Trans 2002;30:935–940. doi: 10.1042/bst0300935.

[20] Fuchs T, Spitzauer S, Vente C, Hevler J, Kapiotis S, Rumpold H, Kraft D, Valenta R. Natural latex, grass pollen, and weed pollen share IgE epitopes. J Allergy Clin Immunol 1997;100:356–364.

[21] Kim KT, Hussain H. Prevalence of food allergy in 137 latex-allergic patients. Allergy Asthma Proc 1999;20(2):95–97.

[22] Amaro C, Goossens A. Immunological occupational contact urticaria and contact dermatitis from proteins: a review. Contact Dermatitis 2008;58:67–75. doi: 10.1111/j.1600-0536.2007.01267.

[23] Davari P, Maibach HI. Contact urticaria to cosmetic and industrial dyes. Clin Exp Dermatol 2011;36:1–5. doi: 10.1111/j.1365-2230.2010.03854.

[24] Williams JD, Lee AY, Matheson MC, Frowen KE, Noonan AM, Nixon RL. Occupational contact urticaria: Australian data. Br J Dermatol 2008;159:125–131. doi: 10.1111/j.1365-2133.2008.08583.

[25] Kanerva L, Toikkanen J, Jolanki R, Estlander T. Statistical data on occupational contact urticaria. Contact Dermatitis 1996;35:229–233.

[26] Niinimäki A, Niinimäki M, Mäkinen-Kiljunen S, Hannuksela M. Contact urticaria from protein hydrolysates in hair conditioners. Allergy 1998;53:1078–1082.

[27] Poltronieri A, Patrini L, Pigatto P, Riboldi L, Marsili C, Previdi M, Margonari M, Marraccini P. Occupational allergic "march". Rapid evolution of contact dermatitis to ammonium persulfate into airborne contact dermatitis with rhinitis and asthma in a hairdresser. Med Lav 2010;101:403–408.

[28] Ortolani C, Ispano M, Pastorello E, Bigi A, Ansaloni R. The oral allergy syndrome. Ann Allergy 1988;61:47–52.

[29] Konstantinou GN, Grattan CE. Food contact hypersensitivity syndrome: the mucosal contact urticaria paradigm. Clin Exp Dermatol 2008;33:383–389. doi: 10.1111/j.1365-2230.2008.02893.x.

[30] Kelso JM. Pollen-food allergy syndrome. Clin Exp Allergy 2000;30(7):905–907.

[31] Miranda-Romero A, Navarro L, Pérez-Oliva N, González-López A, García-Muñoz M. Occupational heat contact urticaria. Contact Dermatitis 1998;38:358–359.

http://dx.doi.org/10.5772/67994

[32] Bourrain JL, Amblard P, Béani JC. Contact urticaria photoinduced by benzophenones. Contact Dermatitis 2003;48:45–46.

[33] Yamazaki S, Katayama I, Kurumaji Y, Yokozeki H, Nishioka K. Contact urticaria induced by mexiletine hydrochloride in a patient receiving iontophoresis. Br J Dermatol 1994;130:538–540.

[34] Katsarou A, Armenaka M, Ale I, Koufou V, Kalogeromitros D. Frequency of immediate reactions to the European standard series. Contact Dermatitis 1999;41:276–279.

[35] Bernstein IL, Li JT, Bernstein DI, Hamilton R, Spector SL, Tan R, Sicherer S, Golden DB, Khan DA, Nicklas RA, Portnoy JM, Blessing-Moore J, Cox L, Lang DM, Oppenheimer J, Randolph CC, Schuller DE, Tilles SA, Wallace DV, Levetin E, Weber R, American Academy of Allergy, Asthma and Immunology, American College of Allergy, Asthma and Immunology. Allergy diagnostic testing: an updated practice parameter. Ann Allergy Asthma Immunol 2008;100(Suppl 3):1–148.

[36] Zuberbier T, Asero R, Bindslev-Jensen C, et al. EAACI/GA2LEN/EDF guideline: management of urticaria. Allergy 2009;64:1427–1443. doi: 10.1111/j.1398-9995.2009.02178.x.

Chapter 6

Urticarial Vasculitis

Erol Koç, Berna Aksoy and Aslı Tatlıparmak

Additional information is available at the end of the chapter

http://dx.doi.org/10.5772/68109

Abstract

Urticarial vasculitis (UV) is a small vessel vasculitis and an immune-complex mediated disease like other leukocytoclastic vasculitis. UV seems similar to common urticaria clinically. Major difference between urticarial vasculitis and urticaria is the duration of lesions. Urticarial lesions regress in 24 hours, but UV lesions persist longer than 24 hours. Residual hyperpigmentation, constitutional symptoms like fever, arthralgia, and abdominal pain are other main clinical differences between these disorders. Upon confirmation of diagnosis, patients are divided into two major categories on the basis of serum complement levels: normocomplementemic UV (NUV) and hypocomplementemic UV (HUV). Consensus meeting in 1996 stated that long lasting (at least 24 hour–5 days) indurated wheals, which may be itchy, painful or tender, be associated with purpura and presence of associated extracutaneous findings, and cutaneous vasculitis confirmed by histopathological examination are defined as UV.

Keywords: hypocomplementemia, normocomplementemic, urticaria, vasculitis

1. Introduction

Urticarial vasculitis (UV) is an entity that is characterized by clinical presence of urticarial lesions and histopathological presence of vasculitis. Major difference between urticarial vasculitis and urticaria is the duration of lesions. Urticarial lesions regress in 24 hours, but UV lesions persist longer than 24 hours. Residual hyperpigmentation, constitutional symptoms like fever, arthralgia, and abdominal pain are other main clinical differences between these disorders [1]. UV lesions can be pruritic but more commonly these lesions are associated with symptom of burning. Skin biopsy shows histopathologic features of leukocytoclastic vasculitis [2]. Lesions usually persist for several months but very rarely they persist for years [3]. UV may be seen as a manifestation of a systemic disease or it may develop into a systemic illness by itself [2].

2. Section

2.1. Epidemiology

UV is a rare condition and the exact incidence is not known as a result of small number of literature reports. UV frequency is reported to be between 2 and 20% in chronic urticaria patients and if histologic definition of vasculitis is used as a criterion for diagnosis then the estimate of the prevalence of UV in chronic urticaria patients becomes approximately 5% [1, 3, 4]. Approximately 80% of UV patients have underlying or associated disease [2]. UV is more common in women and very rare in children [4]. Case report of an infant with UV is the only case report presenting the literature [5]. The peak incidence of the disease is in the fourth decade of life [4].

2.2. Etiopathogenesis

UV is a small vessel vasculitis and an immune-complex mediated disease like other leukocytoclastic vasculitis. Leukocytoclastic vasculitis is an example for type III immune reaction, which is characterized with circulatory immune complexes [6]. Initially antigen-antibody complex is formed in blood and then accumulation of the vessel walls. This complex reaction leads to the activation of complement system by the classical pathway. Anaphylatoxins C3a and C5a induce mast cell degranulation and cytokine synthesis. Mast cells release tumor necrosis factor alpha (TNFα), prostaglandins, histamine, heparin, platelet activating factor, leukotrienes, neutrophil chemotactic factor A, neutral protease, and tryptase [6]. Increase in cytokine and chemokine production results in edema and tissue reaction. Main antibodies in this reaction are IgG or IgM, and rarely IgA. The antigen in the complex may be autologous or it may derive from exogenous origin such as an infection or drugs [4]. But the antigens are mostly not known [1]. Based on the level of complement, UV is divided into two subgroups: normocomplementemic UV (NUV) and hypocomplementemic UV (HUV) [7]. UV is often idiopathic, but in some cases, it can be triggered with drugs, infection (hepatitis B and hepatitis C), connective tissue disease, neoplasia, cold, and exercise. [3, 8–12]. Drugs were found to be responsible for 10% of UV patients. The risk of UV is irrespective of both dose and frequency [8]. Infliximab, procainamide, antidepressants, methotrexate, sulfamethoxazole-trimethoprim, diltiazem, cimetidine, enalaprilin, and nonsteroid anti-inflammatory drugs (NSAIDs) are the main drugs reported in the literature [3, 13]. A patient with UV should also be examined for underlying diseases like viral infections, monoclonal gammopathies, serum sickness, and serum sickness like reactions, SLE, Sjögren's syndrome (SS) or mixed cryoglobulinemia [2, 14, 15]. Polycythaemia rubra vera [16], essential thrombocythemia [17], systemic sclerosis [18], acquired reactive perforating collagenosis [19], lymphoma [20], leukemia [21, 22], and thyroid dysfunction [23] are the other systemic diseases reported in the literature. UV patients with normal serum complement levels have rarely systemic manifestations. By contrast, UV patients with decreased C3 and C4 have systemic diseases including lung, kidney, and eye involvement [14]. At the same time, HUV patients may have extracutaneous symptoms like fever, myalgia, malaise, fatigue, arthralgia, conjunctivitis, episcleritis, nephritis, and cardiac valve involvement [8, 24]. A small group of patients with HUV also

http://dx.doi.org/10.5772/68109

have anti-C1q antibodies (anti-C1q Ab), and this group is considered as a separate entity called HUVS [7]. Ig G autoantibodies to the collagen like region of C1q (anti-C1q Ab) were detected in HUVS patients' serum. Anti-C1q Abs were also detected in patients with systemic lupus erythematosus (SLE) and 85% of these patients had glomerulonephritis. Anti-C1q Ab is associated with glomerulonephritis in SLE patients [2]. However, all HUVS patients have UV lesions and anti-C1q Ab, but only a group of SLE patients have UV lesions [2]. UV occurs in 5–10% of SLE patients and 28–47% of SLE patients have anti-C1q Ab [14]. HUVS patients form a small fraction of idiopathic HUV group (less than 5%), and these patients may have gastrointestinal, neurologic, ophthalmologic, renal, and pulmonary involvement [7]. Pulmonary disease in patients with HUVS was first described in 1982 with an incidence of 50%. However, these patients had history of tobacco exposure. After this report, different incidences (15–50%) were reported in HUVS patients. The exact mechanism of obstructive lung disease is not known but vasculitis of pulmonary capillaries, dysfunction of α 1 antitrypsin and binding of anti-C1q Ab to the surfactant proteins in pulmonary alveoli are the possible hypotheses for pathogenesis [14]. Renal disease was also reported in 20–30% of patients with HUVS [25].

2.3. Clinical features

UV is characterized by widespread urticarial lesions each lasting longer than 24 hours clinically [12, 26]. Classically urticarial plaques of UV are persistent or long lasting (in 64% of patients more than 24 hours) (**Figure 1**) and may resolve with purpura (**Figure 2**) or hyperpigmentation (in up to 35% of patients) in comparison to common urticaria [12]. Lesions may

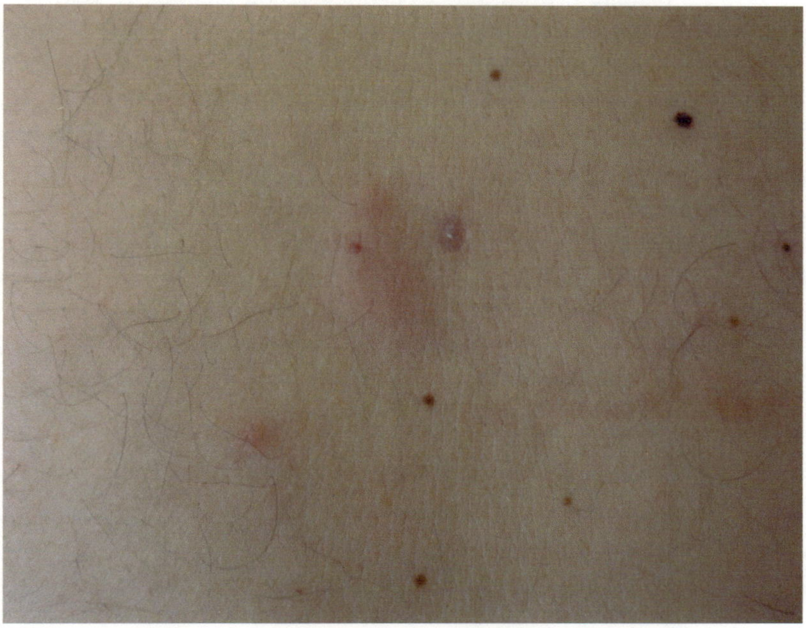

Figure 1. Urticarial lesions on the dorsal trunk of 47 years old male that is present for a month. The histopathological examination revealed lymphocytic vasculitis and laboratory examinations yield a diagnosis of accompanying Sjögren syndrome.

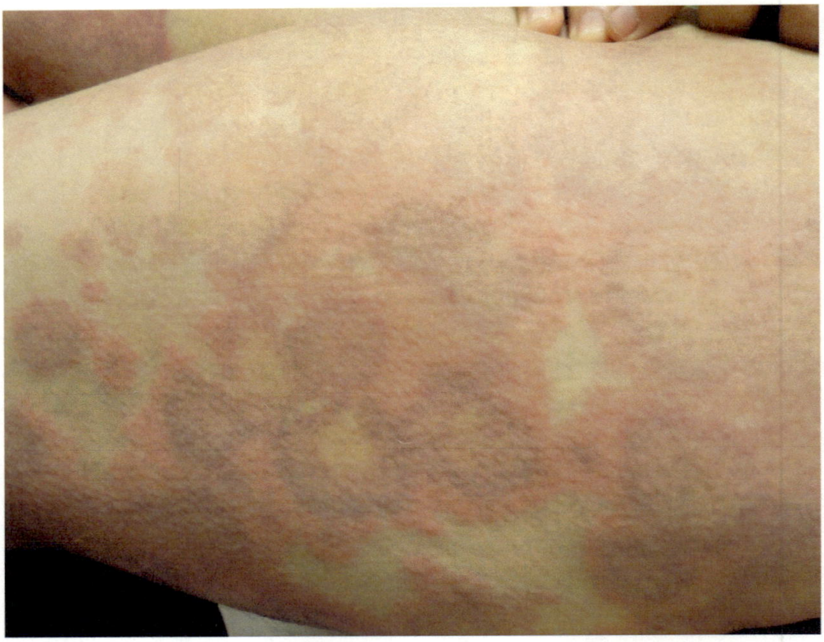

Figure 2. Widespread urticarial lesions with central purpura located on left lateral thigh of 85 years old female patient.

be asymptomatic, are usually pruritic and sometimes painful, tender or burning (in 33% of patients) in comparison to intensely pruritic urticarial lesions (**Table 1**) [12, 27]. UV presents usually with classical wheals but rarely livedo reticularis or even bullae may develop [12]. Angioedema can sometimes accompany urticarial lesions in up to 42% of UV patients [4, 12]. In a study reported it was detected that angioedema was present in 13% of HUV and 23% of NUV cases [28]. Following angioedema, a residual bruising may develop [12]. Typically clinical lesions of UV are recurrent and persist for more than 4–6 weeks even years [27]. As there are different clinical presentations of UV lesions, a biopsy is crucial in establishing a definite diagnosis [12]. All patients show histopathological evidence of leukocytoclastic vasculitis on biopsy [28].

Clinical characteristic	UV	Common urticaria
Lesion predilection	Dependent areas, areas under focal pressure, anywhere	Anywhere
Symptoms	Painful, tender, burning, pruritic	Intensely pruritic
Persistence	More than 24 hours [usually 24–72 hours]	Less than 24 hours [usually 30 minutes–24 hours]
Residual signs	Purpura or hyperpigmentation	None

Table 1. Clinical characteristics of cutaneous lesions of UV in comparison with common urticaria.

http://dx.doi.org/10.5772/68109

Upon confirmation of diagnosis, patients are divided into two major categories on the basis of serum complement levels: normocomplementemic UV (NUV) and hypocomplementemic UV [HUV] cases [28]. Many UV patients have NUV [27]. UV patients also frequently present with systemic manifestations (**Table 2**) [26]. The most commonly observed systemic manifestation of UV is termed as "AHA syndrome": arthralgias and arthritis, hives and angioedema [12]. Like in the situation of cutaneous lesions, common urticariais still in the differential diagnosis of systemic manifestations of UV as common urticariacan rarely has angioedema and systemic symptoms like arthralgia or abdominal pain [12]. Systemic manifestations of UV develop mostly in hypocomplementemic patients [12]. HUV patients frequently have an underlying systemic disease [26, 29]. Systemic manifestations of HUV patients occur regardless of being idiopathic (primary HUV) or associated with an underlying disease (secondary HUV) [12]. Clinical features of UV can exacerbate with some situations like emotional stress, anxiety, exercise, and excessive alcohol consumption [12]. Additionally, heat and spicy foods can increase the pruritus and/or urticarial lesions [30]. UV lesions can develop under pressure of tight and narrow clothing [30]. Smokers can develop more severe respiratory involvement and progression to COPD in HUV patients [31]. UV can sometimes develop in striae distensae and can present a diagnostic challenge in pregnancy [13]. UV can sometimes be a presenting sign of SLE or present with a clinical picture similar to SLE [12, 28]. Some patients have autoimmune idiopathic HUV with a lupus-like clinical picture, hence termed HUVS [2, 27]. HUVS patients usually have accompanying systemic involvement involving more than one organ system [26]. These patients presenting clinically as HUVS are mostly young women and many aspects of the clinical picture are similar to SLE [12, 28]. Schnitzler syndrome is another clinical condition related to UV [32]. It is defined as the presence of UV in association with mostly IgM monoclonal gammopathy and increased markers of systemic inflammation [32].

Occurrence	Systemic features
Common	Musculoskeletal: arthralgia, arthritis
Less common	Respiratory: cough, dyspnea, hemoptysis, COPD, asthma, pleural effusion Renal disease: hematuria, proteinuria, glomerulonephritis Gastrointestinal: substernal pain, abdominal pain, nausea, vomiting, diarrhea
Rare	Cardiac: pericarditis, pericardial effusion, cardiac tamponade Ophthalmologic: conjunctivitis, episcleritis, uveitis, geographic serpiginous choroidopathy, visual loss Other: fever, splenomegaly, lymphadenopathy, cold sensitivity, reversible tracheal stenosis
Very rare	CNS: pseudotumor cerebri, cranial nerve palsies, aseptic meningitis Miscellaneous: transvers myelitis, cardiac valve disease, optic atrophy, Jaccaud's syndrome [chronic postrheumatic fever arthropathy], peripheral neuropathy, pleuritis

Table 2. Clinical features of systemic involvement in UV.

Patients can present with general constitutional symptoms, like fever, arthralgias, malaise, and fatigue [12]. Most UV patients have musculoskeletal involvement presenting as arthralgia or arthritis [12, 26, 28]. Jaccoud's syndrome or arthropathy was defined as joint deformities similar to that of rheumatoid arthritis [12]. It consists of ulnar deviation of the fingers, swan neck deformities and subluxations in the hands [12]. This hand deformity is most commonly associated with SLE and rarely with HUV [12]. Ophthalmologic involvement is rare (10% of UV patients) and can present as conjunctivitis, episcleritis, uveitis, or geographic serpiginous choroidopathy leading to visual loss [12]. Eye involvement in the form of episcleritis and uveitis can develop mostly in HUV patients (21%) [28]. Pulmonary involvement may present clinically as cough, dyspnea, hemoptysis, COPD, asthma, pleuritic, emphysema, or pleural effusion [12]. HUVS patients presenting with COPD are usually young smokers, and the observed COPD is more severe than that seen in heavy smoker patients without HUVS [12]. Emphysema can develop in UV patients as a result of leukocytoclastic vasculitis of pulmonary vessels. Lung involvement may present clinically late in the disease process but is a leading cause of morbidity and mortality [12]. Renal disease can occur in 5–10% of patients with HUVS and is discovered by finding proteinuria and microscopic hematuria [12]. Renal involvement can present as glomerulonephritis in 20–30% of HUV cases [12]. Gastrointestinal involvement can present clinically as nausea, vomiting, substernal pain, abdominal pain, diarrhea, or general feeling of gastrointestinal distress [12]. Cardiac involvement can develop rarely [12]. Recurrent pericarditis, pericardial effusion, cardiac tamponade, and cardiac valvular disease have been reported [12]. Several HUVS patients with Jaccoud's arthropathy were reported to develop valvular heart disease requiring valvular replacement [12, 24, 33, 34]. Central and peripheral nervous systems can rarely be affected [12].

2.4. Diagnosis

Consensus meeting in 1996 stated that long lasting (at least 24 hour–5 days) indurated wheals, which may be itchy, painful, or tender, be associated with purpura and presence of associated extracutaneous findings, and cutaneous vasculitis confirmed by histopathological examination are defined as UV [35]. UV should be suspected in any patient with urticarial lesions lasting more than 24 hours. The prevalence of UV among all patients that present with urticarial lesions is 11% and among patients with chronic urticaria it is 15–20% [23, 36, 37]. To ascertain the exact duration of urticarial lesions, a particular lesion could be encircled with a marking pen and the patient is re-examined 24 hour later to confirm the persistence of urticarial lesions [23]. Diascopy and dermatoscopy can help to suspect UV [23, 38]. The lesions of UV may be non- or partially-blanchable on diascopic examination [23, 38]. It was termed as "disappearing halo test" in which upon diascopy clinically invisible purpura becomes evident as dark red or slightly brown macule in the center of a blanched UV lesion [38]. UV can disclose purpuric dots or globules in a patchy orange-brown background dermatoscopically corresponding to extravasation and degradation of red blood cells due to leukocytoclastic vasculitis [39–41]. These purpuric dots are reddish initially and later they become more purplish [40]. Conversely, urticarial lesions disclose prominent and sometimes reticular red lines corresponding to ectatic and horizontal subpapillary vessels [39–41]. Definitive diagnosis of UV requires a lesion biopsy demonstrating typical histopathological features in addition to the previously described clinical characteristics in a patient presenting with urticarial lesions [4]. Two lesion biopsies, one for routine histopathology and one for direct immunofluorescence, should be obtained [2]. Biopsies should be taken from the early lesions, which are maximum 24–48 hours old [42]. Multiple biopsies may be required to establish a biopsy [42]. In the case, an UV diagnosis is made, the physician should additionally search for the presence of any underlying infectious etiology [43, 44]. The major finding to be searched for is the presence or absence of hypocomplementemia [2]. It was previously reported that 53–82% of UV patients have normal complement levels and hence NUV, 18–47% of UV patients have decreased complement levels and hence HUV [28, 45]. Approximately, 65% of HUV and 45% of NUV patients have systemic involvement [23]. Hypocomplementemic patients are rare (10–20% of all UV patients) and more likely to have systemic involvement and hence they should be appropriately investigated [23, 28, 42, 46]. Optimal classification of UV patients should be done by multiple (two to three) measurements of C1q, C3, C4, and CH50 during clinical observation of several months duration [2]. Measurements should be done during active and quiescent periods [2]. Rare patients with HUVS may have cardiac valvular incompetence with/without Jaccoud's arthropathy [24, 33, 35, 47]. In 1973, criteria to diagnose HUVS have been proposed [48]. A patient is diagnosed to have HUVS if he/she has two major and at least two minor criteria (**Table 3**) [48].

2.5. Laboratory examinations

A patient diagnosed to have UV should be appropriately tested [2]. Complete blood count, ESR, renal and liver functions, urinalysis, ANA, complements, should be examined in all cases with appropriate clinical findings of UV [2]. A scheme would be helpful for planning the laboratory examinations in all patients with clinical UV presentation and specialized tests should be performed in some patients who have clinical clues of systemic involvement [30]. Once

- Two major criteria
- Chronic urticarial eruption
- Low levels of complements

- At least two minor criteria
- Leukocytoclastic vasculitis
- Arthralgia/arthritis
- Ocular involvement [episcleritis or uveitis]
- Renal involvement [glomerulonephritis]
- Recurrent abdominal pain
- Presence of anti-C1q antibody

Table 3. Proposed criteria for diagnosing HUVS.

basic diagnostic evaluation has been performed, additional laboratory examinations should not be so extensive and should be directed with regard to clues in the history and physical examination [30]. Hematologic examinations can reveal anemia and leukocytosis in nearly half of the patients [49]. Patients with positive anti-C1q antibodies have been detected to have more frequent HUVS, angioedema, livedo reticularis, musculoskeletal, ocular and kidney involvement, and less frequent gastrointestinal and pulmonary involvement than patients without anti-C1q antibodies [46]. These anti-C1q autoantibodies may sometimes be detected in patients having SLE, Good-pasture syndrome or idiopathic membranoproliferative glomerulonephritis without showing signs of urticarial vasculitis [4, 50, 51]. A case having circulating immune complexes and a positive autologous serum skin test was also reported [52]. There are numerous reported cases who were associated with gammopaties and so patients should be appropriately evaluated [53–56]. Soluble serum vascular endothelial-cadherin is detected in systemic vasculitis cases in the acute period, and this can be used as a marker for endothelial cell damage and inflammatory response, but this is nonspecific for UV [57].

2.6. Histopathology

A lesional biopsy demonstrating the features of UV is the gold standard for diagnosis [4]. The key histopathologic feature is leukocytoclastic vasculitis affecting dermal capillaries and postcapillary venules (**Figure 3**) [2, 4]. Inflammation is located within the vessel walls and perivascularly [4]. Cellular infiltrate is primarily composed of neutrophils, rarely eosinophils, and lymphocytes may take place (**Figure 4**) [4]. Lymphocytes predominate in lesions older

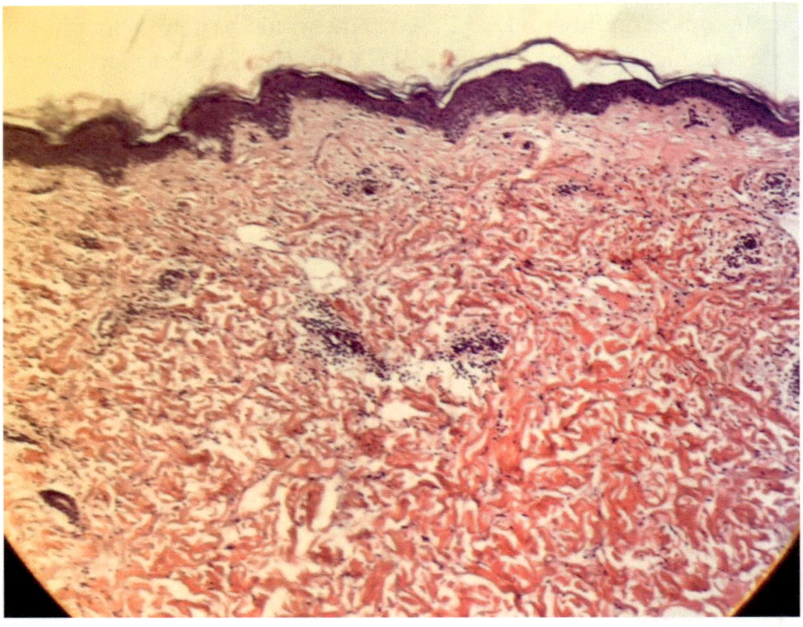

Figure 3. Superficial perivascular infiltration and leukocytoclastic vasculitis [Hemotoxylin & Eosin, original magnification ×100] [Courtesy, Onat Akin, MD].

than 48 hours [23]. In a study, 86% of specimens showed lymphocytic vasculitis, probably due to the age of the lesion biopsied [58]. If these histopathological changes described for UV involve the capillaries and postcapillary venules of the deep dermal layers, subcutaneous tissue, and submucosal connective tissue layers then it is termed as angioedema [2]. Direct immunofluorescence examination shows deposition of immunoglobulins, complement, and/or fibrinogen within and around vessel walls in 58–79% of cases [1, 4, 30, 46]. Basement membrane positive immunofluorescence examination is more frequent in HUV (70–96%) patients than in NUV (1–18%) patients [1]. However, the presence of basement membrane staining in a hypocomplementemic patient may suggest the diagnosis of SLE [30].

2.7. Differential diagnosis

The main differential diagnosis of UV is common urticaria [42]. The lesions in urticaria typically resolves in minutes to hours, migrates continually, and leaves no residual pigmentation after resolving in contrast to UV [42]. The main symptom in urticaria is the presence of intense pruritus, UV lesions may present with a more burning sensation [2]. Indurated urticarial lesions of UV are indistinguishable especially from that of chronic spontaneous urticaria [4]. Urticaria lesions may be huge and are usually larger than those of UV [2]. Chronic urticarial lesions are clinically more indurated than that of acute urticaria [4]. Eleven percent of all patients presenting with urticarial lesions are found to have UV [23]. In cases of chronic and antihistamine unresponsive chronic urticaria, when biopsies of lesions were performed, 15–20% of patients were found to have histopathological features of UV and hence diagnosed as UV [36, 37]. So performing a biopsy is necessary to differentiate exactly these two conditions. When patients

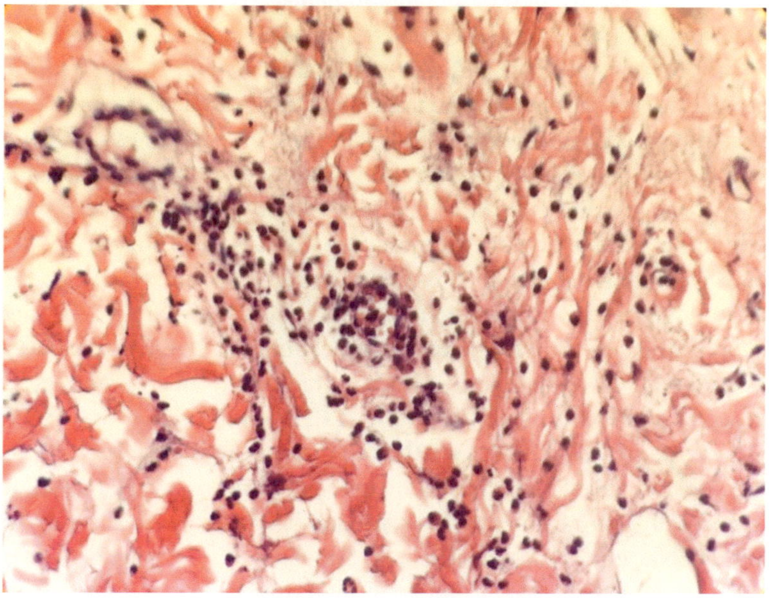

Figure 4. Small vessel vasculitis with neutrophilic infiltration and leukocytoclasia [Hemotoxylin & Eosin, original magnification ×400] [Courtesy, Onat Akin, MD].

with acute urticaria are biopsied, histopathology shows sparse cellular infiltrate and moderate to intense dermal edema [4]. Lesions of UV are usually smaller than ordinary urticaria and never present with annular lesions [38]. Additionally ordinary urticarial lesions are more pinkish than darker reddish lesions of UV [38]. In addition, UV lesions tend to be located more on dependent areas of the body [38]. Serum-sickness is a type-III hypersensitivity reaction that develops for example against horse-serum diphtheria antitoxin and can present with urticarial lesions [59]. Serum-sickness like reaction is a similar clinical entity triggered by drugs or infections [59]. Urticaria multiforme presents with annular lesions and acral edema or angioedema, mostly triggered by viral infections [59]. Both are self-limited and have favorable long-term prognoses [59]. Acute infantile hemorrhagic edema is another self-limited disorder that should be remembered in differential diagnosis of hemorrhagic urticarial lesions in pediatric cases [59]. Henoch-Schönlein purpura can present with urticarial lesions and should be searched for especially in pediatric cases with renal and/or gastrointestinal and/or arthritic involvement [59]. Urticarial arthritis is a condition observed in HLA-B51 positive patients, presenting with arthritis, urticaria (lasting less than 24 hours), and facial angioedema [49]. Some of the patients may show a biopsy with leukocytoclastic vasculitis some only leukocytic infiltration without vasculitis [49]. Acquired angioedema should be differentiated from HUV associated with angioedema and both disorders have decreased complement levels. Pruritic urticarial papules and plaques of pregnancy is the main differential diagnosis when UV develops in the pregnancy, especially in the striae distensae [60]. Likewise erythema multiforme, bullous pemphigoid, sweet's syndrome, and urticarial pigmentosa can be added to the differential diagnoses of UV [27].

Auto-inflammatory diseases are a group of rare hereditary monogenic disorders of innate immunity with presenting symptoms of fever and inflammatory, sometimes urticarial, skin lesions [3, 61, 62]. Auto-inflammatory diseases usually cause a familial life-long disease that starts in childhood in hereditary fever syndromes [62]. Auto-inflammatory syndromes cause flatter wheals and erythematous patches without surrounding flare and they last hours and even up to 24 hours and are accompanied by burning sensation rather than itching and they may be painful [62]. Lesions do not give any response to antihistamines and are associated with systemic symptoms of fever, fatigue, and arthralgia [62]. Very recently, vasculitis has been described histopathologically in three cases of auto-inflammatory diseases [61]. Hence, the clinician should take into account the rare possibility of auto-inflammatory associated vasculitis presenting with urticarial lesions and fever in the differential diagnosis of UV [61]. Some autoimmune disorders like SLE, Sjögren syndrome, dermatomyositis, or rheumatoid arthritis may present clinically with urticarial lesions [3]. Histopathological findings of UV are not specific in general and similar histopathological findings can be seen in SLE [42]. It is still unclear that HUVS is a similar disease to or a subtype of SLE [12, 28, 48, 63]. Both diseases share similar clinical findings and can present together [12, 28, 48, 63]. So when a patient is diagnosed as HUVS, he/she should also be evaluated for SLE [48]. Other systemic vasculitides may present clinically with urticarial lesions [3]. Rarely polyarteritis nodosa and Churg-Strauss syndrome may present clinically with urticarial lesions [3]. Some hematologic malignancies (lymphoma or gammopathies) and hematologic disorders (polycythemia vera and thrombocythemia) can also present clinically with urticarial lesions [3, 16, 17]. Other rare syndromes like PAPA, Blau, or Majeed syndromes can also present clinically with urticarial lesions [3].

2.8. Treatment

In any given patient with UV, if an underlying condition is present, it must be treated initially [2, 42]. Different degrees of clinical severity of the disease preclude proposal of any standard form of therapy [30]. Therefore, there is no universal therapy and variation in individual response to any form of therapy that exist [30]. In general, the more severe the systemic involvement (as in HUVS) is, the more challenging it becomes to treat the disease [42]. The most difficult patient to treat is the one who develops COPD or has established COPD in the setting of HUVS [2]. COPD in HUVS develops more frequently and most severely in patients who smoke, so patients should give up smoking and also avoid inhaling second-hand smoke [31]. One case has been reported to go into remission with an elimination diet [64]. This case may show the possibility of pseudoallergens' role in the etiopathogenesis of UV and similar to chronic urticaria treatment a pseudoallergen-free diet can be tried in selected cases. Antihistamines are helpful for the symptomatic control of pruritus in all patients and may be sufficient for the therapy of mild cutaneous UV without systemic involvement [4, 30]. However, antihistamines do not affect immune-complex-mediated inflammation and hence do not alter the course of the disease [4]. Cinnarizine, an antihistaminic used for Meniere's disease and car sickness, was found to be effective in UV patients [36]. A brief course of systemic corticosteroids may be useful to control intermittent exacerbations of UV, with both cutaneous and systemic involvement [4]. However, a dose of systemic corticosteroids up to 40 mg/day of prednisolone may be needed [30]. Long-term use is limited by the well-known side effects of corticosteroids and they should only be used in cases who are intolerant to or unresponsive to other alternative drugs [30]. A variety of alternatives to corticosteroids are used in the treatment of milder forms of UV [4]. These alternatives include indomethacin, colchicine, and dapsone that are commonly used in the clinical practice [4]. NSAIDs like indomethacin may help approximately half of patients with minimal disease [42]. Indomethacin use is usually discontinued or restricted by its gastrointestinal adverse effect potential, like upset stomach [4, 42]. In some unfortunate patients, NSAIDs can even cause UV or exacerbation of the existing UV [30]. Dapsone is a sulfone and shows more effectiveness than other alternatives in the treatment of UV [4]. Dapsone may work synergistically with pentoxifylline [4]. The mechanism of action of dapsone is poorly understood in the treatment of UV [4]. Before commencing on dapsone treatment, serum levels of glucose-6-phosphate dehydrogenase enzyme should be measured as deficiency of it results in severe hemolysis with dapsone usage [4]. Headache, nonhemolytic mild anemia and most importantly agranulocytosis may develop less frequently [4]. Hence, monitorization of complete blood count should be performed periodically in patients who use dapsone [4]. Patients having UV in the clinical setting of SLE or lupus-like disorder may have a more favorable response to treatment with dapsone [4]. Antimalarials like hydroxychloroquine have been reported to be effective in approximately 50% of patients with only cutaneous involvement [4, 30, 52]. Colchicine is an alkaloid that inhibits neutrophil chemotaxis, generation of lysosomes and stabilizes lysosomal membranes [4, 65]. It has clinical efficacy in selected cases of UV [65]. Reserpine is an alkaloid extracted from the roots of the plant Rauwolfia serpentine [66]. Reserpine was once used for the treatment of psychosis and hypertension [66]. It can be added to the antihistamines /corticosteroids in a dose of 0.3–0.4 mg thrice daily and reported to be helpful in majority of patients with UV [25, 66, 67]. If these alternative drugs do not get enough benefit or intermittent systemic corticosteroids do not control symptoms adequately then chronic systemic corticosteroid usage can be considered in milder forms of disease [4]. Higher dosage systemic corticosteroid treatment is necessary in the presence of hypocomplementemia or systemic involvement [4]. Systemic prednisone or equivalent is usually given at 1 mg/kg dose till clinical remission, later the dose could be slowly tapered [4]. Systemic corticosteroids could be tapered and discontinued without relapse in some patients [4]. However, many patients do experience disease relapse and need chronic corticosteroid treatment [4]. In the case of inadequate systemic corticosteroid response or when unacceptable corticosteroid adverse effects do occur than second line treatment choices should be considered, like azathioprine or cyclophosphamide [4]. In the resistant patients, systemic corticosteroids can even be effectively combined with dapsone, azathioprine, and cyclophosphamide [30]. In the chronic and resistant subset of patients, corticosteroid-sparing immunosuppressive agents such as azathioprine, cyclophosphamide, cyclosporine A, or mycophenolate mofetil have been shown to be effective [4]. Azathioprine has been shown to be a useful adjunct to corticosteroids for stabilization of renal and pulmonary function [4, 68]. Methotrexate has usually inconsistent and disappointing results in the treatment of UV [4, 24, 33, 69]. Methotrexate is typically effective in inflammatory myositis associated with HUVS [70]. Favorable clinical responses have been achieved with cyclophosphamide in corticosteroid-resistant UV cases [4, 71]. Cyclosporine A has provided favorable clinical efficacy in the treatment of HUVS, including cases that are resistant to cyclophosphamide [4]. Cyclosporine A has been shown to improve respiratory involvement in HUVS patients with improvements in the forced expiratory volume in one second (FEV1), the diffusing capacity of the lung for carbon monoxide (DLCO) and regression of leukocytosis in bronchoalveolar lavage (BAL) [2]. Cyclosporine A has also been shown to be effective in renal involvement associated with HUVS [72]. Mycophenolate mofetil has also been shown to be efficacious in the treatment and maintenance of patients with HUV/HUVS [24, 73, 74]. Gold injections were tried and found to be effective in UV as in rheumatoid arthritis, but it is now a historical approach [75]. Plasmapheresis can provide rapid but temporary benefit in recalcitrant cases of UV [4, 76]. Plasma exchange has been shown to control symptoms rapidly during treatment but lesions recurred later in some patients [30, 76, 77]. High dose intravenous immunoglobulin (IVIG) also has been tried and shown to be effective in some recalcitrant HUVS cases [20, 78]. However, there are cases with inefficient response to IVIG [67, 79]. Rituximab can be used in refractory and/or relapsing or severe cases with prolonged duration of efficacy [46, 56, 80]. Anti-IL-1 blockage (anakinra, canakinumab) has shown promising results in the treatment of UV [81, 82]. However, these patients may have UV associated with auto-inflammatory diseases. A therapy-resistant SLE patient with UV lesions showed good response to IL-6 antagonist tocilizumab [83]. Omalizumab was used in a small number of NUV patients with success but some displayed a quick relapse following discontinuance [84, 85]. First line treatments used were determined to be mostly corticosteroids, hydroxychloroquine, and colchicine in decreasing order in a large retrospective study that involved only HUV patients [46]. Second and third line treatments given in this study were corticosteroids, hydroxychloroquine, and immunosuppressive agents in decreasing order [46]. In patients having hepatitis C infection, cryoglobulinemia and resultant UV, effective antiviral therapy (interferon-alpha and ribavirin) should be instituted [2]. Effective antiviral therapy has been shown to control HCV infection and cure UV in nearly half of these patients [2, 86, 87]. However, if the antiviral treatment is stopped the UV lesions do recur [87]. Angioedema may develop at any time in the course of UV [31]. If angioedema develops and involves larynx, the initial treatment may be epinephrine [31].

2.9. Course and prognosis

UV is a complicated disease and it has an unpredictable course [12]. An individual can have lesions for weeks to many years continuously or intermittently [12, 30]. The average duration of the disease was found to be 3 years and disease could last up to 23 years [30, 42]. Response of patients with UV to any given treatment is variable [4]. The course of the idiopathic NUV is favorable overall and patients usually do not develop any other diseases or mortality in the follow up [12, 30]. The course of HUV and HUVS may be less favorable [12, 30]. Patients with HUV may need an additional add-on therapeutic after about a median of 8 months duration [46]. Musculoskeletal, ocular, and renal disease usually responds to systemic treatment without any long-term severe consequences [14]. After adequate therapy serum complements increase to or near to normal values and anti-C1q antibody titers decrease [14]. However, serum C1q levels remained below normal values even in the presence of complete remission [14]. UV presents clinically in a spectrum of disease severity from NUV to HUV to HUVS [42, 46]. However, there is no finding to support the presence of any transition from one to another in follow up of these patients [42]. The main causes of morbidity and mortality are pulmonary manifestations like COPD, cardiac manifestations and laryngeal edema in patients with HUVS [14, 30, 31]. Precocious emphysema and COPD develop in patients with HUVS and especially in those patients who are moderate to heavy smokers [14, 88]. Onset of dyspnea heralds a poor outcome in HUVS patients with pulmonary involvement [14]. Treatment usually did not appear to alter the progression of COPD [14]. Of these HUVS patients with chronic or recurrent dyspnea, 55% die of respiratory failure [14]. In this subset of patients bronchogenic carcinoma can also be seen and adds to the overall morbidity and mortality risk [46, 88]. Cardiac involvement with pericarditis or valvulitis and significant valvular damage may develop in rare cases with HUVS and may be progressive and fatal [24, 33, 34, 46]. As cardiac involvement may cause significant morbidity and mortality and as its frequency is unknown, all patients should be evaluated [89]. Angioedema develops in 51% of cases with HUVS and may be life-threatening if it involves larynx [31, 46]. Pediatric and young adult patients (onset of disease before age of 30) may experience more renal involvement and show severe pulmonary complications and may have graver prognosis [89]. There may be significant morbidity resulting from involvement of other organ systems. Rarely vasculitis can affect optic nerve and retina and hence can threaten vision [90]. All UV patients need to be evaluated ophthalmologically as 15–20% of all UV cases may have ocular involvement in the disease course [90]. A patient with Muckle-Wells disease with associated UV developed sudden bilateral sensorineural hearing loss and had modest outcome following cochlear implantation [91]. Gastrointestinal involvement can lead to ischemic ulceration in the bowel [30]. Renal involvement can lead to renal insufficiency, this is especially common in pediatric cases and should be promptly treated [30, 89].

There are other rare associated cutaneous findings in UV patients reported in the literature. A case with rapidly progressing acquired cutis laxa following involvement of the skin areas with lesions of NUV was reported [92]. A reported pregnant woman developed acquired reactive perforating collagenosis at the sites of resolved UV lesions 3 weeks following the onset and treatment of UV [19]. A reported UV case developed acquired hemophilia following 4.5 years of follow up [93]. Another reported NUV case first presented with acquired hemophilia and developed NUV and angioedema in the following 5 months [94]. Rarely inflammatory myositis can develop in HUVS cases despite ongoing immunosuppressive therapy [70]. Complement deficiency may lead to increased susceptibility to the infections with encapsulated bacteria, especially meningococcus [95]. As a result, a case of meningococcal meningitis that developed in a patient with HUVS was reported [95]. The course of the UV may accompany the course of underlying disease. A paraneoplastic NUV case was reported to clear with chemotherapy for underlying chronic lymphocytic leukemia and disease recurred with the recurrence of underlying hematologic malignancy [21]. Three women with UV were evaluated in a study including 29 systemic vasculitis patients with 51 pregnancies to search for the outcome of pregnancy in systemic vasculitis [96]. The authors have found that the patients with a diagnosis of systemic vasculitis may have exacerbation of the vasculitic disease during pregnancy or following delivery, may have more pregnancy related morbidity like preeclampsia and may have a lower median gestational age [96].

Author details

Erol Koç[1], Berna Aksoy[2] and Aslı Tatlıparmak[3]*

*Address all correspondence to: drasligunaydin@yahoo.com.tr

1 Bahçeşehir University, Ankara Medicalpark Hospital, Department of Dermatology, İstanbul, Turkey

2 Bahçeşehir University, Kocaeli Medicalpark Hospital, Department of Dermatology, İstanbul, Turkey

3 Bahçeşehir University, Fatih Medicalpark Hospital, Department of Dermatology, İstanbul, Turkey

References

[1] Carlson JA, Chen KR. Cutaneous Vasculitis Update: Small Vessel Neutrophilic Vasculitis Syndromes. Am J Dermatopathol. 2006;28:486–506.

[2] Wisnieski JJ. Urticarial Vasculitis. Curr Opin Rheumatol. 2000 Jan;12[1]:24–31.

[3] Peroni A, Colato C, Zanoni G, Girolomoni G. Urticarial Lesions: If Not Urticaria, What Else? The Differential Diagnosis of Urticaria. J Am Acad Dermatol. 2010;62:557–70.

[4] Venzor J, Lee WL, Huston DP. Urticarial Vasculitis. Clin Rev Allergy Immunol. 2002 Oct;23[2]:201–16.

[5] Koch PE, Lazova R, Rosen JR, Antaya RJ. Urticarial Vasculitis in an İnfant. Cutis. 2008 Jan;81[1]:49–52.

[6] Mehregan DR, Gibson LE. Pathophysiology of Urticarial Vasculitis. Arch Dermatol. 1998 Jan;134[1]:88–9.

[7] Chimenti MS, Ballanti E, Triggianese P, Perricone R. Vasculitides and the Complement System: A Comprehensive Review. Clin Rev Allergy Immunol. 2015 Dec;49[3]:333–46.

[8] Mahajan VK, Singh R, Gupta M, Raina R. Telmisartan Induced Urticarial Vasculitis. Indian J Pharmacol. 2015 Sep–Oct;47[5]:560–2.

[9] Pérez-Bustillo A, Sánchez-Sambucety P, García-Ruiz de Morales JM, Rodríguez-Prieto MÁ. Cold-Induced Urticarial Vasculitis. Int J Dermatol. 2012 Jul;51[7]:881–3.

[10] Kano Y, Orihara M, Shiohara T. Cellular and Molecular Dynamics in Exercise-Induced Urticarial Vasculitis Lesions. Arch Dermatol. 1998 Jan;134[1]:62–7.

[11] Sais G, Vidaller A. Pathogenesis of Exercise-Induced Urticarial Vasculitis Lesions: Can the Changes Be Extrapolated to All Leukocytoclastic Vasculitis Lesions? Arch Dermatol. 1999 Jan;135[1]:87–9.

[12] Davis MD, Brewer JD. Urticarial Vasculitis and Hypocomplementemic Urticarial Vasculitis Syndrome. Immunol Allergy Clin North Am. 2004 May;24[2]:183–213.

[13] Koregol S, Naidu V, Rao S, Ankad BS. Enalapril Induced Normocomplementemic Urticarial Vasculitis. Indian J Dermatol Venereol Leprol. 2015 Jan–Feb;81[1]:73–4.

[14] Wisnieski JJ, Baer AN, Christensen J, Cupps TR, Flagg DN, Jones JV, Katzenstein PL, McFadden ER, McMillen JJ, Pick MA, et al. Hypocomplementemic Urticarial Vasculitis Syndrome. Clinical and Serologic Findings in 18 Patients. Medicine [Baltimore]. 1995 Jan;74[1]:24–41.

[15] Ramos-Casals M, Anaya JM, García-Carrasco M, Rosas J, Bové A, Claver G, Diaz LA, Herrero C, Font J. Cutaneous Vasculitis in Primary Sjögren Syndrome: Classification and Clinical Significance of 52 Patients. Medicine [Baltimore]. 2004 Mar;83[2]:96–106.

[16] Farell AM, Sabroe RA, Bunker CB. Urticarial Vasculitis Associated with Polycythaemia Rubra Vera. Clin Exp Dermatol. 1996 Jul;21[4]:302–4.

[17] Scott AD, Francis N, Yarranton H, Singh S. Urticarial Vasculitis Associated with Essential Thrombocythaemia. Acta Derm Venereol. 2014 Mar;94[2]:244–5.

[18] Kato Y, Aoki M, Kawana S. Urticarial Vasculitis Appearing in The Progression of Systemic Sclerosis. J Dermatol. 2006 Nov;33[11]:792–7.

[19] Eriyagama S, Wee JS, Ho B, Natkunarajah J. Acquired Reactive Perforating Collagenosis Associated with Urticarial Vasculitis In Pregnancy. Clin ExpDermatol. 2014 Jan;39[1]:81–3.

[20] Shah D, Rowbottom AW, Thomas CL, Cumber P, Chowdhury MM. Hypocomplementaemic Urticarial Vasculitis Associated with Non-Hodgkin Lymphoma and Treatment with Intravenous Immunoglobulin. Br J Dermatol. 2007 Aug;157[2]:392–3.

[21] Kassim JM, Igali L, Levell NJ. A 14-Year Paraneoplastic Rash: Urticarial Vasculitis and Dermal Binding Bullous Pemphigoid Secondary to Chronic Lymphocytic Leukaemia. Clin Exp Dermatol. 2015 Jun;40[4]:391–4.

[22] Blanco R, Martinez-Taboada VM, Gonzalez-Vela C, Rodriguez-Valverde V. Urticarial Vasculitis as Clinical Presentation of Megakaryocytic Leukemia. J ClinRheumatol. 1996 Dec;2[6]:366.

[23] Dincy CV, George R, Jacob M, Mathai E, Pulimood S, Eapen EP. Clinicopathologic Profile of Normocomplemententemic and Hypocomplemententemic Urticarial Vasculitis: A Study from South India. J Eur Acad Dermatol Venereol. 2008 Jul;22[7]:789–94.

[24] Hauser B, McRorie E, McKay N, Brenn T, Amft N. A case of hypocomplementaemic urticarial vasculitis with cardiac valve involvement successfully treated with cyclophosphamide and high-dose glucocorticoids. Int J Rheum Dis. 2014 Apr 5. Version of Record online DOI: 10.1111/1756-185X.12360

[25] Ashida A, Murata H, Ohashi A, Ogawa E, Uhara H, Okuyama R. A Case of Hypocomplementaemic Urticarial Vasculitis with a High Serum Level of Rheumatoid Factor. Australas J Dermatol. 2013 Aug;54[3]:62–3.

[26] Taillandier J, Alemanni M, Emile JF. Normocomplementemic Urticarial Vasculitis Inaugurating Destructive Polyarthritis. Joint Bone Spine. 2001 Dec;68[6]:510–2.

[27] Brown NA, Carter JD. Urticarial Vasculitis. Curr Rheumatol Rep. 2007 Aug;9[4]:312–9.

[28] Davis MD, Daoud MS, Kirby B, Gibson LE, Rogers RS 3rd. Clinicopathologic Correlation of Hypocomplementemic and Normocomplementemic Urticarial Vasculitis. J Am Acad Dermatol. 1998 Jun;38[6 Pt 1]:899–905.

[29] Napoli DC, Freeman TM. Autoimmunity in Chronic Urticaria and Urticarial Vasculitis. Curr Allergy Asthma Rep. 2001 Jul;1[4]:329–36.

[30] Black AK. Urticarial Vasculitis. Clin Dermatol. 1999;17:565–69.

[31] Jones JM, Reich KA, Raval DG. Angioedema in a 47-Year-Old Woman with Hypocomplementemic Urticarial Vasculitis Syndrome. J Am Osteopath Assoc. 2012 Feb;112[2]:90–2.

[32] Zuberbier T, Maurer M. Urticarial Vasculitis and Schnitzler syndrome. Immunol Allergy Clin North Am. 2014 Feb;34[1]:141–7.

[33] Hong L, Wackers F, Dewar M, Kashgarian M, Askenase PW. Atypical Fatal Hypocomplementemic Urticarial Vasculitis with Involvement of Native and Homograft Aortic Valves in an African American Man. J Allergy Clin Immunol. 2000 Dec;106[6]:1196–8.

[34] Amano H, Furuhata N, Tamura N, Tokano Y, Takasaki Y. Hypocomplementemic Urticarial Vasculitis with Jaccoud's Arthropathy and Valvular Heart Disease: Case Report and Review of The Literature. Lupus. 2008 Sep;17[9]:837–41.

[35] Black AK, Lawlor F, Greaves MW. Consensus Meeting on the Definition of Physical Urticarias and Urticarial Vasculitis. Clin Exp Dermatol. 1996 Nov;21[6]:424–6.

[36] Tosoni C, Lodi-Rizzini F, Cinquini M, Pasolini G, Venturini M, Sinico RA, Calzavara-Pinton P. a Reassessment of Diagnostic Criteria and Treatment of Idiopathic Urticarial Vasculitis: A Retrospective Study of 47 Patients. Clin Exp Dermatol. 2009 Mar;34[2]: 166–70.

[37] Monroe EW, Schulz CI, Maize JC, Jordon RE. Vasculitis in Chronic Urticaria: An İmmunopathologic Study. J Invest Dermatol. 1981 Feb;76[2]:103–7.

[38] Dahl MV. Clinical Pearl: Diascopy Helps Diagnose Urticarial Vasculitis. J Am Acad Dermatol. 1994 Mar;30[3]:481–2.

[39] Vázquez-López F, Fueyo A, Sánchez-Martín J, Pérez-Oliva N. Dermoscopy for the Screening of Common Urticaria and Urticaria Vasculitis. Arch Dermatol. 2008 Apr;144[4]:568.

[40] Suh KS, Kang DY, Lee KH, Han SH, Park JB, Kim ST, Jang MS. Evolution of Urticarial Vasculitis: A Clinical, Dermoscopic and Histopathological Study. J Eur Acad Dermatol Venereol. 2014 May;28[5]:674–5.

[41] Vázquez-López F, Maldonado-Seral C, Soler-Sánchez T, Perez-Oliva N, Marghoob AA. Surface Microscopy for Discriminating Between Common Urticaria and Urticarial Vasculitis. Rheumatology [Oxford]. 2003 Sep;42[9]:1079–82.

[42] Chang S, Carr W. Urticarial Vasculitis. Allergy Asthma Proc. 2007 Jan-Feb;28[1]:97–100.

[43] Dua J, Nandagudi A, Sutcliffe N. Mycoplasma Pneumoniae Infection Associated with Urticarial Vasculitis Mimicking Adult-Onset Still's Disease. Rheumatol Int. 2012 Dec;32[12]:4053–6.

[44] Shaigany S, Dabela E, Teich AF, Husain S, Grossman ME. Resolution of Urticarial Vasculitis After Treatment of Neurocysticercosis. J Am Acad Dermatol. 2015 Jan;72[1]:e32–3.

[45] Moreno-Suárez F, Pulpillo-Ruiz Á, Zulueta Dorado T, Conejo-Mir Sánchez J. Urticarial Vasculitis: A Retrospective Study of 15 Cases. Actas Dermosifiliogr. 2013 Sep;104[7]:579–85.

[46] Jachiet M, Flageul B, Deroux A, Le Quellec A, Maurier F, Cordoliani F, Godmer P, Abasq C, Astudillo L, Belenotti P, Bessis D, Bigot A, Doutre MS, Ebbo M, Guichard I, Hachulla E, Héron E, Jeudy G, Jourde Chiche N, Jullien D, Lavigne C, Machet L, Macher MA, Martel C, Melboucy-Belkhir S, Morice C, Petit A, Simorre B, Zenone T, Bouillet L, Bagot M, Frémeaux-Bacchi V, Guillevin L, Mouthon L, DupinN, Aractingi S, Terrier B. French Vasculitis Study Group. The Clinical Spectrum and Therapeutic Management of Hypocomplementemic Urticarial Vasculitis: Data from a French Nationwide Study of Fifty-Seven Patients. Arthritis Rheumatol. 2015 Feb;67[2]:527–34.

[47] Park C, Choi SW, Kim M, Park J, Lee JS, Chung HC. Membranoproliferative Glomerulon ephritis Presenting as Arthropathy and Cardiac Valvulopathy in Hypocomplementemic Urticarial Vasculitis: A Case Report. J Med Case Rep. 2014 Oct 22;8:352.

[48] Aydogan K, Karadogan SK, Adim SB, Tunali S. Hypocomplementemic Urticarial Vasculitis: A Rare Presentation of Systemic Lupus Erythematosus. Int J Dermatol. 2006 Sep;45[9]:1057–61.

[49] Loricera J, Calvo-Río V, Mata C, Ortiz-Sanjuán F, González-López MA, AlvarezL, González-Vela MC, Armesto S, Fernández-Llaca H, Rueda-Gotor J, González-GayMA, Blanco R. Urticarial Vasculitis in Northern Spain: Clinical Study of 21 Cases. Medicine [Baltimore]. 2014 Jan;93[1]:53–60.

[50] Criado PR, Antinori LC, Maruta CW, Reis VM. Evaluation Of D-Dimer Serum Levels Among Patients with Chronic Urticaria, Psoriasis and Urticarial Vasculitis. Ann Bras Dermatol. 2013 May–Jun;88[3]:355–60.

[51] Wisnieski JJ, Jones SM. Comparison of Autoantibodies to the Collagen-Like Region of C1q in Hypocomplementemic Urticarial Vasculitis Syndrome and Systemic Lupus Erythematosus. J Immunol. 1992 Mar 1;148[5]:1396–403.

[52] Athanasiadis GI, Pfab F, Kollmar A, Ring J, Ollert M. Urticarial Vasculitis with a Positive Autologous Serum Skin Test: Diagnosis and Successful Therapy. Allergy. 2006 Dec;61[12]:1484–5.

[53] Wakamatsu R, Watanabe H, Suzuki K, Suga N, Kitagawa W, Miura N, Nishikawa K, Yokoi T, Banno S, Imai H. Hypocomplementemic Urticarial Vasculitis Syndrome is Associated with High Levels of Serum IGg4: A Clinical Manifestation that MimicsIGg4-Related Disease. Intern Med. 2011;50[10]:1109–12.

[54] Takao M, Hamada T, Kaji T, Ikeda-Mizuno K, Takehara-Yasuhara C, Ichimura K, Yanai H, Yshino T, Iwatsuki K. Hypocomplementemic Urticarial Vasculitis Arisingİn a Patient with Immunoglobulin G4-Related Disease. Int J Dermatol. 2016Apr;55[4]:430–3.

[55] Demierre MF, Winkelman WJ. Idiopathic Cold-İnduced Urticarial Vasculitis and Monoclonal Igg Gammopathy. Int J Dermatol. 1996 Feb;35[2]:151–2.

[56] Swaminath A, Magro CM, Dwyer E. Refractory Urticarial Vasculitis as a Complication of Ulcerative Colitis Successfully Treated with Rituximab. J ClinRheumatol. 2011 Aug;17[5]:281–3.

[57] Chen T, Guo ZP, Cao N, Qin S, Li MM, Jia RZ. Increased Serum Levels of Soluble Vascular Endothelial-Cadherin in Patients with Systemic Vasculitis. RheumatolInt. 2014 Aug;34[8]:1139–43.

[58] Lee JS, Loh TH, Seow SC, Tan SH. Prolonged Urticaria with Purpura: The Spectrum of Clinical and Histopathologic Features in a Prospective Series of 22Patients Exhibiting the Clinical Features of Urticarial Vasculitis. J Am Acad Dermatol. 2007 Jun;56[6]:994–1005.

[59] Mathur AN, Mathes EF. Urticaria Mimickers in Children. Dermatol Ther. 2013 Nov–Dec; 26[6]:467–75.

[60] Kwon CW, Lee CW, Kim YT, Kim JH. Urticarial Vasculitis Developed on the Striae Distensae During Pregnancy. Int J Dermatol. 1993 Oct;32[10]:751–2.

[61] Ginsberg S, Rosner I, Rozenbaum M, Slobodin G, Zilber K, Boulman N, Kaly L, Awisat A, Jiries N, Beyar-Katz O, Rimar D. Autoinflammatory Associated Vasculitis. Semin Arthritis Rheum. 2016 Dec;46[3]:367–71.

[62] Krause K, Grattan CE, Bindslev-Jensen C, Gattorno M, Kallinich T, de Koning HD, Lachmann HJ, Lipsker D, Navarini AA, Simon A, Traidl-Hoffmann C, Maurer M. How not to Miss Autoinflammatory Diseases Masquerading as Urticaria. Allergy. 2012 Dec;67[12]:1465–74.

[63] Roy K, Talukdar A, Kumar B, Sarkar S. Hypocomplementaemic Urticarial Vasculitis Syndrome: A Mimicker of Systemic Lupus Erythematosus. BMJ Case Rep. 2013 May 22;2013.doi:10.1136/bcr-2013-009082.

[64] Epstein MM, Watsky KL, Lanzi RA. The Role of Diet in The Treatment of a Patient with Urticaria and Urticarial Vasculitis. J Allergy Clin Immunol. 1992 Sep;90[3 Pt 1]:414–5.

[65] Asherson RA, Buchanan N, Kenwright S, Fletcher CM, Hughes GR. The Normocomplementemic Urticarial Vasculitis Syndrome – Report of a Case and Response to Colchicine. Clin Exp Dermatol. 1991 Nov;16[6]:424–7

[66] Demitsu T, Yoneda K, Kakurai M, Sasaki K, Hiratsuka Y, Azuma R, Yamada T, Umemoto N. Clinical Efficacy of Reserpine As "Add-On Therapy" to Antihistamines in Patients with Recalcitrant Chronic Idiopathic Urticaria and Urticarial Vasculitis. J Dermatol. 2010 Sep;37[9]:827–9.

[67] Demitsu T, Yoneda K, Iida E, Takada M, Azuma R, Umemoto N, Hiratsuka Y, Yamada T, Kakurai M. Urticarial Vasculitis with Haemorrhagic Vesicles Successfully Treated with Reserpine. J Eur Acad Dermatol Venereol. 2008 Aug;22[8]:1006–8.

[68] Breda L, Nozzi M, Harari S, Torto MD, Lucantoni M, Scardapane A, Chiarelli F. Hypocomplementemic Urticarial Vasculitis [HUVS] with Precocius Emphysema Responsive to Azathioprine. J Clin Immunol. 2013;33:891–5.

[69] Borcea A, Greaves MW. Methotrexate-Induced Exacerbation of Urticarial Vasculitis: An Unusual Adverse Reaction. Br J Dermatol. 2000 Jul;143[1]:203–4.

[70] Chew GY, Gatenby PA. Inflammatory Myositis Complicating Hypocomplementemic Urticarial Vasculitis Despite On-Going İmmunosuppression. Clin Rheumatol. 2007 Aug;26[8]:1370–2.

[71] Worm M, Muche M, Schulze P, Sterry W, Kolde G. Hypocomplementaemic Urticarial Vasculitis: Successful Treatment with Cyclophosphamide-Dexamethasone Pulse Therapy. Br J Dermatol. 1998 Oct;139[4]:704–7.

[72] Soma J, Sato H, Ito S, Saito T. Nephrotic Syndrome Associated with Hypocomplementaemic Urticarial Vasculitis Syndrome: Successful Treatment with Cyclosporin A. Nephrol Dial Transplant. 1999 Jul;14[7]:1753–7.

[73] Al Mosawi ZS, Al Hermi BE. Hypocomplementemic Urticarial Vasculitis Syndrome in an 8-Year-Old Boy: A Case Report and Review of Literature. Oman Med J. 2013 Jul;28[4]:275–7.

[74] Worm M, Sterry W, Kolde G. Mycophenolate Mofetil is Effective for Maintenance Therapy of Hypocomplementaemic Urticarial Vasculitis. Br J Dermatol. 2000 Dec;143[6]:1324.

[75] Handfield-Jones SE, Greaves MW. Urticarial Vasculitis--Response to Gold Therapy. J R Soc Med. 1991 Mar;84[3]:169.

[76] Kartal O, Gulec M, Caliskaner Z, Nevruz O, Cetin T, Sener O. Plasmapheresis in a Patient with "Refractory" Urticarial Vasculitis. Allergy Asthma Immunol Res. 2012 Jul;4[4]:245–7.

[77] Grimbert P, Schulte K, Buisson C, Desvaux D, Baron C, Pastural M, Dhamane D, Remy P, Weil B, Lang P. Renal Transplantation in a Patient with Hypocomplementemic Urticarial Vasculitis Syndrome. Am J Kidney Dis. 2001 Jan;37[1]:144–8.

[78] Yamazaki-Nakashimada MA, Duran-McKinster C, Ramírez-Vargas N, Hernandez-Bautista V. Intravenous Immunoglobulin Therapy for Hypocomplementemic Urticarial Vasculitis Associated with Systemic Lupus Erythematosus in a Child. Pediatr Dermatol. 2009 Jul–Aug;26[4]:445–7.

[79] Filosto M, Cavallaro T, Pasolini G, Broglio L, Tentorio M, Cotelli M, Ferrari S, Padovani A. Idiopathic Hypocomplementemic Urticarial Vasculitis-Linked Neuropathy. J Neurol Sci. 2009 Sep 15;284[1–2]:179–81.

[80] Mukhtyar C, Misbah S, Wilkinson J, Wordsworth P. Refractory Urticarial Vasculitis Responsive to Anti-B-Cell Therapy. Br J Dermatol. 2009Feb;160[2]:470–2.

[81] Botsios C, Sfriso P, Punzi L, Todesco S. Non-Complementaemic Urticarial Vasculitis: Successful Treatment with the IL-1 Receptor Antagonist. Anakinra. Scand J Rheumatol. 2007 May–Jun;36[3]:236–7.

[82] Krause K, Mahamed A, Weller K, Metz M, Zuberbier T, Maurer M. Efficacy and Safety of Canakinumab in Urticarial Vasculitis: An Open-Label Study. J Allergy Clin Immunol. 2013 Sep;132[3]:751–4.

[83] Makol A, Gibson LE, Michet CJ. Successful Use of Interleukin 6 Antagonist Tocilizumab in a Patient with Refractory Cutaneous Lupus and UrticarialVasculitis. J Clin Rheumatol. 2012 Mar;18[2]:92–5.

[84] Kai AC, Flohr C, Grattan CE. Improvement in Quality of Life Impairment Followed by Relapse with 6 Monthly Periodic Administration of Omalizumab for Severe Treatment-Refractory Chronic Urticaria and Urticarial Vasculitis. Clin ExpDermatol. 2014 Jul;39[5]:651–2.

[85] Ghazanfar MN, Thomsen SF. Omalizumab for Urticarial Vasculitis: Case Report and Review of the Literature. Case Rep Dermatol Med. 2015:576893.

[86] Lin RY. Urticarial Vasculitis. Br J Dermatol. 1996 Dec;135[6]:1016.

[87] Hamid S, Cruz PD Jr, Lee WM. Urticarial Vasculitis Caused by Hepatitis C Virüs İInfection: Response to Interferon Alfa Therapy. J Am Acad Dermatol. 1998 Aug;39:278–80.

[88] Jamison SC, Brierre S, Sweet J, de Boisblanc B. A Case of Precocious Emphysema and Lung Cancer in a Woman with a History of Hypocomplementemic Urticarial Vasculitis. Chest. 2008 Mar;133[3]:787–9.

[89] Hauser B. Systemic Manifestations of Hypocomplementemic Urticarial Vasculitis: Comment on the Article by Jachiet et al. Arthritis Rheumatol. 2015 Jul;67[7]:1984–5.

[90] Batioğlu F, Taner P, Aydintuğ OT, Heper AO, Ozmert E. Recurrent Optic Disc and Retinal Vasculitis in a Patient with Drug-Induced Urticarial Vasculitis. Cutan Ocul Toxicol. 2006;25[4]:281–5.

[91] Hall AC, Leong AC, Jiang D, Fitzgerald-O'Connor A. Sudden Bilateral Sensorineural Hearing Loss Associated with Urticarial Vasculitis. J Laryngol Otol. 2013 Jul;127[7]:708–11.

[92] Turner RB, Haynes HA, Granter SR, Miller DM. Acquired Cutis Laxa Following Urticarial Vasculitis Associated with IgA Myeloma. J Am Acad Dermatol. 2009 Jun;60[6]:1052–7.

[93] Patel N, Shovel L, Moran N, Woo K, Stewart G, Tricot T. Acquired Haemophilia in Urticarial Vasculitis Revealed by Injudicious Heparin. J R Soc Med. 2006Mar;99[3]:151–2.

[94] Christiansen J, Kahn R, Schmidtchen A, Berggård K. Idiopathic Angioedema and Urticarial Vasculitis in a Patient with a History of Acquired Haemophilia. Acta Derm Venereol. 2015 Feb;95[2]:227–8.

[95] Alachkar H, Qasim F, Ahmad Y, Helbert M. Meningococcal Meningitis in a Patient with Urticarial Vasculitis: Is There a Link? J Clin Pathol. 2007 Oct;60[10]:1160–1.

[96] Sangle SR, Vounotrypidis P, Briley A, Nel L, Lutalo PM, Sanchez-Fernandez S, Chaib A, Salas-Manzanedo V, Shennan A, Khamashta MA, D'Cruz DP. Pregnancy Outcome in Patients with Systemic Vasculitis: A Single-Centre Matched Case-Control Study. Rheumatology [Oxford]. 2015 Sep;54[9]:1582–6.

Chapter 7

Comorbidities in Chronic Spontaneous Urticaria

Müzeyyen Gönül, Havva Hilal Ayvaz and
Selda Pelin Kartal

Additional information is available at the end of the chapter

http://dx.doi.org/10.5772/67911

Abstract

Chronic spontaneous urticaria (CSU) is a disease that makes people's lives miserable with unknown etiology. In recent years, there have been many studies trying to explain the etiology of CSU, and many of them reported that there are some comorbidities or triggering factors related to CSU. However, it has not been clearly known yet that whether these conditions are true comorbidities associated with CSU or they are coincidentally found at the same time. In this chapter, related comorbidities and conditions have been told.

Keywords: chronic spontaneous urticaria, autoimmunity, infectious diseases, psychological comorbidities, coagulation factors, metabolic syndrome

1. Introduction

Chronic spontaneous urticaria (CSU) is a common mast cell-driven skin disorder characterized by the occurrence of recurrent and spontaneously daily or frequent wheals with or without angioedema, for more than 6 weeks with symptoms present at least three times weekly [1, 2]. CSU affects 0.1–5% of the population, especially during the third and fourth decades and predominantly women [3]. There are many studies that some disorders or conditions may be related to CSU.

2. Comorbidities and possible triggering factors

There are studies showing that CSU affects not only the skin but also the life quality and psychology of the person. At the same time, there has been a relation between CSU and other diseases which can be based on similar pathogenesis such as autoimmune thyroiditis. After these data researches have mainly focused on the relationship between comorbidities and CSU.

The possible mechanisms and triggering factors underlying CSU have been identified as acute or chronic infections, stress, nonallergic hypersensitivity reactions to foods and drugs (pseudoallergic), and autoreactivity including autoimmunity mediated by functional autoantibodies directed against the IgE receptor [4]. Stress is a major triggering and risk factor along CSU patients [5]. Furthermore, several studies revealed that stress can trigger or aggravate some skin diseases by the alternation of the functions of T cells and local neuroimmunoendocrine circuitry [6]. Most of the patients with CSU experience a stressor event within 6 months before the onset of the symptoms [7].

CSU patients have a higher level of stressful life events, perceived stress, and psychiatric comorbidity [7]. And many studies have shown that CSU patients more frequently have psychiatric comorbidities [7–11]. The most common psychiatric situations in these patients are depression, somatoform, and anxiety disorders [11, 12]. Both these disorders and CSU symptoms could affect the quality of life (QoL) of the patients. Also, it was shown that CSU patients had lower social relationship scores compared to healthy controls [8, 11]. CSU patients reportedly suffer more sleep disturbance, fatigue, emotional upset, and physical and mental restrictions at home and work [8]. Furthermore, in a study which compared patients with CSU to patients with psoriasis, physical impairment and effects of the disorder on QoL were found higher in patients with CSU than patients with psoriasis [13]. In a study QoL impairment in CSU patients was found higher than in patients with vitiligo [14]. Interestingly, Staubach et al. reported no significant relation between impact of QoL and age-sex, concurrent angioedema, and duration of CSU condition of the patients [8]. They also reported that the severity of the concomitant depression-anxiety or somatoform disorders in patients with CSU is important, because these patients, with concomitant severe psychiatric conditions, had significant impairment of QoL than patients with CSU who did not exhibit psychiatric comorbidity. Moreover, these psychiatric problems could be the primary factors in these patients or might arise as psychosocial consequences of underlying dermatological disorders [8]. As a result, an interdisciplinary approach that combines dermatological and psychiatric treatments is necessary for the management of CSU.

In recent years, associations between CSU and autoimmunity have been increasingly recognized in many studies [15–19]. Approximately 30–50% of patients with chronic urticaria produce specific IgG antibodies against the alpha subunit of the mast cell IgE receptor, and approximately 5–10% produce IgG antibodies against IgE itself [15]. Autoimmune mechanisms have been proposed as responsible for the development of some of the cases. Especially, intradermal autologous serum injections were applied, and urticarial responses were seen in 60% of patients with CSU [16].

Also, subsequent studies revealed that anti-IgG and anti-IgE autoantibodies, anti-FcεRI targeted at basophils, and mast cells were found in 45–55% of patients with CSU. These autoantibodies bind to mast cell-bound IgE molecules or surface IgE receptors to stimulate and eventually degranulate the cells and cause the urticarial symptoms [17–19]. It was suggested that some CSU patients have an autoimmune mechanism induced by these autoantibodies [20].

Thyroid diseases, especially Hashimoto's disease in which production of thyroid autoantibodies (antithyroid peroxidase antibodies and antithyroglobulin antibodies) and lymphocytic infiltration into the thyroid gland are seen, are the most common autoimmune diseases accompanying patients with CSU [19–21]. The etiology of thyroid autoimmunity is not known, but the genetic susceptibility and environmental factors are thought to initiate the process [22]. Leznoff and Sussman reported that 15% of the CSU patients had thyroid autoantibodies and there has been a relation between CSU and thyroid autoimmunity. The rate of high antithyroid antibodies in the patients with CSU ranges from 6.5% up to 57% in the other reports [23, 24]. The mechanism of these associations is not known. Confino-Cohen et al. hypothesized that the relationship between thyroid diseases and CSU might be based on shared susceptibility to autoimmune or chronic inflammatory processes [21]. Moreover, many small patient series and case reports reported that patients with CSU and thyroid autoimmunity benefit from levothyroxine sodium or antithyroid drug treatment. In these studies, clinical remission of chronic urticaria was seen, whereas no change has been demonstrated in thyroid antibody levels [25–27].

Although autoimmune thyroid disorders have been investigated in CSU, its relation with other autoimmune diseases has been investigated less [20]. But there is a fact that if there is an autoimmune disease in a patient, the second or third autoimmune disease more often appears even if the patient is under immunosuppressive treatment [21]. And rheumatoid arthritis (RA) was found as the second most common autoimmune disease in patients with CSU. Confino et al. reported that RA was found 13 times more in patients with CSU than healthy controls [21]. Rheumatoid factor was found significantly more often in patients with CSU [28].

In a small series of patients or case reports, celiac disease was reported higher in patients with CSU [29]. Several case reports revealed a 1.5–7-fold increased risk of urticaria in patients with celiac disease [30–32]. Also, systemic lupus erythematosus (SLE) and type I diabetes mellitus were each found significantly more prevalent in female patients with CSU [21, 33, 34].

Patients with CSU were found to have a significantly 15 times higher risk of developing SLE as compared to the control group. Furthermore, SLE was found to be 25 times higher in women than in men with CSU or women of the control group [21].

The high prevalence of these autoimmune diseases in patients with CSU makes it thinkable that somehow CSU can be also a member of autoimmunity. But the underlying mechanism of autoimmunity related to urticaria has not been known yet, but as mentioned before, susceptibility to autoimmune and/or chronic inflammatory processes might be the reason [21].

In the last few years, many researches published about the activation of the coagulation system in patients with CSU. A study revealed that the levels of plasma prothrombin fragment (PF)1+2, a marker of thrombin generation, were significantly increased in patients with CSU. They also reported that patients with CSU have more positive autologous plasma skin test result than a positive autologous serum skin test result. This study showed that there should be possible role of clotting factors in flaring symptoms induced by autologous plasma, because autoantibodies are equally present in serum and plasma [35]. Also, a statistically significant relationship between elevated plasma levels of PF1+2 and D-dimer and the severity of CSU was reported in some studies [36, 37].

CSU is characterized by the activation of the coagulation cascade [38, 39]. And it is probable that both intrinsic and extrinsic pathways are affected in CSU patients [40]. The coagulation system factors that most likely involved in the pathogenesis of CSU are tissue factor, thrombin, D-dimer, PF1+2, and activated factor VII [41, 42].

Thrombin activation, which is derived from platelets, directed investigations toward the evaluation of mean platelet volume (MPV) and CSU correlation. MPV is a potential marker of platelet reactivity because larger platelets are metabolically and enzymatically more active. It was shown that platelets secrete a large number of mediators of thrombosis, coagulation, inflammation, and atherosclerosis [43]. And MPV values were found significantly more in patients with CSU than the control group [21, 44]. A suggested possible way in the pathogenesis of CSU is that large activated platelets might activate the coagulation cascade. The activation of the coagulation pathways elicits increase in number of protease-activated receptor-1 on mast cells, mediator degranulation from mast cells and, increase in vascular permeability [45–47]. In many studies, this activated coagulation cascade was found associated with more severe disease [40, 41, 47]. Also, some studies showed that coagulation factors decreased to normal limits after disease remission or during treatment [35, 36, 40]. In contrast to this view, some authors suggest that the activation of the coagulation cascade seems a potential intensifying mechanism in the pathogenesis of CSU but is quite likely not the main trigger of the disease [47].

Chronic persistent infections,(e.g., *Helicobacter pylori* (Hp), streptococci, staphylococci, *yersinia, Giardia lamblia, Mycoplasma pneumoniae,* Hepatitis viruses, *Norovirus, Parvovirus B19, Anisakis simplex, Entamoeba* spp., and *Blastocystis* spp.) have been suspected to be triggering factors in patients with CSU [3]. Especially, Hp infection was popularly investigated in the pathogenesis of CSU [48, 49]. It is thought that Hp infections could be a triggering factor in underlying autoimmune pathology of CSU [50], and there are studies showing that Hp infection is related to production of autoreactive IgM and IgG3 antibodies [51]. Another suggestion is that Hp-associated lipoprotein 20 (lpp20) could act as an antigen that is involved in molecular mimicry to mast cells, T cells, and B cells as well [51–53]. Also in some studies, eradication of Hp infection resulted in remission of CSU symptoms [54, 55].

CSU is histopathologically characterized by infiltrating perivascularT cells, eosinophils, and neutrophils, and neutrophils, and several studies reported that circulating levels of C-reactive protein (CRP), pro-inflammatory cytokines such as interleukin (IL)-6 and TNF-α, and matrix metalloproteinase 9 (MMP-9) have been found increasing in patients with CSU. Also, these markers are thought to appear to correlate with clinical activity score and severity of urticaria [56–58]. Metabolic syndrome (MetS) involves dyslipidemia, central obesity, glucose intolerance, and high blood pressure [59]. Furthermore it has been reported that patients suffering from MetS had higher serum levels of inflammatory markers such as IL-1, IL-6, TNF, and CRP than healthy controls [60].

In a study, the prevalence of MetS was reported higher among the patients with CSU. Thus, systemic inflammation promoted by MetS may play a role in CSU pathogenesis as well. Furthermore, some studies revealed that the levels of TNF and C3 were found significantly higher and correlated with more severe, uncontrolled urticaria symptoms in patients with CSU and MetS at the same time [59, 60].

Some studies showed that activation of eosinophils which are sources of vascular endothelial growth factor and tissue factor in lesional skin of patients with CSU may play a role in the pathogenesis of CSU [61]. Elevated serum eosinophilic cationic protein levels were found correlated with symptoms in patients with CSU and MetS. Both diseases, CSU and MetS, which may mutually trigger or exacerbate each other, have elevated systemic inflammation [60].

3. Conclusion

Studies investigating comorbidities associated with CSU have been increasing in recent years, and new disorders possibly associated with the CSU have been reported. It has not been clearly known yet that whether these conditions are true comorbidities associated with CSU or they are coincidentally found at the same time. This will be clearer as more studies on the subject are added.

Author details

Müzeyyen Gönül[1]*, Havva Hilal Ayvaz[2] and Selda Pelin Kartal[1]

*Address all correspondence to: muzeyyengonul@gmail.com

1 University of Health Sciences, Dışkapı Yıldırım Beyazıt Training and Research Hospital in Ankara, Turkey

2 Polatlı Duatepe State Hospital, Polatlı, Ankara, Turkey

References

[1] Van Der Valk PGM, Moret G, Kiemeney LA. The natural history of chronic urticaria and angioedema in patients visiting a tertiary referral centre. Br J Dermatol. 2002;**146**: 110–113. DOI: 10.1046/j.1365-2133.2002.04582.x.

[2] Vestergaard C, Deleuran M. Chronic spontaneous urticaria: latest developments in aetiology, diagnosis and therapy. Ther Adv Chronic Dis. 2015 Nov;**6**(6):304–313. DOI: 10.1177/2040622315603951.

[3] Zuberbier T. Chronic urticaria. Curr Allergy Asthma Rep. 2012;**12**:267–272. DOI: 10.1007/s11882-012-0270-7.

[4] Zuberbier T, Asero R, Bindslev-Jensen C, Walter Canonica G, Church MK, Gimenez-Arnau A, Grattan CE, Kapp A, Merk HF, Rogala B, Saini S, Sanchez-Borges M, Schmid-Grendelmeier P, Schunemann H, Staubach P, Vena GA, Wedi B, Maurer M. EAACI/GA[2] LEN/EDF/WAO guideline: definition, classification and diagnosis of urticaria. Allergy. 2009;**64**:1417–1426. DOI: 10.1111/j.1398-9995.2009.02179.x.

[5] Malhotra SK, Mehta V. Role of stressful life events in induction or exacerbation of psoriasis and chronic urticaria. Indian J Dermatol Venereol Leprol. 2008 Nov-Dec;**74**(6):594–599. DOI: 10.4103/0378-6323.45100.

[6] Paus R, Theoharides TC, Arck PC. Neuroimmunoendocrine circuitry of the 'brain-skin connection'. Trends Immunol. 2006 Jan;**27**(1):32-39. DOI:10.1016/j.it.2005.10.002.

[7] Staubach P, Dechene M, Metz M, Magerl M, Siebenhaar F, Weller K, Zezula P, Eckhardt-Henn A, Maurer M. High prevalence of mental disorders and emotional distress in patients with chronic spontaneous urticaria. Acta Derm Venereol. 2011 Sep;**91**(5): 557–561. DOI: 10.2340/00015555-1109.

[8] Staubach P, Eckhardt-Henn A, Dechene M, et al. Quality of life in patients with chronic urticaria is differentially impaired and determined by psychiatric comorbidity. Br J Dermatol. 2006;**154**:294–298. DOI: 10.1111/j.1365-2133.2005.06976.x.

[9] Lyketsos CG, Lyketsos GC, Richardson SC, Beis A. Dysthymic states and depressive syndromes in physical conditions of presumably psychogenic origin. Acta Psychiatr Scand. 1987 Nov;**76**(5):529–534. DOI: 10.1111/j.1600-0447.1987.tb02914.x.

[10] Sukan M, Maner F. The problems in sexual functions of vitiligo and chronic urticaria patients. J Sex Marital Ther. 2007 Jan–Feb;**33**(1):55–64. DOI: 10.1080/00926230600998482.

[11] Engin B, Uguz F, Yilmaz E, Özdemir M, Mevlitoglu I. The levels of depression, anxiety and quality of life in patients with chronic idiopathic urticaria. J Eur Acad Dermatol Venereol. 2008 Jan;**22**(1):36–40. DOI: 10.1111/j.1468-3083.2007.02324.x.

[12] Chung MC, Symons C, Gillioam J. The relationship between posttraumatic stress disorder, psychiatric comorbidity, and personality traits among patients with chronic idiopathic urticaria. Compr Psychiatry. 2010;**51**:55–63. DOI: 10.1016/j.comppsych.2009.02.005.

[13] Weldon DR. Quality of life in patients with urticaria. Allergy Asthma Proc. 2006;27:96–99.

[14] Poon E, Seed PT, Greaves MW, et al. The extent and nature of disability in different urticaria conditions. Br J Dermatol. 1999;**140**:667–671. DOI: 10.1046/j.1365-2133.1999.02767.x.

[15] Bernstein JA, Lang DM, Khan DA, et al. The diagnosis and management of acute and chronic urticaria: 2014 update. J Allergy Clin Immunol. 2014;**133**(5):1270–1277. DOI: 10.1016/j.jaci.2014.02.036.

[16] Sabron RA, Grattan CE, Francis DM, Barr RM, Kobza Black A, Greaves MW. The autologous serum skin test: a screening test for autoantibodies in chronic idiopathic urticaria. Br J Dermatol. 1999;**140**:446–452. DOI: 10.1046/j.1365-2133.1999.02707.x.

[17] Kikuchi Y, Kaplan AP. Mechanisms of autoimmune activation of basophils in chronic urticaria. J Allergy Clin Immunol. 2001 Jun;**107**(6):1056–1062. DOI: 10.1067/mai.2001.115484.

[18] Sugiyama A, Nishie H, Takeuchi S, Yoshinari M, Furue M. Hashimoto's disease is a frequent comorbidity and an exacerbating factor of chronic spontaneous urticaria. Allergol Immunopathol [Madr]. 2015 May–Jun;**43**(3):249–253. DOI: 10.1016/j.aller.2014.02.007.

[19] Marone G, Spadaro G, Palumbo C, Condorelli G. The anti-IgE/anti-FcepsilonRIalpha autoantibody network in allergic and autoimmune diseases. Clin Exp Allergy. 1999 Jan;**29**(1):17–27. DOI: 10.1046/j.1365-2222.1999.00441.x.

[20] Kolkhir P, Pogorelov D, Olisova O, Maurer M. Comorbidity and pathogenic links of chronic spontaneous urticaria and systemic lupus erythematosus—a systematic review. Clin Exp Allergy. 2016 Feb;**46**(2):275–287. DOI: 10.1111/cea.12673.

[21] Confino-Cohen R, Chodick G, Shalev V, Leshno M, Kimhi O, Goldberg AA. Chronic urticaria and autoimmunity: associations found in a large population study. J Allergy Clin Immunol. 2012;**129**:1307–1313. DOI: 10.1016/j.jaci.2012.01.043.

[22] Pan XF, Gu JQ, Shan ZY. The prevalence of thyroid autoimmunity in patients with urticaria: a systematic review and meta-analysis. Endocrine. 2015 Apr;**48**(3):804–810. DOI: 10.1007/s12020-014-0367-y.

[23] Leznoff A, Sussman GL. Syndrome of idiopathic chronic urticaria and angioedema with thyroid autoimmunity: a study of 90 patients. J Allergy Clin Immunol. 1989 Jul;**84**(1): 66–71. DOI: http://dx.doi.org/10.1016/0091-6749(89)90180-2.

[24] Turktas I, Gokcora N, Demirsoy S, Cakir N, Onal E. The association of chronic urticaria and angioedema with autoimmune thyroiditis. Int J Dermatol. 1997 Mar;36(3):187–190. DOI: 10.1046/j.1365-4362.1997.00187.x.

[25] Kim DH, Sung NH, Lee AY. Effect of levothyroxine treatment on clinical symptoms in hypothyroid patients with chronic urticaria and thyroid autoimmunity. Ann Dermatol. 2016;**28**(2):199–204. DOI: 10.5021/ad.2016.28.2.199.

[26] Aversano M, Caiazzo P, Iorio G, Ponticiello L, Laganá B, Leccese F. Improvement of chronic idiopathic urticaria with L-thyroxine: a new TSH role in immune response? Allergy. 2005 Apr;**60**(4):489–493. DOI: 10.1111/j.1398-9995.2005.00723.x.

[27] O'Donnell BF, Francis DM, Swana GT, Seed PT, Kobza Black A, Greaves MW. Thyroid autoimmunity in chronic urticaria. Br J Dermatol. 2005 Aug;**153**(2):331–335. DOI: 10.1111/j.1365-2133.2005.06646.x.

[28] Tobón GJ, Youinou P, Saraux A. The environment, geo-epidemiology, and autoimmune disease: rheumatoid arthritis. J Autoimmun. 2010 Aug;**35**(1):10–14. DOI: 10.1016/j.jaut.2009.12.009.

[29] Meneghetti R, Gerarduzzi T, Barbi E, Ventura A. Chronic urticaria and celiac disease. Arch Dis Child. 2004;**89**:293. DOI: 10.1136/adc.2003.037259.

[30] Ludvigsson JF, Lindelöf B, Rashtak S, Rubio-Tapia A, Murray JA. Does urticaria risk increase in patients with celiac disease? A large population-based cohort study. Eur J Dermatol. 2013 Sep–Oct;**23**(5):681–687. DOI: 10.1684/ejd.2013.2158.

[31] Caminiti L, Passalacqua G, Magazzù G, Comisi F, Vita D, Barberio G, Sferlazzas C, Pajno GB. Chronic urticaria and associated coeliac disease in children: a case-control study. Pediatr Allergy Immunol. 2005 Aug;**16**(5):428–432. DOI: 10.1111/j.1399-3038.2005.00309.x.

[32] Gabrielli M, Candelli M, Cremonini F, Ojetti V, Santarelli L, Nista EC, Nucera E, Schiavino D, Patriarca G, Gasbarrini G, Pola P, Gasbarrini A. Idiopathic chronic urticaria and celiac disease. Dig Dis Sci. 2005 Sep;**50**(9):1702–1704. DOI: 10.1007/s10620-005-2919-8.

[33] Borchers AT, Naguwa SM, Shoenfeld Y, Gershwin ME. The geoepidemiology of systemic lupus erythematosus. Autoimmun Rev. 2010;**9**:277–287. DOI: 10.1016/j.autrev.2009.12.008.

[34] Asero R, Orsatti A, Tedeschi A, Lorini M. Autoimmune chronic urticaria associated with type 1 diabetes and Graves' disease. J Allergy Clin Immunol. 2005 May;**115**(5):1088–1089. DOI: 10.1016/j.jaci.2004.12.009.

[35] Asero R, Tedeschi A, Riboldi P, Cugno M. Plasma of patients with chronic urticaria shows signs of thrombin generation, and its intradermal injection causes wheal-and-flare reactions much more frequently than autologous serum. J Allergy Clin Immunol. 2006;**117**:1113–1117. DOI: 10.1016/j.jaci.2005.12.1343.

[36] Takeda T, Sakurai Y, Takahagi S, Kato J, Yoshida K, Yoshioka A, Hide M, Shima M. Increase of coagulation potential in chronic spontaneous urticaria. Allergy. 2011;**66**: 428– 433. DOI: 10.1111/j.1398-9995.2010.02506.x.

[37] Takahagi S, Mihara S, Iwamoto K, Morioke S, Okabe T, Kameyoshi Y, Hide M. Coagulation/fibrinolysis and inflammation markers are associated with disease activity in patients with chronic urticaria. Allergy. 2009;**65**:649–656. DOI: 10.1111/j.1398-9995.2009.02222.x.

[38] Asero R, Tedeschi A, Coppola R, Griffini S, Paparella P, Riboldi P, Marzano AV, Fanoni D, Cugno M. Activation of the tissue pathway of blood coagulation in patients with chronic urticaria. J Allergy Clin Immunol. 2007;**119**:705–710. DOI: 10.1016/j.jaci.2006.08.043.

[39] Asero R, Tedeschi A, Riboldi P, Griffini S, Bonanni E, Cugno M. Severe chronic urticaria is associated with elevated plasma levels of D-dimer. Allergy. 2008;**63**:176–180. DOI: 10.1111/j.1398-9995.2007.01514.x.

[40] Triwongwaranat D, Kulthanan K, Chularojanamontri L, Pinkaew S. Correlation between plasma D-dimer levels and the severity of patients with chronic urticaria. Asia Pac Allergy. 2013 Apr;**3**(2):100–105. DOI: 10.5415/apallergy.2013.3.2.100.

[41] Cirino G, Cicala C, Bucci MR, Sorrentino L, Maraganore JM, Stone SR. Thrombin functions as an inflammatory mediator through activation of its receptor. J Exp Med. 1996;183:821–827.

[42] Cugno M, Tedeschi A, Borghi A, et al. Activation of Blood Coagulation in Two Prototypic Autoimmune Skin Diseases: A Possible Link with Thrombotic Risk. Picardo M, ed. PLoS ONE. 2015;**10**(6):e0129456. DOI: 10.1371/journal.pone.0129456.

[43] Coppinger JA, Cagney G, Toomey S, Kislinger T, Belton O, McRedmond JP, et al. Characterization of the proteins released from activated platelets leads to localization of novel platelet proteins in human atherosclerotic lesions. Blood. 2004;**103**:2096–2104. DOI: 10.1182/blood-2003-08-2804.

[44] Magen E, Mishal J, Zeldin U, Feldman V, Kidon M, Schlesinger M, et al. Increased mean platelet volume and C-reactive protein levels in patients with chronic urticaria with a positive autologous serum skin test. Am J Med Sci. 2010;**339**:504–508. DOI: 10.1097/MAJ.0b013e3181db6ed5.

[45] Nobe K, Sone T, Paul RJ, Honda K. Thrombin-induced force development in vascular endothelial cells: contribution to alteration of permeability mediated by calcium-dependent and -independent pathways. J Pharmacol Sci. 2005 Nov;**99**(3):252–263. http://doi.org/10.1254/jphs.FP0050679. (Bunun DOI numarası boyle site adresi seklinde verilmiş, başka bulamadım :S Denedim açılıyor makale direk bu şekilde).

[46] Asero R, Tedeschi A, Cugno M. Heparin and tranexamic acid therapy may be effective in treatment-resistant chronic urticaria with elevated d-dimer: a pilot study. Int Arch Allergy Immunol. 2010;**152**(4):384-389. DOI: 10.1159/000292947.

[47] Asero R, Tedeschi A, Riboldi P, Griffini S, Bonanni E, Cugno M. Coagulation cascade and fibrinolysis in patients with multiple-drug allergy syndrome. Ann Allergy Asthma Immunol. 2008 Jan;**100**(1):44–48. DOI:10.1016/S1081-1206(10)60403-6.

[48] Ojetti V, Armuzzi A, De Luca A, Nucera E, Franceschi F, Candelli M, et al. *Helicobacter pylori* infection affects eosinophilic cationic protein in the gastric juice of patients with idiopathic chronic urticaria. Int Arch Allergy Immunol. 2001;**125**(1):66–72. DOI: 10.1159/000053798.

[49] Akelma AZ, Cizmeci MN, Mete E, Tufan N, Bozkurt B. A neglected cause for chronic spontaneous urticaria in children: *Helicobacter pylori*. Allergol Immunopathol (Madr). 2015 May–Jun;**43**(3):259–263. DOI: 10.1016/j.aller.2013.12.001.

[50] Chiu YC, Tai WC, Chuah SK, Hsu PI, Wu DC, Wu KL, Huang CC, Ho JC, Ring J, Chen WC. The clinical correlations of *Helicobacter pylori* virulence factors and chronic spontaneous urticaria. Gastroenterol Res Pract. 2013;**2013**:436727. DOI:10.1155/2013/436727.

[51] Yamanishi S, Iizumi T, Watanabe E, Shimizu M, Kamiya S, Nagata K, et al. Implications for induction of autoimmunity via activation of B-1 cells by *Helicobacter pylori* urease. Infect Immun. 2006;**74**(1):248–256. DOI: 10.1128/IAI.74.1.248-256.2006.

[52] Curth HM, Dinter J, Nigemeier K, Kütting F, Hunzelmann N, Steffen HM. Effects of *Helicobacter pylori* eradication in chronic spontaneous urticaria: results from a retrospective cohort study. Am J Clin Dermatol. 2015 Dec;**16**(6):553–558. DOI: 10.1007/s40257-015-0152-6.

[53] Magen E, Mishal J. Possible benefit from treatment of Helicobacter pylori in antihistamine-resistant chronic urticaria. Clin Exp Dermatol. 2013 Jan;**38**(1):7–12. DOI: 10.1111/j.1365-2230.2012.04467.x.

[54] Fukuda S, Shimoyama T, Umegaki N, Mikami T, Nakano H, Munakata A. Effect of *Helicobacter pylori* eradication in the treatment of Japanese patients with chronic idiopathic urticaria. J Gastroenterol. 2004;**39**(9):827–830. DOI: 10.1007/s00535-004-1397-7.

[55] Magen E, Mishal J, Schlesinger M, Scharf S. Eradication of *Helicobacter pylori* infection equally improves chronic urticaria with positive and negative autologous serum skin test. Helicobacter. 2007 Oct;**12**(5):567–571. DOI: 10.1111/j.1523-5378.2007.00522.x.

[56] Kasperska-Zajac A, Sztylc J, Machura E, Jop G. Plasma IL-6 concentration correlates with clinical disease activity and serum C-reactive protein concentration in chronic urticaria patients. Clin Exp Allergy. 2011;**41**:1386–1391. DOI: 10.1111/j.1365-2222.2011.03789.x.

[57] Tedeschi A, Asero R, Lorini M, Marzano AV, Cugno M. Plasma levels of matrix metalloproteinase-9 in chronic urticaria patients correlate with disease severity and C-reactive protein but not with circulating histamine-releasing factors. Clin Exp Allergy. 2010;**40**:875–881. DOI: 10.1111/j.1365-2222.2010.03473.x.

[58] Ye YM, Jin HJ, Hwang EK, Nam YH, Kim JH, Shin YS, Park HS. Co-existence of chronic urticaria and metabolic syndrome: clinical implications. Acta Derm Venereol. 2013 Mar;**93**(2):156–160. DOI: 10.2340/00015555-1443.

[59] da Silva VN, Fiorelli LN, da Silva CC, Kurokawa CS, Goldberg TB. Do metabolic syndrome and its components have an impact on bone mineral density in adolescents? Nutr Metab [Lond]. 2017 Jan;**14**:1. DOI: 10.1186/s12986-016-0156-0.

[60] Devaraj S, Rosenson RS, Jialal I. Metabolic syndrome: an appraisal of the pro-inflammatory and procoagulant status. Endocrinol Metab Clin North Am. 2004;**33**:431–453. DOI: 10.1016/j.ecl.2004.03.008.

[61] Cugno M, Marzano AV, Tedeschi A, Fanoni D, Venegoni L, Asero R. Expression of tissue factor by eosinophils in patients with chronic urticaria. Int Arch Allergy Immunol. 2009;**148**:170–174. DOI: 10.1159/000155748.

Chapter 8

Urticaria and Angioedema Treatment

Emel Erdal Çalıkoğlu, Didem Mullaaziz and
Asli Kaptanoğlu

Additional information is available at the end of the chapter

http://dx.doi.org/10.5772/intechopen.68676

Abstract

Chronic urticaria (CU), one of the most frequent skin disorders, is defined as the repeated occurrence of red, swollen, itchy and sometimes painful hives (wheals), and/or angioedema (swellings in the deeper layers of the skin), for more than 6 weeks [1, 2]. CU has an estimated worldwide prevalence of approximately 1% [3], which includes spontaneous and inducible types. In chronic spontaneous urticaria (CSU), the most common type of CU, symptoms occur without a specific trigger [1, 3]. In contrast, in chronic inducible urticaria (CIndU), symptoms occur in response to specific stimuli, such as exposure to cold, heat or pressure [4]. Patients may suffer from CSU and CIndU in parallel [2]. Chronic urticaria (CU) is defined as the repeated occurrence of red, swollen, itchy and sometimes painful wheals, and/or angioedema, for more than 6 weeks. CU includes spontaneous and inducible types. In chronic spontaneous urticaria (CSU), the most common type of CU, symptoms occur without a specific trigger. Treatment of urticaria and/or angioedema mainly consist of antihistamines, short courses of corticosteroids, other immunosuppressive, and anti-inflammatory agents. Angioedema is a deeper expression of urticaria which is classified by allergic, hereditary, acquired, and angiotensin-converting enzyme inhibitor (ACEI)-induced forms.

Keywords: urticaria, treatment, management, angioedema

1. Introduction

H1 antihistamines are usually effective in the majority of urticaria and/or angioedema patients but might be insufficient in some patients. Second-generation antihistamines are safe and effective in patients with urticaria and are the first-line agents in all guidelines. For patients not responding to monotherapy with a second-generation antihistamine in the second step, several treatments can be used including higher doses of second-generation antihistamines, addition of H2 antagonist, or leukotriene receptor antagonists. First-generation antihistamines like hydroxyzine or doxepin can be considered in patients whose symptoms remain uncontrolled in bed time. Systemic corticosteroids are frequently used for refractory patients with urticaria and might be considered in some patients for only short-time use. Alternative therapies including omalizumab are approved by the Food and Drug Administration (FDA) for patients with chronic refractory urticaria and cyclosporine. Anti-inflammatory agents including dapsone, sulfasalazine, hydroxychloroquine, and colchicine have been used in some patients with limited evidence for efficacy in chronic urticaria.

Acute attacks of HAE are unresponsive to antihistamines or corticosteroids. C1-INH replacement, plasma kallikrein inhibitor, bradykinin receptor antagonist, and fresh frozen plasma have been approved for the treatment of acute attacks. Angioedema caused by ACE inhibitors can be an acute emergency with laryngeal or tongue edema. There is no response to antihistamines or corticosteroids. Fresh frozen plasma, C1 inhibitor, and bradykinin receptor antagonist appear to be safe and effective therapeutic options for the management of ACEI-induced angioedema.

2. Management of urticaria

Urticaria is commonly defined as the sudden appearance of wheals that are typically pruritic and resolve within 24 h without any skin changes, although some lesions may last up to 48 h [1]. The updated classification of urticaria distinguishes acute and chronic urticaria. Acute urticaria is defined as the one persisting less than 6 weeks, whereas chronic urticaria (CU) persists for at least 6 weeks [1]. Chronic urticaria is spontaneous (CSU) or inducible (CIU) [2]. CSU is a common disorder with a prevalence of 1% that is characterized by recurrent wheals, angioedema, or both for more than 6 weeks (with or without free intervals). CSU is self-limited but in many patients, symptoms recur for several years and can be refractory to standard therapies [3, 4].

The international urticaria guidelines advise standard dose, second-generation H1-antihistamines as first-line therapy [5]. However, H1 antihistamine treatment leads to absence of symptoms in fewer than 50% of patients, and in about 10% of cases, they fail to control the disease even at higher than licensed doses [5, 3]. Up-dosing of second-generation H1 antihistamines (up to fourfold), as recommended by the urticaria guideline as second-line therapy, can improve response, but many patients remain symptomatic. The urticaria guideline recommends add-on omalizumab, cyclosporin A (CsA) or montelukast third line in patients with an inadequate response to high-dose H1 antihistamines [5]. In refractory patients, short courses of oral steroids may induce a remission in about 50% of cases [3]. Other approaches include intravenous immunoglobulin, rituximab, dapsone, and anticoagulants are also limited by paucity of data on their efficacy and adverse effect profile [3, 6].

According to guidelines prepared in accordance with data obtained mostly in adult studies, the primarily preferred drug in acute and chronic urticaria exacerbations in children is second-generation H1 antihistamines. Guidelines recommend that the dose should be increased three

http://dx.doi.org/10.5772/intechopen.68676

or fourfold in cases where response to H1 antihistamines treatment is not obtained at normal doses. If success of therapy cannot be achieved with H1 antihistamines used at the usual dose, high-dose H1 antihistamines is recommended. It has been reported that corticosteroids may be used short term (up to 10 days) in periods of urticaria exacerbations. However, guidelines also state that a definite recommendation cannot be made because there are insufficient randomized controlled studies in this area. The primary treatment option in long-term treatment of chronic urticaria is again second-generation nonsedative H1 antihistamines. However, the number of randomized controlled studies is substantially low for evidence-based recommendations in children. In patients who do not respond to high-dose H1 antihistaminic treatment, corticosteroid, omalizumab, cyclosporin A, and montelukast constitute tertiary treatment options. However, these drugs are recommended only in eligible patients because of the adverse effects and costs of these drugs [7].

It is clear that the current evidence-based treatment algorithm does not fit every urticaria patient. It is important that physicians do not just consult the algorithm but read the guideline line by line and employ an individualized approach for the care of each patient.

2.1. H1 antihistamines

Current international guidelines recommend a licensed dose of second- or third-generation (non-sedating) antihistamines for the treatment of all forms of urticaria as the first-line therapeutic option. Second-generation H1 antihistamines include fexofenadine, loratadine, and cetirizine. Third-generation antihistamines include desloratadine and levocetirizine. These medications should be taken continuously at the lowest necessary dose rather than on demand. This treatment with licensed doses of H1 antihistamines leads to an absence of symptoms in fewer than 50% of patients with CSU [5].

If CSU symptoms persist after 2 weeks of treatment with licensed doses of second-generation H1 antihistamines, it is recommended to increase the dose up to four times the licensed dose instead of combining different H1 antihistamines to obtain control as a second-line treatment. But there are only few controlled studies that have assessed the efficacy and safety of non-sedating antihistamines [5, 6]. This dose increase results in a higher degree of efficacy in some, but not all, patients, with up to one-third of patients remaining symptomatic [5].

First-generation H1 antihistamines (diphenhydramine and hydroxyzine) are lipophilic compounds which cross the blood-brain barrier and therefore sedating and anticholinergic side effects. They impair cognitive function, learning, and performance. First-generation H1 antihistamines have been advocated for use by the US guidelines as step two therapy at night and can be titrated up to higher doses as step three therapy if tolerated by the patient. Non-sedating second- and third-generation H1 antihistamines have lower propensity to cross the blood-brain barrier. Because of this, non-sedating H1 antihistamines are favored [6].

In studies mentioned above, higher-than-standard doses of antihistamines were not associated with an increase in adverse effects in most cases. Antihistamines also have anti-inflammatory effects in the treatment of urticaria when used at higher doses than licensed doses. Anti-inflammatory activity may result from the activation of genes responsible for the synthesis and/or synthesis of pro-inflammatory mediators [6].

2.2. H2 antihistamines

H2 antihistamines such as cimetidine and ranitidine are more typically used as add-on therapy in combination with H1 antihistamines and leukotriene receptor antagonists (LTRAs). A review of the Global Urticaria Forum's attendees' opinions suggested that although these agents are old and generally well tolerated by patients, they are unlikely to be used in clinical practice [8].

2.3. Leukotriene receptor antagonists

Cysteinyl leukotrienes are potent pro-inflammatory mediators, the effects of which can be blocked by LTRAs such as montelukast, zafirlukast, and pranlukast. LTRAs are recommended as add-on step two therapies by the US guidelines and in the third step in the Europe Union's (EU) guidelines. LTRAs have been found to significantly improve CU symptoms when used in conjunction with H1 antihistamines but are not as effective as H1 antihistamines when used as monotherapy. Combination therapy of antihistamines plus LTRAs may be more effective in patients with aspirin and nonsteroidal anti-inflammatory drug-exacerbated CSU. LTRAs appear to be well tolerated, with a good side-effect profile. Montelukast is not currently licensed for the treatment of CSU [1, 5, 9, 10].

2.4. Third-line treatments

If a patient's CSU symptoms persist after 1–4 weeks of second-line treatment, add-on omalizumab, CsA, or montelukast are recommended as third-line options. Both omalizumab and CsA are effective third-line CSU treatments; montelukast appears to have lower efficacy in this setting.

2.5. Omalizumab

Omalizumab, a humanized recombinant immunoglobin (Ig) G1 kappa monoclonal anti-IgE, is effective in antihistamine-unresponsive patients although optimal treatment duration needs to be defined [3]. Omalizumab is currently the only agent licensed for the third-line treatment of CSU [8]. The FDA approved the omalizumab for CU is 150 to 300 mg subcutaneously every 4 weeks. The clinical response starts after 1 week at the earliest, and the complete response can be prolonged up to 4–6 months. Studies found that complete control in approximately one-third of patients, partial control in another one-third, and one-third were unresponsive [1].

Omalizumab carries a label warning for anaphylaxis, although no cases of anaphylaxis were reported in the phase III trials of omalizumab in CSU. Other known risks associated with omalizumab include increased risks of cardiac and neurovascular events and a controversial increased risk of lymphoma. Omalizumab is generally well tolerated in patients with CSU and is rated as pregnancy category B [5, 1].

2.6. Cyclosporin A

Cyclosporin A (CsA) could be a suitable drug for the treatment of CSU as it directly inhibits mast cell degranulation as well as targeting T-cells. Similarly, CsA directly inhibits part of the basophil histamine release assay (BHRA) [5]. Response of autoreactive CSU to CsA has been associated with disappearance of autoantibodies and CsA may be disease-modifying in these patients [5]. A low-dose CsA treatment (3 mg/kg per day or less) has been shown to cause full remission of symptoms in a number of different randomized controlled trials and real-world studies [11–14].

CsA is also effective in the majority of antihistamine-resistant CSU patients, but its use is limited by potential side effects [3]. The most common adverse events associated with the use of CsA include hypertension, fatigue, gastrointestinal problems, and headache [15]. It is also thought that long-term use of CsA may be responsible for the development of non-melanoma skin cancer [16]. In patients receiving CsA therapy, monitoring of blood pressure and renal function is particularly important [13]. CsA is not currently licensed for the treatment of CSU and should be preferred only as a short-term treatment option [5].

Cyclosporin has been reported to be effective in some studies of CSU, including three double-blind [12–18], and one study reported that 40% of patients achieved complete remission in 9 months [18].

2.7. Other treatment options

Other possible options for the treatment of CSU are anti-inflammatory medications (hydroxychloroquine, dapsone, sulfasalazine, and colchicine) and immunosuppressants (mycophenolate, tacrolimus, azathioprine, and methotrexate) supported by low levels of evidence as defined by the Grading of Recommendations Assessment, Development, and Evaluation (GRADE) system (**Table 1**).

Drug	Quality of evidence	Strength of recommendation
H2 antihistamines	Moderate	Weak (+)
Oral corticosteroids (short course)	Low	Weak (+)
Oral corticosteroids	Very low	Strong (−)
Anti-inflammatory agents (dapsone, sulfasalazine, hydroxychloroquine, colchines, mycophenolate mofetil)	Low–very low	Weak (+)
Immunosuppressive agents	Very low	Weak (+)
Methotrexate		
Cyclophosphamide		
Intravenous Ig	Low	Weak (+)

(+) recommendation for medication, (−) recommendation against medication, and Ig: immunoglobulin

Table 1. Quality of evidence and strength of recommendation for use of intervention in CSU based on the GRADE system.

2.8. Dapsone

In the current international urticaria guideline, the use of dapsone and its effectivity is still unclear. However, in a double-blind, placebo-controlled study, dapsone has been reported as a promising agent in patients with CSU unresponsive to antihistamines [19]. Supportive evidence is needed to recommend the use of dapsone in urticaria patients [8].

2.9. Azathioprine

Additional new therapies such as azathioprine are under investigation for use in urticaria, although the evidence supporting their use is currently limited and not robust enough to warrant a change in current guidance [8].

2.10. Corticosteroids

Oral corticosteroids are commonly used in management of acute urticaria, and prednisone has been shown to significantly improve control of symptoms compared to antihistamines alone. Short courses (10 days–3 weeks) of corticosteroids may be used at any time if disease exacerbations are required in CU [5, 1].

3. Management of angioedema

Although both urticaria and allergic angioedema are associated with mast cell activation, there are many differences between them. While urticaria affects the skin, angioedema usually affects the mucosal tissue as well. In addition, middle and papillary dermis are involved in urticaria, whereas reticular dermis and submucosal tissues are involved in angioedema. Angioedema usually resolves in less than 24–48 h, disappear without aftereffects and are more painful than itchy [20, 2, 1].

Most cases of angioedema are attributable to the histamine and bradykinin. Histamine-mediated (allergic) angioedema occurs through a type I hypersensitivity reaction, whereas bradykinin-mediated (non-allergic) angioedema is iatrogenic or hereditary in origin. Bradykinin-mediated angioedema is divided into three distinct types: hereditary angioedema (HAE), angiotensin-converting enzyme inhibitor (ACEI)-induced angioedema, and acquired angioedema (AAE) [20] (**Table 2**). Although their clinical presentations bear similarities, the treatment algorithm differs significantly from each other. Corticosteroids and epinephrine are effective only in the management of histamine-mediated angioedema [20].

Priority of the treatment of angioedema is to provide airway protection. Intramuscular epinephrine may be required in the presence of acute laryngeal edema or anaphylaxis. It is administered in adult patients at doses of 1:1000 mg 0.2–0.5 mg and in children at doses of 0.01 mg/kg (up to 0.03 mg). These doses may be repeated at intervals of 5–15 min and if necessary with monitoring [20].

Angioedema type	Clinical and diagnostic features
Histamine mediated	
Allergic angioedema	Angioedema is usually accompanied by urticaria and sometimes anaphylaxis, may be pruritic, and is associated with exposure to allergens; attacks last for 24–48 h; it is responsive to antihistamines and corticosteroids
Angioedema with urticarial vasculitis	Angioedema may accompanied by urticaria; there may be petechiae or purpura after swelling resolves; symptoms of underlying vasculitis
Bradykinin mediated	
Hereditary angioedema types I and II	Recurrent attacks without urticaria; erythema marginatum is a cardinal finding; onset of the disease in childhood or young adulthood, worsens at puberty; family history in 75% of patients; attacks unresponsive to antihistamines or corticosteroids
Hereditary angioedema type III	Associated with mutations in factor XII, more common in women, may be estrogen dependent, typical onset after childhood, face and tongue extremity involvement is more frequent than abdominal, recurrent tongue swelling is a cardinal symptom, more disease-free intervals than in HAE types I and II, family history of angioedema, and attacks are unresponsive to antihistamines or corticosteroids
Acquired angioedema	Attacks are similar to HEA, onset in middle age or later, no family history, attacks unresponsive to antihistamines or corticosteroids
ACE inhibitor-induced angioedema	History of ACE inhibitor use, no urticaria, face and tongue are the most frequent sites, more common in blacks and smokers, patients usually can tolerate ARBs
Not mediated by histamine or bradykinin	
Idiopathic angioedema	Angioedema sometimes accompanied by urticaria, swelling may persist for up to 48 h, attacks may occur daily, patients are responsive to antihistamines or corticosteroids
Pseudoallergic angioedema	Urticaria is typically present, usually a class-specific reaction thought to be mediated by cysteinyl-leukotriens and includes NSAİD-induced angioedema, which occurs because of cyclooxygenase inhibition and subsequent release of cysteinyl-leukotriens

ACE, angiotensin-converting enzyme; ARB, angiotensin receptor blocker; NSAID, nonsteroidal anti-inflammatory drug.

Table 2. Clinical and diagnostic features of various types of angioedema.

3.1. Hereditary angioedema

Hereditary angioedema (HEA) is a rare, autosomal dominant disorder characterized by a quantitative (type I) or qualitative (type II) deficiency of C1 esterase inhibitor (C1-INH) protein. HAE with normal C1-INH (type III) occurs because of one of two known mutations in the gene for factor XII [20].

3.2. C1-INH replacement therapy

C1-INH replacement therapy maintains a central role for the treatment of angioedema attacks in patients with HAE. Berinert is a purified, pasteurized, and lyophilized form of C1-INH concentrate which is derived from human plasma. It was approved by the US FDA in 2009 for the treatment of acute abdominal, facial, and, more recently, laryngeal attacks of HAE in adult and adolescent patients [20]. It is approved in the European Union and the USA for adults and adolescents (≥13 years of age) for the treatment of acute angioedema attacks in patients with HEA due to C1-INH deficiency [21] (**Table 3**).

3.3. Plasma kallikrein inhibitor

Ecallantide (Kalbitor) received FDA approval in 2009 for use in the treatment of acute exacerbations of HEA in people aged 16 years and more. However, the EU rendered a negative opinion regarding its approval. Ecallantide can be used against attacks of HAE at any anatomical location, including abdominal/gastrointestinal, laryngeal, and peripheral attacks [22] (**Table 3**).

3.4. Bradykinin receptor antagonist

Icatibant (Firazyr) is a highly selective competitive bradykinin β2 receptor antagonist, and it is available as 30 mg in 3-ml solution as a ready-to-use syringe for immediate subcutaneous injection in an HAE attack [20] (**Table 3**).

Therapy and indication	Dosage	Monitoring tests
C1 esterase inhibitor [human] (Berinert; CSL Behring)	20U/kg body weight IV at a rate of 4 ml/min	Monitor patients with known risk factors for thrombotic events
Indicated for the treatment of acute abdominal or facial attacks of HEA in adult and adolescent patients		Epinephrine should be immediately available to treat any acute severe hypersensitivity reactions following discontinuation of administration
Plasma kallikrein inhibitor (kalbitor [ecallantide]; Dyax Corb)	30 mg (3 ml) SC in three 10-mg (1 ml) injections	Given the similarity in hypersensitivity symptoms and acute HAE symptoms, monitor patients closely for hypersensitivity reactions
Indicated for attacks at all anatomic sites	If attack persists, additional dose of 30 mg (3 ml) may be administered within a 24-h period	Administer in a setting equipped to manage anaphylaxis and HEA
Fresh frozen plasma	2U at 1–12 h before the event (only for use when C1-INH concentrate is not available)	Baseline, liver function test, hepatitis virology
Bradykinin β2 receptor antagonist	30 mg (3 ml) injected SC in the abdominal area.	For patients who never received Firazyr previously, the first treatment should be given in a medical institution or under the guidance of a physician
(Fizary [Icatıbant] Shire Orphan Therapies)	If attack persists, additional injections of 30 mg (3 ml) may be administered at intervals of ≥ 6h	
Indicated for attacks at all anatomic sites	No more than 3 injections in 24 h	

C1-INH, C1 esterase inhibitor; IV, ıntravenously; SC, subcutaneously.

Table 3. Treatment options of hereditary angioedema.

3.5. ACE inhibitor-induced angioedema

ACEI-induced angioedema is due to excessive accumulation of bradykinin. ACEI-induced angioedema is most commonly present with swelling of face, lips, tongue, and larynx and rarely involves visceral organs. Urticaria and itching are notably absent. Life-threatening edema of the upper airway is present in 25–39% of cases of ACEI-induced angioedema. Although ACEI-induced angioedema most commonly occurs shortly after treatment is initiated, it can develop long after treatment has started [20]. The nonallergic nature of the reaction renders traditional therapies (corticosteroids and antihistamines) as ineffective. Fresh frozen plasma, C1 inhibitor, and icatibant appear to be safe and effective therapeutic options for the management of ACEI-induced angioedema [22].

4. Management of anaphylaxis

Anaphylactic findings may include diffuse urticarial plaques, angioedema, gastrointestinal symptoms, and hypotension. In severe forms of anaphylaxis, loss of consciousness due to vascular collapse may develop. Pulmonary symptoms such as hyperinflation, peribronchial obstruction, and submucosal edema are frequently observed during anaphylaxis [20].

Elevation of lower extremities and placing in a supine position of the patient (semi-reclining if dyspneic or vomiting) are recommended [23]. An important component of acute management of anaphylaxis is volume expansion. The largest catheter possible should be placed on the largest peripheral vessel, and the rate should be titrated according to pulse and blood pressure. Adults are infused with 1–2 L iv of normal saline (5–10 mL/kg in the first 5 min) and 30 mL/kg iv in the first h in children. Antihistamines act slower than epinephrine and should not be administered alone in the treatment of anaphylaxis or acute allergic angioedema. The combined use of H1 and H2 blockers is more effective than the H1 antihistamines alone. Diphenhydramine should be administered to 25–50 mg iv in adults and 1 mg/kg iv (up to 50 mg) in children. Similar oral doses may be sufficient for mild episodes. Ranitidine should be infused 1 mg/kg iv in adults, 12.5–50 mg, iv for 10 min, in children. Inhaled β2 agonists are useful when bronchospasm is resistant to epinephrine injection alone. Systemic corticosteroids are not sufficient to prevent anaphylaxis. Although the use of parenteral corticosteroids (iv methylprednisolone) provides a benefit in histamine-mediated angioedema, the therapeutic effect is not immediate [20]. Epinephrine is the first choice as recommended in all guidelines. It is recommended to inject from an autoinjector IM in the mid-outher of the thigh. The first-aid dose of epinephrine is 0.01 mg/kg of a 1 mg/mL (1:1000) dilution to a maximum dose of 0.5 mg in an adult or 0.3 mg in a child. This dose can be repeated every 5–15 min as needed [24]. Intravenous epinephrine (0.1 mg in 100 mL saline, 1:100.000 solution, initially at a rate of 30–100 mL/h) may be administered in cases that do not respond to recurrent epinephrine injection and fluid therapy. Hemodynamic monitoring is recommended during intravenous epinephrine therapy [23].

Author details

Emel Erdal Çalıkoğlu[1], Didem Mullaaziz[1]* and Asli Kaptanoğlu[2]

*Address all correspondence to: didem_mullaaziz@yahoo.com

1 Department of Dermatology and Venereology, Faculty of Medicine, Near East University, Nicosia, Cyprus

2 Department of Dermatology and Venereology, Faculty of Medicine, Marmara University, İstanbul, Turkey

References

[1] Fine LM, Bernstein JA. Guideline of chronic urticaria beyond. Allergy, Asthma & Immunology Research. 2016;**8**(5):396–403.

[2] Boccon-Gibod I, Bouillet L. Angioedema and urticaria. Annales de dermatologie et de vénéréologie. 2014;**141** Suppl 3:S586–595.

[3] Asero R, Pinter E, Marra AM, Tedeschi A, Cugno M, Marzano AV. Current challenges and controversies in the management of chronic spontaneous urticaria. Expert Review of Clinical Immunology. 2015;**11**(10):1073–1082.

[4] Wieder S, Maurer M, Lebwohl M. Treatment of severely recalcitrant chronic spontaneous urticaria: a discussion of relevant issues. American Journal of Clinical Dermatology. 2015;**16**(1):19–26.

[5] Vestergaard C, Toubi E, Maurer M, Triggiani M, Ballmer-Weber B, Marsland A, Ferrer M, Knulst A, Giménez-Arnau A. Treatment of chronic spontaneous urticaria with an inadequate response to H1-antihistamines: an expertopinion. European Journal of Dermatology.2017; **27**(1):10–19.

[6] Godse K, Bhattar P, Patil S, Nadkarni N, Gautam M. Updosing of nonsedating anti-histamines in recalcitrant chronic urticaria. Indian Journal of Dermatology. 2016;**61**(3):273–278.

[7] Uysal P, Avcil S, Erge D. High-dose anti-histamine use and risk factors in children with urticaria. Turk Pediatri Arsivi. 2016;**51**(4):198–203.

[8] Staubach P, Zuberbier T, Vestergaard C, Siebenhaar F, Toubi E, Sussman G. Controversies and challenges in the management of chronic urticaria. Journal of the European Academy of Dermatology and Venereology. 2016;**30** Suppl 5:16–24.

[9] De Silva NL, Damayanthi H, Rajapakse AC, Rodrigo C, Rajapakse S. Leukotriene receptor antagonists for chronic urticaria: a systematic review. Allergy Asthma Clinical Immunology. 2014;**10**:24.

[10] Di Lorenzo G, D'Alcamo A, Rizzo M et al. Leukotriene receptor antagonists in monotherapy or in combination with antihistamines in the treatment of chronic urticaria: a systematic review. Journal of Asthma and Allergy. 2008;**2**:9–16.

[11] Toubi E, Blant A, Kessel A, Golan TD. Low-dose cyclosporin A in the treatment of severe chronic idiopathic urticaria. Allergy. 1997;**52**:312–316.

[12] Grattan CE, O'Donnell BF, Francis DM, et al. Randomized doubleblind study of cyclosporin in chronic 'idiopathic' urticaria. British Journal of Dermatology. 2000;**143**:365–372.

[13] Kessel A, Toubi E. Cyclosporine-A in severe chronic urticaria: the option for long-term therapy. Allergy. 2010;**65**:1478–1482.

[14] Vena GA, Cassano N, Colombo D, Peruzzi E, Pigatto P. Cyclosporine in chronic idiopathic urticaria: a double-blind, randomized, placebo-controlled trial. Journal of the American Academy of Dermatology. 2006;**55**:705–709.

[15] Savic S, Marsland A, McKay D et al. Retrospective case note review of chronic spontaneous urticaria outcomes and adverse effects in patients treated with omalizumab or cyclosporin in UK secondary care. Allergy, Asthma & Clinical Immunology. 2015;**11**:21.

[16] Kaplan AP. Treatment of chronic spontaneous urticaria. Allergy, Asthma & Immunology Research. 2012;**4**:326–331.

[17] Vena GA, Cassano N, Colombo D, Peruzzi E, Pigatto P. Cyclosporine in chronic idiopathic urticaria: a double-blind, randomized, placebo-controlled trial. Journal of the American Academy of Dermatology. 2006;**55**:705–709.

[18] Di Gioacchino M, Di Stefano F, Cavallucci E et al. Treatment of chronic idiopathic urticaria and positive autologous serum skin test with cyclosporine: clinical and immunological evaluation. Allergy, Asthma & Proceedings. 2003;**24**:285–290.

[19] Morgan M, Cooke A, Rogers L, Adams-Huet B, Khan DA. Double-blind placebo-controlled trial of dapsone in antihistamine refractory chronic idiopathic urticaria. Journal of Allergy and Clinical Immunology In Practice. 2014;**2**:601–606.

[20] Bernstein JA, Moellman J. Emerging concepts in the diagnosis and treatment of patients with undifferentiated angioedema. International Journal of Emergency Medicine. 2012;**5**:39.

[21] Riedl M. Recombinant human C1 esterase inhibitor in the management of hereditary angioedema. Clinical Drug Investigation. 2015;**35**(7):407–417.

[22] Scalese MJ, Reinaker TS. Pharmacologic management of angioedema induced by angiotensin-converting enzyme inhibitors. American Journal of Health-System Pharmacy. 2016;**73**(12):873–879.

[23] Dhami S, Panesar SS, Roberts G, Muraro A, Worm M, Bilò MB, Cardona V, Dubois AE, DunnGalvin A, Eigenmann P, Fernandez-Rivas M, Halken S, Lack G, Niggemann B, Rueff F, Santos AF, Vlieg-Boerstra B, Zolkipli ZQ, Sheikh A, EAACI Food Allergy and Anaphylaxis Guidelines Group. Management of anaphylaxis: a systematic review. Allergy. 2014;**69**(2):168–175.

[24] Simons FE. Anaphylaxis. Journal of Allergy and Clinical Immunology. 2010;**125**(2 Suppl 2):S161–181.

Chapter 9

Anti IgE Therapy in Chronic Urticaria

Ragıp Ertaş

Additional information is available at the end of the chapter

http://dx.doi.org/10.5772/68015

Abstract

The crucial position of IgE within the pathogenesis of allergic diseases made it a key target for therapy. The inhibition of the allergic inflammatory cascade by anti-immunoglobulin E (IgE) therapy is a new and promising concept in the treatment of these diseases. Currently available anti-IgE agent omalizumab has been started to be used in past 3 years in the cases of chronic spontaneous urticaria (CSU) and chronic inducible urticaria (CINDU), resistant to the first-, second-, and some third-line treatments. The use of omalizumab as an effective and safe biological therapy for inadequately controlled severe, persistent patients with CSU and CINDU provided a valuable new treatment option for these patients. However, the data about possible mechanisms of anti-IgE therapy in these patients, treatment strategies and dose regimens of anti-IgE therapy are different, and special patient groups and possible side effects are still insufficient. Also, studies about possible future anti-IgE treatment options are ongoing in CSU.

Keywords: chronic urticaria, anti-IgE therapy, omalizumab, management, new anti-IgE agents

1. Introduction

Chronic spontaneous urticaria (CSU) is defined as the spontaneous occurrence of itchy wheals, angioedema, or both for more than 6 weeks [1, 2]. More than 5 million people only in Europe suffer from CSU, especially its negative effects are on quality of life and sleep, school and work performance and daily life activities, and social relationships [3]. Recently, inside the EAACI/GA(2) LEN/EDF/WAO Guideline, it has been endorsed that nonsedating H1 antihistamines ought to be used for the first-line treatment of CSU and doses of H1 antihistamines can be increased by four-fold as the second-line treatment till symptoms can be kept under control completely [1, 4]. When these increased doses of H1 antihistamines fail, one of the recommended therapies as the third-line treatment is omalizumab. It is the only available agent of anti-immunoglobulin E (IgE) at the current time [3, 4].

2. Role of IgE in CSU

IgE has an important role in the pathogenesis of many allergic disorders including asthma, allergic rhinitis, latex allergy, hyper-IgE syndrome, chronic rhinosinusitis, atopic dermatitis, food allergy, drug allergy, and CSU. However, the role of IgE levels has different mechanisms in pathogenesis and diagnosis of the leading allergic disorders. In support of this, IgE levels are not correlated with CSU severity [5].

Measurements of total IgE levels during anti-IgE therapy with conventional methods show increases by nearly 3- to 11-fold [6]. The increase in monthly IgE levels is explained by the fact that total IgE measured during therapy is made up of free IgE and IgE binds free IgE and forms a complex and that, daily IgE production continues [3]. This is explained in the literature that commercial kits used to determine IgE levels measure both free IgE and IgE-anti-IgE complex together [3, 7]. Therefore, it is recommended that total IgE should not be used for measurement of free IgE during omalizumab treatment [8].

It is known that immunocomplexes do not cause tissue damage or complement fixation. In addition, it is proposed that accumulation of immunocomplexes in the extravascular space (mucosal epithelial lining) and the inability of anti-IgE forming a complex with IgE to go back to capillary space creates a local space, protective against allergens [7].

The role of IgE measurements in planning treatment for chronic urticaria and adjustment of the dose of omalizumab is not clear yet [9]. A recent study has shown that basal IgE levels do not play a role in responses to treatment [3].

Serum total IgE levels are regulated by several factors in the absence of anti-IgE therapy. It is known that the baseline IgE can predict the clearance and rate of production of IgE [10], and baseline IgE levels have a greater dependence on IgE production than IgE clearance [11]. Thus, in patients with high IgE levels and high IgE production, separately omalizumab, relevant IgE levels will come back after omalizumab loses its action as compared to patients with low IgE production and low IgE levels [6, 12]. Also, it was shown that, during the therapy, decrease in the serum concentration of free IgE is negatively correlated to the baseline IgE [6].

On the other hand, Lowe postulated that longer administration of omalizumab (1 year) decrease 56% of the IgE production [13]. Further studies with longer omalizumab administration may be highlighted in this topic.

The clearance of IgE is dependent on serum levels itself [10]. The half-life of serum free IgE is short (1 day) and changes in half-life of IgE are probably not very common and more likely an insignificant effect on regulation of IgE levels [14].

In a study, a different anti-IgE antibody (CGP 51901) was assessed in patients with another allergic disease rather than CSU. The half-life of the drug was negatively correlated to the free baseline IgE levels. Also, the time for free IgE to return to baseline after anti-IgE treatment was negatively correlated with baseline IgE levels [15]. This issue may be summarized as higher IgE levels predict shorter half-life of anti-IgE antibody. However, the overall results from the studies are difficult to interpret in terms of their relevance because the administration of anti-IgE was different, the observation period was different, and many other aspects of the subjects and the protocols were different. Also, Casale showed that serum concentration of free IgE is correlated to administrated doses of omalizumab. It was claimed that high doses administration of omalizumab, decreases the free IgE to the most stable levels [6].

3. Omalizumab therapy in CSU

It has been known since 2005 that omalizumab, a humanized immunoglobulin G1 (IgG1) monoclonal antibody which binds IgE, is well tolerated by patients with severe atopic asthma [16]. In 2014, as a first anti-IgE agent, omalizumab's marketing authorization for CSU was approved first by European Medicines Agency and then by Food and Drug Administration [17].

Before 2014, there were few case reports on effects of omalizumab used; although not indicated in patients with chronic urticaria, few studies on patients' experiences with omalizumab and omalizumab phase studies in larger groups of patients; however, there is still a limited number of studies on the use of omalizumab for the treatment of CSU in a real life context [4].

The characterization of the response to omalizumab treatment has been previously reported both in the controlled trials and in the case series [3, 4, 18]. But it is still unclear about the long-term management of anti-IgE therapy and possible side effects for the clinician. And, it is also unclear that when will patients show relapse after discontinuation of omalizumab treatment. Omalizumab discontinuation must be taken into consideration every 3–6 months [3, 19]. Patients who have relapsed after discontinuation of omalizumab, the reinitiation of omalizumab therapy is primarily based on modifications in medical factors and doctor's discretion [20]. Metz et al. have reported that, in the case of possible retreatment, resistance to omalizumab does not develop readily in most patients with CSU [20, 21].

It is not often found that an external trigger or any factors that can initiate the symptoms of CSU patients. Most patients with CSU have an autoimmune cause; therefore, autoimmunity can be considered firstly [22]. Some patients produce IgE autoantibodies (against thyroperoxidase or double-stranded DNA) and IgG autoantibodies (against FcεRI and/or IgE), which lead to activate mast cells and basophils. Current reports have demonstrated that IgE, by means of binding to FcεRI on mast cells without FcεRI cross-linking, can boost the proliferation and survival of mast cells [23, 24]. Also, IgE and FcεRI engagement can also lower the release of mast cells and cause high sensitivity to various stimuli through both FcεRI and other receptors. Eventually, in a case of stimuli, this process can give rise to degranulation of mast cells [23]. It is known that anti-IgE therapy shows its effect on urticaria through lowering unfastened IgE levels and mast and basophil cell activations. It also downregulates an IgE receptor FceR1 in the mast, basophil, and dendritic cells [23].

Finally, there are three different mechanisms of omalizumab in patients with CSU [22, 23];

i. Omalizumab sequesters monomeric IgE to lessen its priming effect on mast cells;

ii. In CSU patients with IgG autoantibodies in opposition to IgE or FcεRI, the depletion of mast cell IgE with the aid of omalizumab and the following downregulation of FcεRI on mast cells and basophils might lead to their reduced state of hyperexcitability;

iii. In those sufferers with IgE autoantibodies against autoallergens, the inhibition of IgE binding to FcεRI via omalizumab and the downregulation of FcεRI would represent a significant mechanism of omalizumab.

However, it is quite difficult to explain the mode of action of omalizumab based on elimination of IgE and the other three mechanisms. It is clear that further studies are needed to elucidate its mode of action in CSU.

3.1. The usage of omalizumab in chronic inducible urticaria (CINDU)

Chronic urticaria can also be spontaneous and/or inducible, though the triggers of inducible urticaria [25]. CINDU emerges when triggered by physical stimuli including scratch, cold, heat, pressure, friction, exercise, sun exposure, water exposure, and exercise [19]. The term CINDU includes cold urticaria, delayed pressure urticaria, heat urticaria, solar urticaria, symptomatic dermographism, vibratory angioedema, aquagenic urticaria, cholinergic urticaria, and contact urticaria [19, 25].

The suggested dosing and indications of therapy are not different from that used for CSU in the patients with CINDU. It is either 150 or 300 mg/4 weeks given subcutaneously [3]. Even though, there are many large studies currently underway for CINDU [25], there are individual cases and smaller studies assessing the efficacy of omalizumab in various types of CINDU, while the number of overall cases is low. The results of these studies have shown that efficacy of omalizumab treatment is similar in CSU and CINDU patients [3, 9, 20, 21]. All recent studies and case reports have shown notable and optimistic outcome results in patients with CINDU [9].

3.2. The selection of patients and indications of omalizumab therapy

CSU patients who are planning to use omalizumab should meet the following conditions [1, 3, 19]:

1. Patients who are older than 12 years of age.
2. Patients who are underneath expert care (dermatologists and/or immunologists).
3. Cause of urticaria is not identifiable with the aid of further investigations and CBC, ANA, and urine analysis outcomes are not abnormal.
4. Patients are recognized with the aid of professionals as moderate to severe CSU that is not responsive to standard treatment.

5. Disease period is longer than 3 months and the symptoms stay persistent notwithstanding using guideline primarily-based treatment.

3.3. Dose regimens and assessment of patients

The preliminary and continuation dosing is not similar to that used for asthma. Doses of omalizumab for asthma are adjusted based on weight and serum IgE levels [7]. The role of basal IgE levels in planning treatment for CSU and adjusting doses of omalizumab are not yet clear [26, 27]. Metz et al. have noted that basal IgE levels do not play a part in response to treatment [3]. Also in CSU patients, omalizumab is given 300 mg or 150 mg (sc) every 4 weeks and is not decided with the baseline serum IgE levels or patient's weight [1].

Two doses of omalizumab (150 mg or 300 mg/4 weeks) have been accepted by the USA Food and Drug Administration (FDA) for CSU refractory to H1 antihistamines. Uysal et al. introduced an algorithm for defining dose, dose interval, and clinical response in CSU patients. Due to this set of rules, it is affordable to start omalizumab with a dose of 300 mg every 4 weeks, and if the patient is good enough, taper to a lower dose (e.g., 150 mg every 4 weeks), or much less frequent injections (every 6 weeks) [27] (**Figure 1**). However, in a current meta-analysis, wherein seven randomized, placebo-controlled studies determined substantial proof

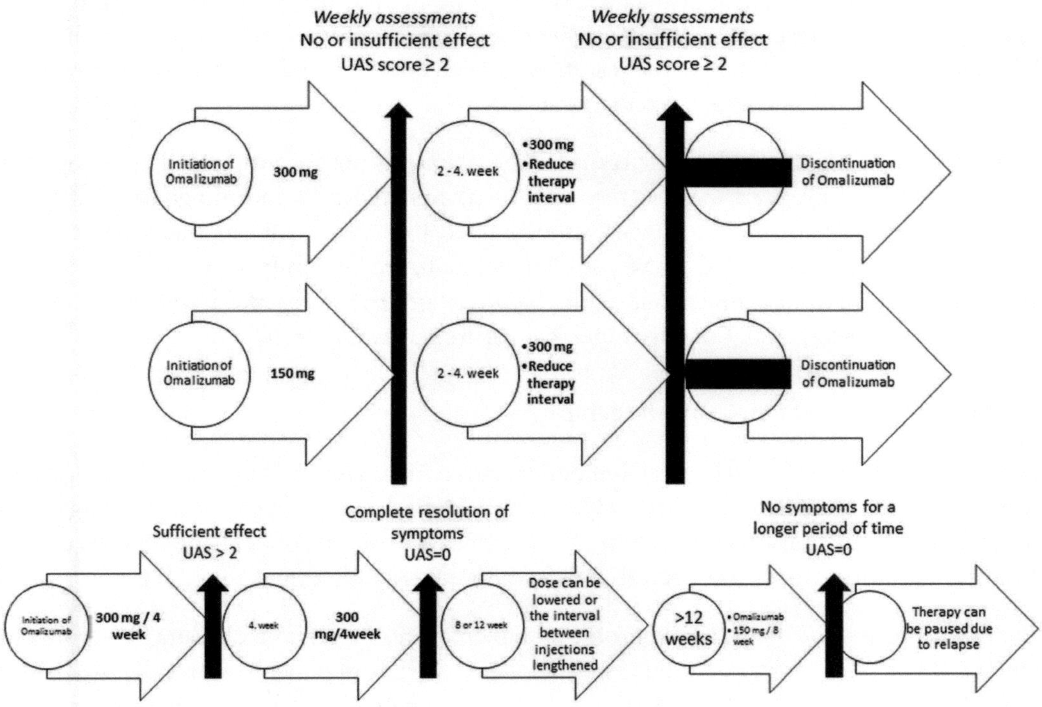

Figure 1. A practical individualization of omalizumab doses during the therapy.

for the efficacy and safety of omalizumab in patients with CSU and to treat patients with CSU with 300 mg of omalizumab for 4 weeks [18].

3.4. Omalizumab therapy in special populations

Current guidelines of CSU consist of tips for special populations, especially children, the elderly, and pregnant or lactating women [1]. They suggest the similar management and treatment algorithms as adults but pay attention to factors such as age, dosage, and availability of toddler-pleasant approaches [1].

3.5. Omalizumab therapy in children and elderly patients

Omalizumab is available as a third-line treatment for CSU in adolescent sufferers (≥12 years) with an insufficient response to antihistamine therapy, and is likewise approved for kids aged ≥6 years with severe persistent allergic asthma [27]. Its efficacy and safety profile have been also shown in a case study in patients with CU aged <12 years [28]. There are no safety warnings about omalizumab in the geriatric population [29].

3.6. Omalizumab therapy in pregnant and lactating women

There are limited posted records at the safety of omalizumab in pregnant women with CSU [30], despite the fact that available data about anti-IgE therapy are reassuring with other diseases; however, the research in asthma patients showed no obvious increase or major anomalies have been observed [31, 32]. The results have been now not distinct from those in women receiving placebo and other asthma therapies [33, 34].

The initiation of omalizumab in the course of pregnancy is not recommended, although if a woman turns into pregnant even as receiving omalizumab, it's far recommended that treatment can persevere if the advantages are estimated to outweigh the possible harms [34]. Immunoglobulin G molecules, along with omalizumab, are known to pass the placenta. IgG is also excreted in human milk, so it would be predicted that a breastfeeding baby might be uncovered to omalizumab. Data in human beings are not available [34].

3.7. Adverse effects of omalizumab therapy

The most common unfavorable reaction derived from omalizumab is injection site reactions, including induration, itching, pain, and bruising. The package insert contains warnings concerning about parasitic infections. While there are not any reports of fatal anaphylaxis due to omalizumab, a few cases have been serious and doubtlessly life-threatening [17].

Available information on the safety profile and tolerability of omalizumab therapy in patients with CSU has been mainly derived from the phase III trials in patients with CSU. ASTERIA I, ASTERIA II, and GLACIAL trials showed a good tolerability profile, which was similar to those with placebo and without any anaphylactic reactions [4, 5, 35].

Limb et al. evaluated anaphylaxis and angioedema profiles of patients with asthma receiving omalizumab [36]. Polysorbate, a part of the drug used to increase its solubility, is very likely to be responsible for adverse reactions [36, 37]. In a report on two cases of atopic asthma on the long-term omalizumab therapy, the intradermal test showed that anaphylaxis is developed due to omalizumab [38]. Anaphylaxis due to omalizumab can be diagnosed; there should be at least two of the following symptoms: angioedema in the throat or in the tongue, bronchospasm, hypotension, syncope, and/or urticaria [39].

In a study performed by omalizumab joint task force (OJTF) in 2006, 0.09% of the asthmatic patients administered omalizumab had anaphylaxis. They reported that anaphylaxis due to omalizumab developed within 2 h of the administration, and after three injections of the drug in most of the patients (78%). Based on this finding, they recommended that patients should be monitored in the clinic for 2 h after the first three injections of omalizumab administration and for 30 min after the following injections [37].

Due to exacerbation of urticaria or angioedema normally appearing in the course of the CSU, the diagnosis of an adverse reaction can be overlooked. Therefore, possibilities of an adverse reaction, lack of a response to omalizumab, and exacerbations due to discontinuation of other medications should be kept in mind because a decision about whether the treatment is effective and should be continued has to be made.

In addition, since delayed adverse reactions due to omalizumab can appear, patients may think that these reactions are independent of the drug. They may not tell their doctors about them due to clinical benefits they receive from their treatment. Therefore, it is necessary that patients should be informed about possible adverse reactions before treatment and observed for a long time after treatment.

According to data we collected in the dermatology clinic in Education and Research Hospital, from 2014 to 2016, about 100 patients diagnosed as CSU were treated with omalizumab. One of these patients, after a long period of time without angioedema, had the first angioedema attack on the tongue within 30 min of omalizumab administration. The reaction appearing was regarded as an adverse effect or flare-up of urticaria. One patient had urticarial exacerbation and angioedema; hypotension, 30 min after the first omalizumab administration, and lack of any other symptoms were proposed to be a nonspecific adverse reaction. Exacerbation of urticaria and angioedema occurring after the second administration in the same patient were indicative of an adverse reaction. One patient had urticarial exacerbation; late-onset urticaria exacerbation after the first dose in was thought to be a delayed adverse reaction due to omalizumab or exacerbation of the disease because the previous cyclosporine therapy was discontinued [17]. Except those, two patients had localized urticarial plaque on the site of omalizumab application. One patient had a mild and one had a moderate headache, three patients had acneiform eruption and two patients had widespread foot pain and myalgia, which can be considered as the flu-like syndrome. One patient had dizziness. Omalizumab changed into discontinued within the patients experiencing urticarial exacerbation and/or angioedema, but the treatment became persevered within the patients located to have other adverse reactions and necessary precautions toward the side effects had been taken.

4. Newly introduced anti-IgE therapies

As a third-line therapy in patients with CSU, omalizumab is an effective and safe biological therapy option for both antihistamine-resistant CSU patients and physicians dealing with CSU [40]. However, there are nonetheless many patients who do not tolerate or benefit from existing and the other third-line therapies including omalizumab [41].

MEDI-4212, ligelizumab (QGE031), and mAbs targeting the extracellular segment (M1′) of membrane IgE: quilizumab is a new anti-IgE reagents that is currently undergoing phase II trial testings [42, 43].

4.1. Ligelizumab (QGE031)

Ligelizumab is a completely humanized IgG1 monoclonal antibody directed in opposition to human IgE that binds with excessive affinity to the Cε3 area of IgE. It also binds to Cε3 area of IgE with much more affinity than omalizumab [41]. Compared to omalizumab, ligelizumab suggests sixfold to ninefold more suppression of allergen-induced skin prick exams *in vivo*. It also affords more and longer suppression of free IgE and IgE on the surface of circulating basophils compared to omalizumab [44].

Current findings suggest that ligelizumab can be more potent than omalizumab within the treatment of CSU. The advent of an even stronger anti-IgE mAb-ligelizumab is developing; in addition, possibilities for anti-IgE therapy to improve the symptoms and life quality of patients with chronic urticaria [40, 41].

4.2. Quilizumab

Quilizumab is a humanized monoclonal antibody that targets the M1 prime of membrane-expressed IgE on IgE-switched B cells and plasmablasts. Quilizumab is in the medical development for the remedy of allergic diseases. By inflicting the depletion of IgE-switched B cells and plasmablasts, it reduces serum IgE [45].

A currently achieved multicenter, double-blind observe with 32 CSU patients showed that there was no significant difference between quilizumab and placebo group in terms of decreases in disease scores [46]. But its longer period use in CSU patients or its combination with omalizumab may enhance treatment effects and lead to sustained responses. This has to be revealed in future studies [41].

These findings suggest that quilizumab may be an effective treatment of CSU. Quilizumab and ligelizumab are still under investigation in CSU [41].

Author details

Ragıp Ertaş

Address all correspondence to: ragipertas@yahoo.com

Kayseri Education and Research Hospital, Dermatology Clinic, Kayseri, Turkey

References

[1] Zuberbier T, Aberer W, Asero R, Bindslev-Jensen C, Brzoza Z, Canonica GW, et al. The EAACI/GA(2) LEN/EDF/WAO Guideline for the definition, classification, diagnosis, and management of urticaria: The 2013 revision and update. Allergy. 2014;**69**:868–887. doi: 10.1111/all.12313

[2] Colgecen E, Ozyurt K, Irfan Gul A, Utas S. Evaluation of etiological factors in patients with chronic urticaria. Acta Dermatovenerologica Croatica. 2015;**23**:36–42

[3] Metz M, Ohanyan T, Church MK, Maurer M. Omalizumab is an effective and rapidly acting therapy in difficult-to-treat chronic urticaria: A retrospective clinical analysis. Journal of Dermatological Science. 2014;**73**:57–62. doi: 10.1016/j.jdermsci.2013.08.011

[4] Kaplan A, Ledford D, Ashby M, Canvin J, Zazzali JL, Conner E, et al. Omalizumab in patients with symptomatic chronic idiopathic/spontaneous urticaria despite standard combination therapy. The Journal of Allergy and Clinical Immunology. 2013;**132**:101–109. doi: 10.1016/j.jaci.2013.05.013

[5] Maurer M, Rosén K, Hsieh HJ, Saini S, Grattan C, Gimenéz-Arnau A, et al. Omalizumab for the treatment of chronic idiopathic or spontaneous urticaria. The New England Journal of Medicine. 2013;**368**:924. doi: 10.1056/NEJMoa1215372

[6] Casale TB, Bernstein IL, Busse WW, LaForce CF, Tinkelman DG, Stoltz RR, et al. Use of an anti-IgE humanized monoclonal antibody in ragweed-induced allergic rhinitis. The Journal of Allergy and Clinical Immunology. 1997;**100**:110–121

[7] Miller CW, Krishnaswamy N, Johnston C, Krishnaswamy G. Severe asthma and the omalizumab option. Clinical and Molecular Allergy. 20 May 2008;**6**:4. doi: 10.1186/1476-7961-6-4

[8] Korn S, Haasler I, Fliedner F, Becher G, Strohner P, Staatz A, et al. Monitoring free serum IgE in severe asthma patients treated with omalizumab. Respiratory Medicine. 2012;**106**:1494–1500. doi: 10.1016/j.rmed.2012.07.010

[9] Saini S, Rosen KE, Hsieh HJ, Wong DA, Conner E, Kaplan A, et al. A randomized, placebo-controlled, dose-ranging study of single-dose omalizumab in patients with H1-antihistamine-refractory chronic idiopathic urticaria. The Journal of Allergy and Clinical Immunology. 2011;**128**:567–573.e1. doi: 10.1016/j.jaci.2011.06.010

[10] Hayashi N, Tsukamoto Y, Sallas WM, Lowe PJ. A mechanism-based binding model for the population pharmacokinetics and pharmacodynamics of omalizumab. British Journal of Clinical Pharmacology. 2007;**63**:548–561. doi: 10.1111/j.1365-2125.2006.02803.x

[11] Lowe PJ, Tannenbaum S, Gautier A, Jimenez P. Relationship between omalizumab pharmacokinetics, IgE pharmacodynamics and symptoms in patients with severe persistent allergic (IgE-mediated) asthma. British Journal of Clinical Pharmacology. 2009;**68**:61–76. doi: 10.1111/j.1365-2125.2009.03401.x

[12] Corren J, Shapiro G, Reimann J, Deniz Y, Wong D, Adelman D, et al. Allergen skin tests and free IgE levels during reduction and cessation of omalizumab therapy. The Journal of Allergy and Clinical Immunology. 2008;**121**:506–511. doi: 10.1016/j.jaci.2007.11.026

[13] Lowe PJ, Renard D. Omalizumab decreases IgE production in patients with allergic (IgE-mediated) asthma; PKPD analysis of a biomarker, total IgE. British Journal of Clinical Pharmacology. 2011;**72**:306–320. doi: 10.1111/j.1365-2125.2011.03962.x

[14] Fick RB Jr, Fox JA, Jardieu PM. Immunotherapy approach to allergic disease. Immunopharmacology. 2000;**48**:307–310

[15] Corne J, Djukanovic R, Thomas L, Warner J, Botta L, Grandordy B, et al. The effect of intravenous administration of a chimeric anti-IgE antibody on serum IgE levels in atopic subjects: Efficacy, safety, and pharmacokinetics. The Journal of Clinical Investigation. 1997;**99**:879–887. doi: 10.1172/JCI119252

[16] McKeage K. Omalizumab: A review of its use in patients with severe persistent allergic asthma. Drugs. 2013;**73**:1197–1212. doi: 10.1007/s40265-013-0085-4

[17] Ertaş R, Özyurt K, Yıldız S, Ulaş Y, Turasan A, Avcı A. Adverse reaction to omalizumab in patients with chronic urticaria: Flare up or ineffectiveness?. Iranian Journal of Allergy, Asthma and Immunology. 2016;**15**:82–86

[18] Zhao Z, Ji C, Yu W, Meng L, Hawro T, Wei JF, et al. Omalizumab for the treatment of chronic spontaneous urticaria: A meta-analysis of randomized clinical trials. The Journal of Allergy and Clinical Immunology. 2016;**137**:1742–1750. doi: 10.1016/j.jaci.2015.12.1342

[19] Kulthanan K, Tuchinda P, Chularojanamontri L, Chanyachailert P, Korkij W, Chunharas A, et al. Clinical practice guideline for diagnosis and management of urticaria. Asian Pacific Journal of Allergy and Immunology. 2016;**34**:190–200

[20] Metz M, Ohanyan T, Church MK, Maurer M. Retreatment with omalizumab results in rapid remission in chronic spontaneous and inducible urticaria. JAMA Dermatology. 2014;**150**:288–290. doi: 10.1001/jamadermatol.2013.8705

[21] Ghazanfar MN, Sand C, Thomsen SF. Effectiveness and safety of omalizumab inchronic spontaneous or inducible urticaria: Evaluation of 154 patients. The British Journal of Dermatology. 2016;**175**:404–406. doi: 10.1111/bjd.14540

[22] Yalcin AD. Advances in anti-IgE therapy. Biomed Research International. 2015;**2015**:317465. doi: 10.1155/2015/317465

[23] Chang TW, Chen C, Lin CJ, Metz M, Church MK, Maurer M. The potential pharmacologic mechanisms of omalizumab in patients with chronic spontaneous urticaria. Journal of Allergy and Clinical Immunology. 2015;**135**:337–342. doi: 10.1016/j.jaci.2014.04.036

[24] Saini SS, MacGlashan DW, Sterbinsky SA, Togias A, Adelman DC, Lichtenstein LM, et al. Down-regulation of human basophil IgE and FceR1 alpha surface densities and mediator release by anti-IgE infusions is reversible in vitro and in vivo. The Journal of Immunology. 1999;**162**:5624–5630

[25] Moolani Y, Lynde C, Sussman G. Advances in understanding and managing chronic urticaria. F1000Research. 2016;16:**5**. pii: F1000 Faculty Rev-177. doi: 10.12688/f1000research.7246.1

[26] Chicharro P, Rodríguez P, de Argila D. Omalizumab in the treatment of chronic inducible urticaria. Actas Dermo-sifiliograficas. 2016 Oct 5. pii: S0001-7310(16)30286-1. doi: 10.1016/j.ad.2016.07.018 [Epub ahead of print]

[27] Uysal P, Eller E, Mortz CG, Bindslev-Jensen C. An algorithm for treating chronic urticaria with omalizumab: Dose interval should be individualized. The Journal of Allergy and Clinical Immunology. 2014;**133**:914–915.e2. doi: 10.1016/j.jaci.2013.10.015

[28] Asero R, Casalone R, Iemoli E. Extraordinary response to omalizumab in a child with severe chronic urticaria. European Annals of Allergy and Clinical Immunology. 2014;**46**:41–42

[29] Maurer M, Church MK, Marsland AM, Sussman G, Siebenhaar F, Vestergaard C, et al. Questions and answers in chronic urticaria: Where do we stand and where do we go? Journal of the European Academy of Dermatology and Venereology. 2016;**30**(Suppl 5):7–15. doi: 10.1111/jdv.13695

[30] Kuprys-Lipinska I, Tworek D, Kuna P. Omalizumab in pregnant women treated due to severe asthma: Two case reports of good outcomes of pregnancies. Postepy Dermatologii i Alergologii. 2014;**31**:104–107. doi: 10.5114/pdia.2014.40975

[31] Hirashima J, Hojo M, Iikura M, Hiraishi Y, Nakamichi S, Sugiyama H, et al. A case of an asthma patient receiving omalizumab during pregnancy. Arerugi. 2012;**61**:1683–1687

[32] Namazy J, Cabana MD, Scheuerle AE, Thorp JM Jr, Chen H, Carrigan G, et al. The Xolair Pregnancy Registry (EXPECT): The safety of omalizumab use during pregnancy. The Journal of Allergy and Clinical Immunology. 2015;**135**:407–412. doi: 10.1016/j.jaci.2014.08.025

[33] Corren J, Casale TB, Lanier B, Buhl R, Holgate S, Jimenez P. Safety and tolerability of omalizumab. Clinical and Experimental Allergy. 2009;**39**:788–797. doi: 10.1111/j.1365-2222.2009.03214.x

[34] Grunewald S, Jank A. New systemic agents in dermatology with respect to fertility, pregnancy, and lactation. Journal der Deutschen Dermatologischen Gesellschaft. 2015;**13**:277. doi: 10.1111/ddg.12596

[35] Saini SS, Bindslev-Jensen C, Maurer M, Grob JJ, Bülbül Baskan E, Bradley MS, et al. Efficacy and safety of omalizumab in patients with chronic idiopathic/spontaneous urticaria who remain symptomatic on H1 antihistamines: A randomized, placebo-controlled study. Journal of Investigative Dermatology. 2015;**135**:925. doi: 10.1038/jid.2014.512

[36] Limb SL, Starke PR, Lee CE, Chowdhury BA. Delayed onset and protracted progression of anaphylaxis after omalizumab administration in patients with asthma. The Journal of Allergy and Clinical Immunology. 2007;**120**:1378–1381. doi: 10.1016/j.jaci.2007.09.022

[37] Cox L, Platts-Mills TA, Finegold I, Schwartz LB, Simons FE, Wallace DV; American Academy of Allergy, Asthma & Immunology; American College of Allergy, Asthma and Immunology. American Academy of Allergy, Asthma & Immunology/American College of Allergy, Asthma and Immunology Joint Task Force Report on omalizumab-associated anaphylaxis. The Journal of Allergy and Clinical Immunology. 2007;**120**:1373–1377. doi: 10.1016/j.jaci.2007.09.032

[38] Price KS, Hamilton RG. Anaphylactic reactions in two patients after omalizumab administration after successful long-term therapy. Allergy & Asthma Proceedings. 2007;**28**:313–319

[39] Kim HL, Leigh R, Becker A. Omalizumab: Practical considerations regarding the risk of anaphylaxis. Allergy, Asthma & Clinical Immunology. 2010;**6**:32. doi: 10.1186/1710-1492-6-32

[40] Giménez-Arnau AM. Omalizumab for treating chronic spontaneous urticaria: An expert review on efficacy and safety. Expert Opinion on Biological Therapy. 2017;**17**:375-385. doi:10.1080/14712598.2017.1285903

[41] Kocatürk E, Maurer M, Metz M, Grattan C. Looking forward to new targeted treatments for chronic spontaneous urticaria. Clinical & Translational Allergy. 2017;**7**:1. doi: 10.1186/s13601-016-0139-2

[42] Gauvreau GM, Harris JM, Boulet LP, Scheerens H, Fitzgerald JM, Putnam WS, et al. Targeting membrane-expressed IgE B cell receptor with an antibody to the M1 prime epitope reduces IgE production. Science Translational Medicine. 2014;**6**:243ra85. doi: 10.1126/scitranslmed.3008961

[43] Boyman O, Kaegi C, Akdis M, Bavbek S, Bossios A, Chatzipetrou A, et al. EAACI IG biologicals task force paper on the use of biologic agents in allergic disorders. Allergy. 2015;**70**:727–754. doi: 10.1111/all.12616

[44] Arm JP, Bottoli I, Skerjanec A, Floch D, Groenewegen A, et al. Pharmacokinetics, pharmacodynamics and safety of QGE031 (ligelizumab), a novel high-affinity anti-IgE antibody, in atopic subjects. Clinical and Experimental Allergy. 2014;**44**:1371–1385. doi: 10.1111/cea.12400

[45] Harris JM, Maciuca R, Bradley MS, Cabanski CR, Scheerens H, Lim J, et al. A randomized trial of the efficacy and safety of quilizumab in adults with inadequately controlled allergic asthma. Respiratory Research. 2016;**17**:29. doi:10.1186/s12931-016-0347-2

[46] Harris JM, Cabanski CR, Scheerens H, Samineni D, Bradley MS, Cochran C, et al. A randomized trial of quilizumab in adults with refractory chronic spontaneous urticaria. Journal of Allergy and Clinical Immunology. 2016;**138**:1730–1732. doi:10.1016/j.jaci.2016.06.023

Chapter 10

Urticarial Syndromes

Hilal Gokalp and Isil Bulur

Additional information is available at the end of the chapter

http://dx.doi.org/10.5772/67993

Abstract

Urticaria is a common dermatological condition that can occur in acute and chronic forms. Common urticaria is generally easy to diagnose; however, urticarial syndromes should be considered in cases where lesions persist for greater than 24–36 h, the location of lesions has bilateral symmetry, urticarial lesions are accompanied by additional elementary lesions, and/or the patient presents with additional systemic symptoms. Additionally, urticarial syndromes should be considered for patients with typical urticarial lesions that do not respond to systemic antihistamine treatment. Hyperpigmentation or bruising can be observed following resolution of urticarial syndromes. Many cutaneous and systemic diseases can cause urticarial syndromes. Systemic causes of urticarial syndromes can affect multiple organ systems and may be accompanied by systemic symptoms such as fever, asthenia, and arthralgia. Clinicopathologic correlation is essential for the accurate diagnosis of urticarial syndromes. In this chapter, cutaneous and systemic etiologies of urticarial syndromes are reviewed.

Keywords: urticaria, common urticaria, urticarial syndromes, cutaneous urticarial syndromes, systemic urticarial syndromes

1. Introduction

Urticaria is a disease with a lifetime prevalence of 25–30% and is characterized by itchy urticarial lesions and/or angioedema [1, 2]. Although its physiopathology is not well understood, cutaneous mast cells are the main causative factor that is responsible for the release of histamine and other mediators [3, 4]. The disease is divided into acute and chronic depending on whether the duration is less or more than 6 weeks. While acute urticaria is often limited and the cause can be determined in most patients, chronic urticaria is a long-term disease, and further investigation is required in terms of accompanying disorders or autoimmunity [5]. The diagnosis of common urticaria is usually made easily. However, some difficulties in terms of response to treatment, accompanying lesions, and systemic findings can be seen in some patients. Various disorders, both cutaneous and systemic, are included in the spectrum called urticarial syndrome (**Table 1**). In general, lesions lasting longer than 24–36 h, showing bilateral symmetric involvement, with elementary lesions other than urticaria and accompanying systemic symptoms should bring urticarial syndromes to mind. Clinicopathologic correlation is essential in the diagnosis of urticarial syndromes [1, 5]. Cutaneous and systemic disorders that may cause the urticarial syndrome will be reviewed in this section.

Cutaneous urticarial syndromes	**Systemic urticarial syndromes**
Urticarial dermatitis	Vasculitides
Contact dermatitis	• Urticarial vasculitis
Papular urticaria	• Other vasculitides
Mastocytosis	Immunologic disorders
Exanthematous drug eruption	• Connective tissue diseases
Autoimmune bullous disorders	• SLE, Sjogren syndrome, dermatomyositis
• Bullous pemphigoid	• Juvenile rheumatoid arthritis
• Gestational pemphigoid	Hematologic diseases
• Linear IgA dermatosis	• Waldenstrom macroglobulinemia
• Dermatitis herpetiformis	• Schnitzler syndrome
• Epidermolysis bullosa acquisita	• Hypereosinophilic syndromes
Pruritic urticarial papules and plaques of pregnancy	• Polycythemia vera
Rare cutaneous urticarial syndromes	• Non-Hodgkin lymphoma (B cell)
• Autoimmune progesterone/estrogen dermatitis	Autoinflammatory syndromes
• Wells syndrome	• Hereditary periodic fever syndromes
• Interstitial granulomatous dermatitis	• Cryopyrin-associated periodic syndromes
• Neutrophilic eccrine hidradenitis	• Other autoinflammatory syndromes
• Urticaria-like follicular mucinosis	

Table 1. Cutaneous and systemic urticarial syndromes.

2. Cutaneous urticarial syndromes

Various skin disorders can cause urticarial lesions and can be confused with common urticaria.

2.1. Urticarial dermatitis

Urticarial dermatitis is a clinical picture where urticarial plaques and edematous lesions are combined and is usually seen in the elderly. Urticarial dermatitis is quite itchy and often characterized by diffuse and symmetrical involvement of the body and proximal extremities. Facial and palmoplantar region involvement is usually not present. Existing lesions may persist for days or even weeks. Excoriations and lichenification due to the severe itching may be observed in time. It usually has a chronic relapsing course and spontaneous regression is very rare [5, 6]. Most pathologists describe urticarial dermatitis as a "dermal hypersensitivity reaction." Papillary dermal edema and minimal epidermal spongiosis with superficial perivascular lymphocytic and eosinophilic infiltration are seen on histopathologic examination [6, 7]. While the etiologic agents most commonly held responsible are drugs, detecting the triggering agent can sometimes be difficult [6]. Low to moderate doses of systemic steroids can provide relief in patients' resistant to topical steroids and systemic antihistamines [5, 8].

2.2. Contact dermatitis

Contact dermatitis (CD) develops after contact with allergic and/or irritant agents and is fairly common. The sensitizers that most commonly cause allergic CD are poison ivy, nickel, formaldehyde, and fragrances that are included in many cosmetics. Irritant CD is also called nonimmunologic contact dermatitis and is most commonly due to fragrances, flavoring agents, and preservatives [9–11]. While CD usually causes itchy eczematous lesions, urticarial lesions may rarely be seen due to dermal edema. The border between CD and contact urticaria is not clear. Dermal edema is seen more commonly in contact urticaria, and this is accepted as the most important difference with CD. Histopathologic investigation is usually not required in CU as it develops in the region that contacts the allergic and/or irritant agent. However, if performed, a spongiotic dermatitis picture characterized by a mixed inflammatory infiltrate formed of lymphocytes, histiocytes, and eosinophils is often observed in CD. Only dermal changes are seen in CU and epidermal spongiosis is not seen [12, 13]. A patch test and/or specific IgE investigation is recommended to detect the agent causing the problem.

2.3. Papular urticaria

Papular urticaria is a kind of allergic hypersensitivity reaction developing after arthropod bites. It is most common in children at the age of 2–10 years [14]. It usually develops in open regions of the body such as the arms, lower leg, and face due to insect bites from fleas, mosquitoes, or bedbugs especially in the summer [15]. The genital, perianal, and axillary regions are generally protected. Vesicles, excoriation, and post-inflammatory hyperpigmentation can be gradually observed in the middle of the lesion that starts as an itchy papule. Mostly, acute-type localized insect bites have urticarial features [16]. Diagnosis is usually clinical but can rarely be confused with other disease such as varicella, miliaria rubra, and Gianotti-Crosti syndrome [17]. Nonsedating antihistamines and moderate-potency topical corticosteroids for itching are usually adequate for treatment [14].

2.4. Exanthematous drug eruptions

Exanthematous drug eruptions, also called morbilliform or maculopapular drug eruptions, are the most common drug hypersensitivity reaction [18]. They are present in form of erythematous fixed macules, papules, or wheal-like lesions with a bilateral and symmetrical distribution especially on the body after an average of 1 week following drug administration. The lesions become confluent in time and improve by leaving transient hyperpigmentation while regressing [5]. The mucous membranes are usually not involved. However, the mucous membranes (oral, conjunctival, nasal, or anogenital) and skin appendages (hair and nails) may be involved in patients with severe drug eruption. Mild fever can be seen. The medication history is essential in the diagnosis. Histopathologic diagnosis is not always required. Biopsy sometimes does not help in the diagnosis because it does not contain specific signs. Skin biopsy is generally recommended in the case of drug use that may cause a drug eruption, fever >38°C, and the presence of erythroderma, blisters, and purpura or pustules and mucous membrane involvement [19]. Discontinuing the suspected drug immediately is recommended in the treatment. Topical corticosteroids and systemic antihistamines are recommended for symptomatic treatment. However, short-term moderate-high dose (prednisone 1–2 mg/kg/day) systemic corticosteroid treatment can be recommended in those with a severe exanthematous drug reaction [20].

2.5. Cutaneous mastocytosis (Urticaria pigmentosa)

Mastocytosis is a group of disorders characterized by the accumulation of mast cells in one or more organs. It is divided into two main groups as cutaneous and systemic [21]. Urticaria pigmentosa (UP) is the most common type of cutaneous mastocytosis both in childhood and adulthood. It presents with brown macules and papules, especially in the trunk or limbs. However, it can be seen as an urticarial rash that can affect the entire body in children. Dermographism-urticaria (Darier finding) development after skin rubbing is present in most cases [21, 22]. Healing is usually with post-inflammatory hyperpigmentation. The number of lesions is variable. The most common symptoms are itching and flushing. However, bulla development, recurrent syncope, and even anaphylaxis can be seen. Regression in symptoms is seen in the majority of the patients until adolescence with full improvement in 50% [23]. Although clinicopathologic correlation is recommended for the diagnosis, histopathologic characteristics may not always be obvious. The treatment is usually symptomatic in children. Phototherapy is the primary treatment in widespread maculopapular lesions seen in adults [24].

2.6. Autoimmune bullous disorders

Bullous pemphigoid, gestational pemphigoid, linear IgA dermatosis, and epidermolysis bullosa acquisita are disorders due to autoantibodies toward various basal membrane components and characterized by subepidermal bulla formation related to these antigens. Another common characteristic of these disorders is the possibility of urticarial lesions.

2.6.1. Bullous pemphigoid

Bullous pemphigoid (BP) is an autoimmune bullous disorder that is especially observed in elderly people and often accompanied by severe itching. It presents with tense bullae following a prodromal stage lasting weeks or even months. Bulla development may not be observed in some patients. Pruritic eczematous and papular or urticaria-like skin lesions are commonly observed in the prodromal period [25–27]. They may develop on a non-inflammatory base or an urticarial-erythematous base [28]. The body, extremity flexures, and axillary and inguinal folds are the main regions involved. Bilateral symmetrical involvement is usually present [25, 26, 28]. BP may not be considered in patients with a long-term prodromal period. The gold standard in the diagnosis is histopathology and direct immunofluorescence. Detection of autoantibodies in the serum with indirect immunofluorescence has become the standard for the diagnosis at many centers [29].

2.6.2. *Gestational pemphigoid*

Gestational pemphigoid is a rare autoimmune skin disorder seen during pregnancy. It is characterized by a severe itchy and bullous eruption due to damage in the basement membrane of the skin by autoantibodies developing against placental BP180 (BPAG2/collagen XVII) [30]. However, urticarial and eczematous lesions may be seen before and/or during bulla development in some cases. The onset is usually with severe itching around the belly. Red papules, urticarial plaques, or erythema multiforme-like targetoid lesions develop. However, cases where the urticarial or targetoid lesions lasted longer have also been reported. Histopathology, direct immunofluorescence, and indirect immunofluorescence are important in the diagnosis [5, 29, 31].

2.6.3. *Linear IgA bullous dermatosis*

Linear IgA bullous dermatosis (LABD) is a mucocutaneous autoimmune subepidermal vesiculobullous disorder. Although the etiopathogenesis is not fully known, it is thought to be associated with drugs, infections, autoimmune diseases, gastrointestinal diseases, and malignancies [32, 33]. There can be clear or hemorrhagic lesions, tense vesicles, or bullae appearing on an erythematous or urticarial base [34]. When erythematous or urticarial lesions last a long time, the diagnosis of bullous disorders can be missed. The diagnosis is made with clinical, histopathologic, and immunologic data as in other autoimmune disorders.

2.6.4. *Epidermolysis bullosa acquisita*

Epidermolysis bullosa acquisita (EBA) is a rare acquired, chronic subepidermal bullous disease of the skin and mucous membranes. It is characterized by antibodies developing against type VII collagen, which is the major component of anchoring fibrils. Clinical presentation is usually in the form of non-inflammatory bullous lesions that improve with scarring and milia formation in trauma-prone acral regions. However, in addition to the classic presentation, BP-like presentation, cicatricial pemphigoid-like presentation, Brunsting-Perry pemphigoid presentation, and LABD-like disease can also be seen. Urticarial lesions can be observed with various durations, especially with a BP-like and LABD-like presentation. Clinical, histopathologic, and immunologic investigations are required in the diagnosis. Colchicine, dapsone, plasmapheresis, photopheresis, infliximab, and intravenous immunoglobulin are the most commonly used treatment agents. However, treatment satisfaction is usually low [5, 35].

2.7. Pruritic urticarial papules and plaques of pregnancy

Pruritic urticarial papules and plaques of pregnancy (PUPPP) is the itchiest dermatosis of pregnancy. PUPPP is seen in the form of erythematous, urticarial plaques, and papules and usually starts from the abdomen and extends to the thighs, legs, back, buttocks, arms, and breasts. However, the periumbilical region is protected. The lesions usually regress within 6 weeks in the postpartum period [36, 37]. In addition to erythematous and urticarial plaques, targetoid and vesicular lesions can be seen in approximately half of the patients as the disease progresses. Moisturizers, topical corticosteroids, and antihistamines can be recommended for symptomatic relief in patients with severe itching [36].

2.8. Rare cutaneous urticarial syndromes

Autoimmune progesterone/estrogen dermatitis, interstitial granulomatous dermatitis, eosinophilic cellulitis (Wells syndrome), neutrophilic eccrine hidradenitis (NEH), and urticaria-like follicular mucinosis are rare cutaneous urticarial syndromes.

2.8.1. Autoimmune progesterone/estrogen dermatitis

Autoimmune progesterone dermatitis (APD) is a rare dermatosis that causes inflammation at the luteal phase of the menstrual cycle and presents with several skin findings. Skin signs include urticarial, eczematous and vesiculopustular eruption, targetoid lesions, and angioedema [38, 39]. Urticaria is seen in about half of patients [5]. There is no specific diagnostic test. A history of premenstrual exacerbation, prevention of lesions with ovulation inhibition, and a positive reaction to intradermal progesterone injection are helpful in the diagnosis [39]. Autoimmune estrogen dermatitis has also been identified in the literature but only in low numbers [5].

2.8.2. Interstitial granulomatous dermatitis

Interstitial granulomatous dermatitis (IGD) is a rare dermatosis and accepted as a separate histopathologic entity [40]. Papules, nodules, plaques, and an urticarial rash can be observed in the disorder that is more common in women and the elderly people. Of the cases identified until today, two-thirds have had a chronic course and the remaining a recurrent and episodic course. Recognizing IGD is quite important in order to indicate the underlying autoimmune disorders [5, 40]. Clinicopathological correlation is essential for the diagnosis.

2.8.3. Wells syndrome (eosinophilic cellulitis)

Wells syndrome is a rare dermatosis that presents as acute, recurrent, itchy, erythematous, and edematous lesions [41]. Although it brings bacterial cellulitis to mind first in the clinic, not responding to systemic antibiotics is an important indicator in the diagnosis. Another differential diagnosis is urticaria due to the presence of urticarial lesions. In addition to bacterial cellulitis and urticaria, it can be confused with insect bite, contact dermatitis, angioedema, and hypereosinophilic syndrome [42]. Clinicopathologic correlation is important in the diagnosis.

http://dx.doi.org/10.5772/67993

Dermal edema, eosinophilic dermal infiltration, and free eosinophilic granules coating collagen bundles ("flame figures") are observed histopathologically. However, the histopathologic signs change in time. Peripheral eosinophilia may also be present in the acute phase [41, 42].

2.8.4. *Neutrophilic eccrine hidradenitis*

Neutrophilic eccrine hidradenitis (NEH) is a very rare dermatosis seen in patients with malignancy or those receiving chemotherapy. The majority of the cases are acute myelogenous leukemia patients receiving chemotherapy [43]. It clinically presents with fixed erythematous and edematous papules and plaques. It is usually accompanied by fever. Histopathologic signs are important in the diagnosis. It is histopathologically characterized by neutrophilic infiltration accompanied by necrosis around eccrine glands and secretory coils. No specific treatment is required as it is usually self-limiting. However, systemic corticosteroid treatment has been reported to shorten the duration of the lesions and the fever [5, 44].

2.8.5. *Urticaria-like follicular mucinosis*

Urticaria-like follicular mucinosis (ULFM) is a very rare disease that presents with itching, urticarial papules, and plaques on an erythematous base, usually in the head and neck. It is usually seen in middle-aged men. Spontaneous improvement is common. However, recurrence can be seen. Histopathological characteristics are important in the diagnosis. Cystic spaces filled with mucin in the outer sheath of hair follicles are histologically seen [45].

3. Systemic urticarial syndromes

In addition to skin disorders, many systemic diseases can cause urticarial lesions. The differential diagnosis with ordinary urticaria should consider that systemic urticarial syndromes may cause elementary skin lesions such as papules, vesicles, hemorrhages, necrosis, and crusts in addition to urticarial skin lesions and also many systemic symptoms such as fever, asthenia, and arthralgia. Lesions usually last longer than 24–36 h, show bilateral and symmetrical distribution, and recover with hyperpigmentation and bruising [46, 47]. Systemic diseases causing urticarial skin lesions will be reviewed in this section.

3.1. Vasculitides

3.1.1. *Urticarial vasculitis*

Urticarial vasculitis (UV) is a separate clinicopathologic entity characterized by recurrent urticarial episodes, histopathologically showing leukocytoclastic vasculitis characteristics [48]. It is the most common clinical picture causing systemic urticarial syndrome. UV has been reported in 2–20% of the patients diagnosed with chronic urticaria [49]. It causes painful and burning skin lesions rather than itching. Urticarial lesions continue longer than 24–36 h. Central clearing of lesions is seen in time and they are accompanied by palpable purpura. Necrosis and ulceration are less common skin findings [50]. The lesions regress with a residual hyperpigmentation [47, 51]. Histopathology is essential in the diagnosis. The correct choice of the lesion is important in order to reveal true vasculitic changes. Leukocytoclastic vasculitis of the small dermal vessels characterized by a neutrophilic perivascular infiltrate, the typical findings for UV, is observed in fully developed lesions. Additionally, neutrophil fragmentation, nuclear dust, erythrocyte extravasation, and fibrin deposition in and around the vessels are observed [50, 52].

Urticarial vasculitis is mostly idiopathic. However, an association with various drugs, sun, cold, connective tissue diseases, infections, and various malignancies (paraneoplastic) has been identified [50, 51, 53]. Among connective tissue diseases, it is most commonly seen with systemic lupus erythematosus (SLE) [53]. The most common laboratory findings in idiopathic UV are elevation of the erythrocyte sedimentation rate and reduction of serum complement levels [48]. UV is divided into two groups as mainly normocomplementemic UV (NUV) and hypocomplementemic UV (HUV), based on complement levels [51, 54]. Systemic involvement is usually absent or minimal and the prognosis is better in NUV patients. However, there is a propensity to more severe multi-organ involvement in HUV patients [48]. The most common systemic manifestations are in the joints, kidneys, and lungs [52, 54]. Gastrointestinal and neurologic involvement can also be seen [50, 52]. Antinuclear antibody (ANA) positivity has also been reported in up to 78% of HUV patients [52, 54].

Several agents are used for UV treatment and the treatment response is variable. Systemic corticosteroids are the basis of the treatment in UV where antihistamines are usually not sufficient. UV can be controlled with prednisone at a dose of 1 mg/kg/day but can recur after the dose is decreased. Steroid-sparing agents are used in the treatment to avoid the side effects of long-term corticosteroids. Dapsone, colchicine, hydroxychloroquine, mycophenolate mofetil, interferon-alpha, cyclosporine A, azathioprine, cyclophosphamide, rituximab, intravenous immunoglobulins, anakinra, and plasmapheresis are treatment agents that can be used alone or in combination with corticosteroids [50–52].

3.1.2. Other vasculitides

Urticarial lesions can be seen in the Churg-Strauss syndrome, Wegener granulomatosis, and polyarteritis nodosa, which are characterized by vasculitis.

The Churg-Strauss syndrome is a rare allergic granulomatous polyangiitis that usually affects middle-aged men. The most common sign is asthma. However, hay fever, rash, gastrointestinal bleeding, and pain can also be seen. Urticarial lesions have been identified in less than 10% of the patients [55].

Polyarteritis nodosa (PAN) is a vasculitis affecting medium-sized vessels and is very rare. Although it can affect any tissue in the body, it most commonly affects the muscles, joints, intestines, nerves, and skin. Urticarial lesions have been identified in about 6% of PAN patients [56].

3.2. Immunologic disorders

Many immunologic disorders can cause urticarial lesions. Connective tissue diseases and mainly SLE, Sjogren syndrome, dermatomyositis, and mixed connective tissue disease are

http://dx.doi.org/10.5772/67993

important among these. It is important to know that urticarial lesions can also be seen in addition to the existing lesions in connective tissue diseases. Although rare, urticarial lesions can also be present in juvenile rheumatoid arthritis [51].

3.3. Hematologic diseases

A wide variety of hematologic diseases can cause urticarial lesions.

3.3.1. Schnitzler syndrome

Schnitzler syndrome is characterized by an urticarial rash and monoclonal gammopathy clinically and neutrophil-mediated inflammation histologically [57]. An urticarial rash and usually IgM but rarely IgG monoclonal gammopathy are present with a chronic pattern in all the patients. Recurrent fever, bone or joint pain, increased bone density, hepato- or splenomegaly, lymphadenopathy, and elevated acute-phase reactants are also accepted as minor criteria [58]. Approximately, 300 cases have been identified in the literature [57]. Risk of developing a lymphoproliferative disorder at an approximate rate of 15% has been reported in the 10-year follow-up, although the syndrome usually has a benign course. The most commonly developing lymphoproliferative disease is Waldenstrom macroglobulinemia. Treatment is usually unsatisfactory, but high doses of corticosteroids, systemic antihistamines, oral cyclosporine, intravenous pulse cyclophosphamide, and pefloxacin mesylate are the therapeutic agents used [58].

3.3.2. Waldenstrom macroglobulinemia

Waldenstrom macroglobulinemia is a chronic indolent lymphoproliferative disorder [59]. Increased levels of IgM paraprotein in the circulation and infiltration of the bone marrow with lymphocytes and plasma cells are seen. Urticarial lesions can be seen in addition to purpura, edema, and ulceration [60].

3.3.3. Hypereosinophilic syndromes

This is a group of myeloproliferative disorders characterized by multiple organ damage caused by persistent eosinophilia. It is more common in young and middle-aged patients but can be seen at any ages. Their classification is complicated. Three factors are mainly included in the diagnostic criteria. These are eosinophilia longer than 6 months (>1500/μl), no identifiable etiology for eosinophilia, and signs and symptoms of organ involvement. The most commonly involved organs are the skin, heart, lungs, and the central and peripheral nervous systems. Skin findings are usually common and are in the form of eczematous, urticarial, and angioedema-like findings [61, 62].

3.4. Autoinflammatory syndromes

Autoinflammatory syndromes are a group of heterogeneous single-gene disorders causing recurrent febrile episodes and inflammatory cutaneous, mucosal, serosal, and osteoarticular manifestations [63, 64]. No infectious, autoimmune, or neoplastic reason has been shown. Excessive activation of the interleukin 1 beta (IL-1β) pathway is most commonly held responsible in the etiopathogenesis [64].

Many syndromes such as familial Mediterranean fever (FMF), Tumor necrosis factor (TNF) receptor-associated periodic syndrome, hyperimmunoglobulinemia D with periodic fever syndrome (HIDS), and cryopyrin-associated periodic syndromes have been identified among the autoinflammatory syndromes. A monogenic defect has been found but only in some of these disorders. However, all have been included within the autoinflammatory syndromes as they show similar inflammatory features [63].

Autoinflammatory syndromes mostly start in infancy or during childhood. Although most cases are familial, some are sporadic. Recurrent episodes of inflammation with fever, elevation in acute-phase reactants, and skin rash can be seen in the absence of an infectious or autoimmune etiology. Although joint and skin involvement can be seen in various forms, fever is almost always present. These symptoms can also be accompanied by systemic findings such as abdominal pain, myalgia, ocular involvement, serositis, amyloidosis, and neurological signs [63, 65].

The skin signs show variety. Urticarial lesions are the predominant skin signs, especially in cryopyrinopathies, and occur in the first year of life. They are more commonly seen as erysipelas-like plaques in the lower extremities in FMF. Erythematous macules and urticarial lesions are seen in HIDS [51, 65].

Autoinflammatory disorders can pose a significant challenge for primary care physicians, pediatricians, dermatologists, rheumatologists, and infectious disease specialists in terms of wide-ranging clinical spectrum. A perivascular and interstitial neutrophil-rich infiltration suggesting neutrophilic urticarial dermatoses is observed in the histopathologic evaluation of skin lesions. Leukocytoclastic vasculitis-like signs can also be seen [65, 66]. However, these signs are not specific. The diagnosis of autoinflammatory disorders is usually made with the clinical features and then supported by either genetic testing or the patient's response to IL-1 inhibition or other specific therapies [63].

4. Conclusion

Ordinary urticaria is a clinical picture frequently encountered by dermatologists and usually presents no diagnostic difficulty. However, cutaneous and systemic urticarial syndromes should be considered in the case of persistence of urticarial lesions, bilateral and symmetrical location, healing with hyperpigmentation or bruising, the presence of other elementary lesions, not responding to systemic antihistamines, and being accompanied by systemic findings. The differential diagnosis of ordinary urticaria and urticarial syndromes is not easy. A detailed clinical evaluation should therefore be performed. Clinicopathologic correlation and, if necessary, further studies should be conducted in the presence of findings suggesting urticarial syndromes.

http://dx.doi.org/10.5772/67993

Author details

Hilal Gokalp[1]* and Isil Bulur[2]

*Address all correspondence to: hilalgklp@gmail.com

1 Department of Dermatology, Koç University School of Medicine, Istanbul, Turkey

2 Department of Dermatology, Memorial Sisli Hospital, Istanbul, Turkey

References

[1] Kaplan A. Urticaria and angioedema. In: Adkinson NFYJ, Buss WW, Bochner BS, et al., editors. Middleton's allergy principles and practice. 6th ed. Phaledelphia (PA): Mosby; 2003. pp. 1537–1558.

[2] Gaig P, Olona M, Muñoz Lejarazu D, Caballero MT, Domínguez FJ, Echechipia S, et al. Epidemiology of urticaria in Spain. J Investig Allergol Clin Immunol. 2004;14:214–220.

[3] Schocket AL. Chronic urticaria: pathophysiology and etiology, or the what and why. Allergy Asthma Proc. 2006;27:90–95.

[4] Kaplan AP, Greaves M. Pathogenesis of chronic urticaria. Clin Exp Allergy. 2009;39: 777–787.

[5] Peroni A, Colato C, Schena D, Girolomoni G. Urticarial lesions: if not urticaria, what else? The differential diagnosis of urticaria: part I. Cutaneous diseases. J Am Acad Dermatol. 2010;62:541–555.

[6] Kossard S, Hamann I, Wilkinson B. Defining urticarial dermatitis: a subset of dermal hypersensitivity reaction pattern. Arch Dermatol. 2006;142:29–34.

[7] Kossard S, Hamann I. A clinician's view of urticarial dermatitis. Reply. Arch Dermatol. 2006;142:932–933.

[8] Fung MA. The clinical and histopathologic spectrum of "dermal hypersensitivity reactions," a nonspecific histologic diagnosis that is not very useful in clinical practice, and the concept of a "dermal hypersensitivity reaction pattern". J Am Acad Dermatol. 2002;47:898.

[9] Belsito DV. Occupational contact dermatitis: etiology, prevalence, and resultant impairment/disability. J Am Acad Dermatol. 2005;53:303–313.

[10] Templet JT, Hall S, Belsito DV. Etiology of hand dermatitis among patients referred for patch testing. Dermatitis. 2004;15:25–32.

[11] Mowad CM. Contact dermatitis: practice gaps and challenges. Dermatol Clin. 2016; 34:263–267.

[12] Mowad CM, Marks JG Jr. Allergic contact dermatitis. In: Bolognia JL, Jorizzo JL, Rapini RP, editors. Dermatology. St Louis: Mosby; 2003. pp. 227–240.

[13] Cohen DE, Bassiri-Tehrani S. Irritant contact dermatitis. In: Bolognia JL, Jorizzo JL, Rapini RP, editors. Dermatology. St Louis: Mosby; 2003. pp. 241–249.

[14] Hernandez RG, Cohen BA. Insect bite-induced hypersensitivity and the SCRATCH principles: a new approach to papular urticaria. Pediatrics. 2006;118:189–196.

[15] Steen CJ, Carbonaro PA, Schwartz RA. Arthropods in dermatology. J Am Acad Dermatol. 2004;50:819–842.

[16] Moffit JE, Golden DBK, Reisman RE, Lee R, Nicklas R, Freeman T, et al. Stinging insect hypersensitivity: a practice parameter update. J Allergy Clin Immunol. 2004;114:869–886.

[17] Steen CJ, Janniger CK, Schutzer SE, Schwartz RA. Insect sting reactions to bees, wasps, and ants. Int J Dermatol. 2005;44:91–94.

[18] Valeyrie-Allanore L, Sassolas B, Roujeau JC. Drug-induced skin, nail and hair disorders. Drug Saf. 2007;30:1011–1030.

[19] Justiniano H, Berlingeri-Ramos AC, Sánchez JL. Pattern analysis of drug-induced skin diseases. Am J Dermatopathol. 2008;30:352–369.

[20] Schneck J, Fagot JP, Sekula P, Sassolas B, Roujeau JC, Mockenhaupt M. Effects of treatments on the mortality of Stevens-Johnson syndrome and toxic epidermal necrolysis: a retrospective study on patients included in the prospective EuroSCAR Study. J Am Acad Dermatol. 2008;58:33–40.

[21] Briley LD, Phillips CM. Cutaneous mastocytosis: a review focusing on the pediatric population. Clin Pediatr. 2008;47:757–761.

[22] Yanagihori H, Oyama N, Nakamura K, Kaneko F. C-kit mutations in patients with childhood-onset mastocytosis and genotype-phenotype correlation. J Mol Diagn. 2005; 7:252–257.

[23] Akoglu G, Erkin G, Cakir B, Boztepe G, Sahin S, Karaduman A, et al. Cutaneous mastocytosis: demographic aspects and clinical features of 55 patients. J Eur Acad Dermatol Venereol. 2006;20:969–973.

[24] Gobello T, Mazzanti C, Sordi D, Annessi G, Abeni D, Chinni ML, et al. Medium versus high dose ultraviolet A1 phototherapy for urticaria pigmentosa: a pilot study. J Am Acad Dermatol. 2003;49:679–684.

[25] Kneisel A, Hertl M. Autoimmune bullous skin diseases. Part 1: clinical manifestations. J Dtsch Dermatol Ges. 2011;9:844–856.

[26] Schmidt E, della Torre R, Borradori L. Clinical features and practical diagnosis of bullous pemphigoid. Dermatol Clin. 2011;29:427–438.

[27] Kasperkiewicz M, Zillikens D, Schmidt E. Pemphigoid diseases: pathogenesis, diagnosis, and treatment. Autoimmunity. 2012;45:55–70.

[28] Di Zenzo G, Marazza G, Borradori L. Bullous pemphigoid: physiopathology, clinical features and management. Adv Dermatol. 2007;23:257–288.

[29] Karpati S. Dermatitis herpetiformis: close to unraveling a disease. J Dermatol Sci. 2004;34:83–90.

[30] Huilaja L, Mäkikallio K, Tasanen K. Gestational pemphigoid. Orphanet J Rare Dis. 2014;9:136.

[31] Boulinguez S, Bedane C, Prost C, Bernard P, Labbe L, Bonnetblanc JM. Chronic pemphigoid gestationis: comparative clinical and immunopathological study of 10 patients. Dermatology. 2003;206(2):113–119.

[32] Chanal J, Ingen-Housz-Oro S, Ortonne N, Duong TA, Thomas M, Valeyrie-Allanore L, et al. Linear IgA bullous dermatosis: comparison between the drug-induced and spontaneous forms. Br J Dermatol. 2013;169:1041–1048.

[33] Chen S, Mattei P, Fischer M, Gay JD, Milner SM, Price LA. Linear IgA bullous dermatosis. Eplasty. 2013;13:49.

[34] Guide SV, Marinokovich MP. Linear IgA bullous dermatosis. Clin Dermatol. 2001; 19:719–727.

[35] Gupta R, Woodley DT, Chen M. Epidermolysis bullosa acquitsita. Clin Dermatol. 2012;30:60–69.

[36] Rudolph CM, Al-Fares S, Vaughan-Jones SA, Mullegger RR, Kerl H, Black MM. Polymorphic eruption of pregnancy: clinicopathology and potential trigger factors in 181 patients. Br J Dermatol. 2006;154:54–60.

[37] Matz H, Orion E, Wolf R. Pruritic urticarial papules and plaques of pregnancy: polymorphic eruption of pregnancy (PUPPP). Clin Dermatol. 2006;24:105–108.

[38] Baptist AP, Baldwin JL. Autoimmune progesterone dermatitis in a patient with endometriosis: case report and review of the literature. Clin Mol Allergy. 2004;2:10.

[39] Stranahan D, Rausch D, Deng A, Gaspari A. The role of intradermal skin testing and patch testing in the diagnosis of autoimmune progesterone dermatitis. Dermatitis. 2006;17:39–42.

[40] Ahmed ZS, Joad S, Singh M, Bandagi SS. Interstitial granulomatous dermatitis successfully treated with etanercept. Am J Case Rep. 2014;15:94–96.

[41] Gandhi RK, Coloe J, Peters S, Zirwas M, Darabi K. Wells syndrome (eosinophilic cellulitis): a clinical imitator of bacterial cellulitis. J Clin Aesthet Dermatol. 2011;4:55–57.

[42] Weiss G, Shemer A, Confino Y, Kaplan B, Trau H. Wells' syndrome: report of a case and review of the literature. Int J Dermatol. 2001;40:148–152.

[43] Bachmeyer C, Aractingi S. Neutrophilic eccrine hidradenitis. Clin Dermatol. 2000;18: 319–330.

[44] Bhanu P, Santosh KV, Gondi S, Manjunath KG, Rajendaran SC, Raj N. Neutrophilic eccrine hidradenitis: a new culprit-carbamazepine. Indian J Pharmacol. 2013;45:91–92.

[45] Crovato F, Nazzari G, Nunzi E, Rebora A. Urticaria-like follicular mucinosis. Dermatologica. 1985;170:133–135.

[46] Zuberbier T, Asero R, Bindslev-Jensen C, Walter Canonica G, Church MK, Gimenez-Arnau A, et al. EAACI/GA(2)LEN/EDF/WAO guideline: definition, classification and diagnosis of urticaria. Allergy. 2009;64:1417–1426.

[47] Buck A, Christensen J, McCarty M. Hypocomplemententemic urticarial vasculitis syndrome: a case report and literature review. J Clin Aesthet Dermatol. 2012;5:36–46.

[48] Venzor J, Lee WL, Huston DP. Urticarial vasculitis. Clin Rev Allergy Immunol. 2002;23: 201–216.

[49] Grotz W, Baba H, Becker J, Baumgartel MW. Hypocomplemententemic urticarial vasculitis syndrome. An interdisciplinary challenge. Dtsch Arztebl Int. 2009;106:756–763.

[50] Brown NA, Carter JD. Urticarial vasculitis. Curr Rheumatol Rep. 2007;9:312–319.

[51] Peroni A, Colato C, Schena D, Girolomoni G. Urticarial lesions: if not urticaria, what else? The differential diagnosis of urticaria: part II. Systemic diseases. J Am Acad Dermatol. 2010;62:557–570.

[52] Dincy CVP, George R, Jacob M, Mathai E, Pulimood S, Eapen EP. Clinicopathologic profile of normocomplemententemic and hypocomplemententemic urticarial vasculitis: a study from South India. J Eur Acad Dermatol. 2008;22:789–794.

[53] DeAmicis T, Mofid MZ, Cohen B, Nousari HC. Hypocomplemententemic urticarial vasculitis: report of a 12-year-old girl with systemic lupus erythematosus. J Am Acad Dermatol. 2002;47:273–274.

[54] Tosoni C, Lodi-Rizzini F, Cinquini M, Pasolini G, Venturini M, Sinico RA, et al. A reassessment of diagnostic criteria and treatment of idiopathic urticarial vasculitis: a retrospective study of 47 patients. Clin Exp Dermatol. 2009;34:166–170.

[55] Tlacuilo-Parra A, Soto-Ortiz JA, Guevara-Gutierrez E. Churg-Strauss syndrome manifested by urticarial plaques. Int J Dermatol. 2003;42:386–388.

[56] Chang S, Carr W. Urticarial vasculitis. Allergy Asthma Proc. 2007;28:97–100.

[57] Gusdorf L, Asli B, Barbarot S, Masseau A, Puechal X, Gottenberg JE, et al. Schnitzler syndrome: validation and applicability of diagnostic criteria in real-life patients. Allergy. 2017;72:177–188.

[58] Eiling E, Schröder JO, Gross WL, Kreiselmaier I, Mrowietz U, Schwarz T. The Schnitzler syndrome: chronic urticaria and monoclonal gammopathy—an autoinflammatory syndrome? J Dtsch Dermatol Ges. 2008;6:626–631.

[59] Vogt RF, Marti GE. Overview of monoclonal gammopathies of undetermined significance. Br J Haematol. 2007;139:687–689.

[60] Chan I, Calonje E, Whittaker SJ. Cutaneous Waldenstrom's macroglobulinaemia. Clin Exp Dermatol. 2003;28:491–492.

[61] Simon HU, Rothenberg ME, Bochner BS, Weller PF, Wardlaw AJ, Wechsler ME, et al. Refining the definition of hypereosinophilic syndrome. J Allergy Clin Immunol. 2010;126:45–49.

[62] Liao W, Long H, Chang CC, Lu Q. The eosinophil in health and disease: from bench to bedside and back. Clin Rev Allergy Immunol. 2016;50:125–139.

[63] Cush JJ. Autoinflammatory syndromes. Dermatol Clin. 2013;31:471–480.

[64] Lachmann HJ, Lowe P, Felix SD, Rordorf C, Leslie K, Madhoo S, et al. In vivo regulation of interleukin 1a in patients with cryopyrin-associated periodic syndromes. J Exp Med. 2009;206:1029–1036.

[65] Farasat S, Aksentijevich I, Toro JR. Autoinflammatory diseases. Clinical and genetic advances. Arch Dermatol. 2008;144:392–402.

[66] Kanazawa N, Furukawa F. Autoinflammatory syndromes with a dermatological perspective. J Dermatol. 2007;34:601–618.

Chapter 11

Hereditary Angioedema

Asli Gelincik and Semra Demir

Additional information is available at the end of the chapter

http://dx.doi.org/10.5772/intechopen.68208

Abstract

Hereditary angioedema (HAE) is an autosomal dominantly inherited orphan disease manifested by recurrent unpredictable nonpitting and nonpruritic swelling attacks without urticarial plaques. HAE is caused by a deficiency of the C1 esterase inhibitor (C1-inh) or decreased function of C1-inh. Type 1 HAE, the most common form, occurs due to C1-inh deficiency and is seen with low-serum C1-inh levels. In type 2 HAE, the function of C1-inh is impaired, and in HAE with normal C1-inh serum levels, the function of C1-inh is normal. HAE episodes can affect various sites in the body such as the larynx, face, extremities, gastrointestinal tract, and urogenital area. Acute episodes can be treated with C1-inh concentrates, a kallikrein inhibitor, called ecallantide and bradykinin B2 receptor antagonist, icatibant. Depending on the frequency, severity, and location of the episodes, long-term prophylaxis regimens with plasma-derived C1-inh concentrates, antifibrinolytics, or 17α-alkylated androgens can be used. C1-inh concentrates or 17α-alkylated androgens should be administered before dental procedures and minor or major surgical interventions to provide short-term prophylaxis. In conclusion, HAE is a rare life-threatening disease of which clinical presentation is highly variable and early accurate diagnosis significantly prevents mortality and morbidity.

Keywords: hereditary angioedema, C1-inhibitor, bradykinin, complement, orphan disease

1. Introduction

Hereditary angioedema (HAE) is a rare disease, clinically characterized by recurrent unpredictable nonpitting and nonpruritic swelling episodes involving different mucosal or cutaneous surfaces of the body such as the larynx, face, extremities, gastrointestinal tract, and urogenital area [1]. In the late 1880s, Osler described the hereditary feature of angioedema for the first time [2]. In the 1960s, a deficiency in a type of serine proteinase inhibitor, C1 esterase inhibitor (C1-inh), was discovered as the cause of HAE, and a few years later, the second form was defined as non-functioning C1-inh. These diseases are called type I and type II HAE, respectively [3, 4]. These laboratory abnormalities in C1-inh are the result of the mutations found in the C1-inh gene called SERPING1 [5]. In the 2000s, a third form of HAE was defined and in these patients characteristic clinical signs and symptoms are seen; however, the level and the function of C1-inh are normal with no mutations on the SERPING1 gene [6, 7]. However, mutations in the F12 gene were found in approximately 25% of these patients. A strong association between this type of HAE and conditions causing increased levels of estrogen such as pregnancy and the usage of oral contraceptives was determined [7, 8]. Therefore, at first, this type was called estrogen-dependent or type III hereditary angioedema [6]. After affected male relatives were reported, it was renamed as hereditary angioedema with normal C1-inh [9].

HAE is rarely seen, and its estimated prevalence ranges from 1:30,000 to 1:80,000 in the general population [10]. The most common form of HAE is the first type, which is responsible for 85% of the patients [10]. HAE is an autosomal dominant disease generally affecting all generations in a family, although a quarter of patients do not have a family history. Patients are similarly affected independent of gender and ethnicity [11]. Mortality rates range from 14 to 33% mostly because of poorly treated laryngeal episodes, which indicates the significance of early diagnosis and appropriate management [12, 13].

2. Clinical presentation

Symptoms primarily develop when the serum level of C1-inh is below 35% but are not usually correlated with serum C1-inh levels. Symptoms can be expected from birth in a heterozygote individual with a serum level of C1-inh around 50% [14]. Although signs and symptoms can start at any age, including after 70, they are primarily seen starting around the second decade of life when the level of C1-inh usually decreases and then continues to occur lifelong [14, 15].

Angioedema episodes can affect any cutaneous or mucosal sites of the body such as the face, larynx, extremities, gastrointestinal tract, and urogenital area [1]. A typical HAE episode worsens within the first 24 h, begins to improve after 48–72 h, and lasts approximately 72–96 h [11, 14]. Apart from visible angioedema, fluid extravasation on the gastrointestinal tractus through the intestinal wall or peritoneum leads to abdominal pain attacks. Nausea and emesis may accompany them [16]. The majority of the patients experience gastrointestinal angioedema during their lives and the abdominal attacks accompany 50% of the overall attacks [17]. Due to these abdominal attacks, unnecessary operations like appendectomy and diagnostic laparotomy are sometimes performed [16]. Fever or leucocytosis is not observed during a typical attack unless the cause is an infection [18]. Sometimes, fluid extravasation can be so severe that it causes hypotension or ascites [19]. The most severe complication is angioedema in the larynx and/or oropharynx, which can prevent air passage leading to asphyxiation or even death. Fortunately, this seems less frequent [16]. More than 50% of the patients experience laryngeal edema at least once in their lifetime [20].

Although the precipitating factors of attacks are not well determined in all attacks, some episodes of HAE can be triggered by factors such as stress, trauma, infection, angiotensin-converting enzyme inhibitors (ACEIs), estrogen-containing hormones, oropharyngeal surgery, and minor medical procedures like tooth extraction [21–23]. Sometimes, the usage of ACEI or estrogen-containing drugs can trigger the symptoms in patients with a silent disease [14]. Prodromal symptoms can precede the attacks; the most frequent symptoms are erythema marginatum, which is a nonurticarial erythematous rash and tingling on the angioedema site. Fatigue, malaise, irritability, hyperactivity, mood changes, and nausea are other preceding factors [21, 24].

The severity of HAE is variable and usually unpredictable. While some patients do not experience any attacks in their lives, others experience swelling up to twice a week. Similarly, the attacks of some patients can be so severe that treatment in an intensive care unit may be needed while the attacks of other patients can be so mild that treatment is unnecessary [15, 17]. The disease severity and the course of the disease cannot be predicted according to the initial symptoms [9].

Types I and II HAE are very similar in their clinical presentation; however, HAE with normal C1-inh differs from the other two types with respect to some features. In HAE with normal C1-inh, abdominal attacks are less frequently seen and angioedema on the face, lips, and tongue are the major symptoms. It predominantly affects females, rarely starts under the age of 10, symptoms recur less frequently, and asymptomatic intervals are more common [21].

3. Pathogenesis

C1-inh is a broad-spectrum serine proteinase inhibitor, which regulates the activity of various proteases comprising those of the contact system, the intrinsic coagulation pathway, and the fibrinolytic pathway [5]. C1-inh is produced primarily in the liver and inhibits the plasma kallikrein, a type of protease that cleaves high-molecular-weight kininogen (HMWK) to produce bradykinin and also inhibits activated coagulation factor XII (FXII), which in turn enhances the activation of the contact system by activating the plasma kallikrein [10].

Trauma as well as surgical interventions causing a negatively charged endothelial surface and a deficiency in the serum level of C1-inh leads to the development of FXIIa in significant amounts. FXIIa induces the transformation of prekallikrein to kallikrein, which in turn leads to the cleavage of high-molecular-weight kininogen to bradykinin [10, 14] (**Figure 1**).

The major mediator responsible for angioedema is a type of nanopeptide called bradykinin. Bradykinin is formed secondary to the activation of the contact system. It leads to an increase in vascular permeability by binding to the B2 receptor on the vascular endothelial cells, and this in turn causes the development of edema, ascites, and hypotension [25, 26].

C1-inh is encoded by the SERPING1 gene which is located on the 11th chromosome. Around 300 different mutations of the SERPING1 gene were identified in both type I and type II HAE patients. Approximately a quarter of patients with C1-inh deficiency do not have a family history, indicating the occurrence of de novo mutations. In type I HAE, various types of mutations involving nonsense, missense, insertion, or deletion mutations developed throughout SERPING1 leading to a decrease in the serum level of C1-inh [10, 27]. By contrast, almost all

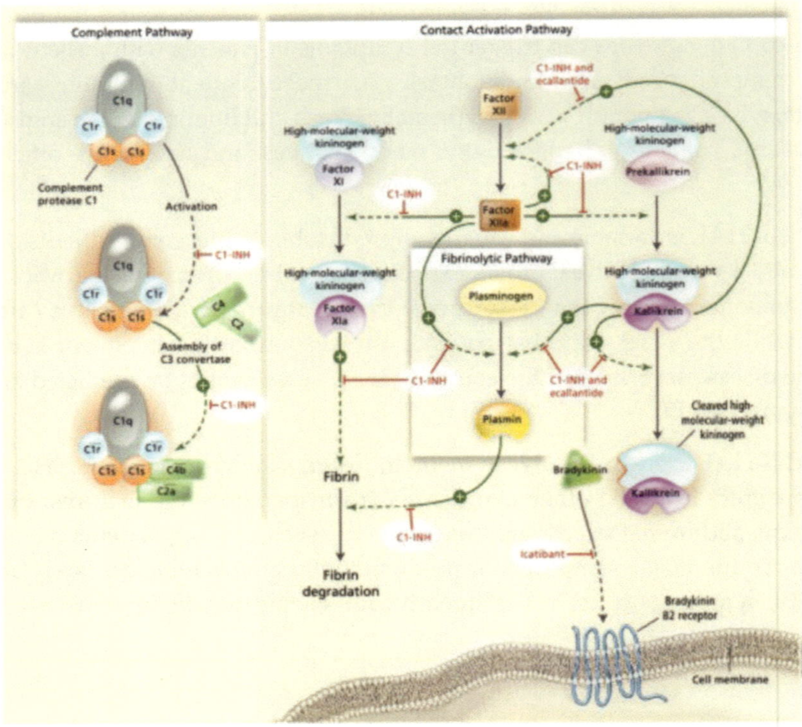

Figure 1. The role of C1-inh in the plasma cascade and complement pathway and the pathogenesis of the HAE [14]. (With permission from Massachusetts Medical Society).

of the mutations in type II HAE are missense at or near the active site causing the production of a defective protein, which cannot act properly [10]. In patients with HAE with normal C1-inh, the SERPING1 gene is not mutated, but in some of these patients mutations on the FXII gene, which is located on the fifth chromosome, can be detected. The pathomechanism of angioedema in these patients is not well defined. One of the detected mutations on factor XII leads to a gain of function, which is thought to cause the increase in the production of bradykinin [28]. However, this hypothesis was not confirmed in another study [29]. Since bradykinin antagonist drugs are effective in uncontrolled patients, it can be assumed that this type of angioedema is also bradykinin mediated [10].

4. Diagnosis

Low awareness of the disease among both doctors and the public can lead to more than a 10-year delay in the diagnosis and also result in a misdiagnosis such as allergies, systemic lupus erythematosus, and appendicitis [30–32]. HAE patients usually have a typical medical history with episodes of angioedema without urticarial plaques on their skin and/or abdominal pain attacks without inflammatory signals. Such a clinical presentation accompanied by a family history is highly suggestive of the diagnosis, but laboratory tests are recommended to confirm the diagnosis [9]. Serum C4 level is the screening test for HAE, which is decreased both during and between episodes in almost all of patients (98%). Interestingly, C4 can seldom be observed at a normal level between episodes [20]. Serum C1 and C3 levels are not affected by the disease. If C4 levels are normal during an episode, the diagnosis of type I, type II HAE, and acquired angioedema is excluded. After measuring C4, C1-inh must be measured in the serum to accurately diagnose the HAE type. In type I HAE, both serum C1-inh and C4 levels are detected below the normal ranges (the reference range of C4 is 15–50 mg/dl and of C1-inh is 16–33 mg/dl), whereas in type II HAE serum C1-inh is normal but the function of C1-inh is impaired. These tests can indicate a false negative in children younger than one, so the tests must be repeated to confirm the diagnosis [9]. In the third HAE type, HAE with normal C1-inh, serum C4- and C1-inh levels are normal and the diagnosis is challenging. Its diagnosis depends on recurrent angioedema attacks without urticaria or abdominal pain attacks and possibly a family history. However, clinical presentation is highly variable, which often leads to a misdiagnosis, and genetic tests including FXII mutations rarely support the diagnosis [33]. In **Table 1**, differential diagnoses of angioedema including both hereditary and sporadic diseases based on laboratory are shown.

Type of angioedema	C1-inh antigenic level	C1-inh functional level	C4 level	C1q level
HAE-1	Low	Low	Low	Normal
HAE-2	Normal	Low	Low	Normal
HAE with normal C1-inh	Normal	Normal	Normal	Normal
ACID	Low	Low	Low	Low
Angioedema due to ACEI	Normal	Normal	Normal	Normal
Nonclassified angioedema[a]	Normal	Normal	Normal	Normal

ACEI, angiotensin-converting enzyme inhibitor; ACID, acquired angioedema due to C1-inh deficiency; HAE-1, hereditary angioedema type I (due to C1-inh deficiency); HAE-2, hereditary angioedema type II (due to C1-inh defect); C1-inh, C1 inhibitor.

[a]Nonclassified implies that no cause has been identified [34]. http://dx.doi.org/10.1016/j.anai.2012.10.008

Table 1. Differential diagnosis of angioedema according to laboratory results [34].

5. Management

Angioedema and abdominal pain episodes do not respond to antihistamines, corticosteroids, and epinephrine, which are effectively used in histaminergic angioedema. The management of HAE comprises prophylaxis and treatment of acute attacks [35]. Moreover, patients should be educated about their disease and some preventive measures must be taken, such as avoiding known triggering factors like estrogen-containing pills and ACEI [30]. All patients are at risk for life-threatening episodes independent from their previous attacks. Therefore, all patients should have a written action plan that includes what to do in a severe attack [21].

5.1. Treatment of acute attacks (on-demand treatment)

For the treatment of acute attacks, C1 inhibitor concentrates, B2 receptor antagonist, icatibant, and an inhibitor of kallikrein synthesis, ecallantide, are used (**Table 2**, **Figure 1**) [34].

The faster intervention leads to a quicker response; therefore, patients should be treated as early as possible in attacks [21]. If these drugs cannot be provided in a health-care facility, fresh-frozen plasma can be substituted. However, it can possibly worsen an attack because of the presence of bradykinin in the plasma [36]. Furthermore, symptomatic treatment including intravenous fluid replacement, anti-emetics, and analgesics can be effective in relieving the symptoms [14]. Patients experiencing angioedema in the oropharyngeal or laryngeal region should be closely observed for the possibility of the impairment of the air passage since tracheostomy or intubation may be needed [21].

Drug	EMA and FDA indications	Recommended dosage	Mechanism	Potential adverse effects
Plasma-derived nanofiltered C1-inh				
Berinert-P®	Acute attacks	20 U/kg IV	Deficiency replacement	Theoretical: transmission of infectious agent
Cinryze®	Long-term prophylaxis in the US and Europe Short-term prophylaxis and on demand in Europe	1000 U IV every 3–4 days	Deficiency replacement	Theoretical: transmission of infectious agent
Recombinant human C1-inh (Rhucin®)	Acute attacks	50 U/kg IV	Deficiency replacement	Uncommon: risk of anaphylaxis in rabbit-sensitized individuals
Ecallantide	Acute attacks	30 mg SC (administered as three injections of 10 mg/ml each)	Inhibits plasma kallikrein	Uncommon: antidrug antibodies, injection-site reactions, risk of anaphylaxis
Icatibant	Acute attacks	30 mg SC	Bradykinin B2-receptor antagonist	Common: injection-site reactions

EMA, European Medicines Agency; FDA, Food and Drug Administration; IV, intravenous; SC, subcutaneous [34]. http://dx.doi.org/10.1016/j.anai.2012.10.008.

Table 2. Drugs used for acute attacks in HAE [34].

5.2. C1-inh concentrates

There are three kinds of C1-inh concentrates: Cinryze® (Shire ViroPharma Inc., Lexington, USA) and Berinert® (CSL Behring GmbH, Marburg, Germany) are both plasma-derived C1-inh, and Ruconest® (Pharming, Leiden, Netherlands) is a recombinant human C1-inh and was approved in 2014 by the Food and Drug Administration (FDA). Plasma-derived C1-inh concentrates have been widely used for many years and carry the potential risk of contamination of pathogens as in the case with other plasma-derived products [37]. The recombinant human C1-inh was produced as an alternative and has been used to treat angioedema attacks for a few years in some countries. The studies evaluating the efficacy of this drug in acute attacks of HAE showed that it rapidly improves the episodes and it is well tolerated with headache and nausea as the most common adverse effects [38–41].

In a recently published review, it was observed that weight-adjusted doses of 20-U/kg plasma-derived C1-inh concentrates lead to more rapid improvement in symptoms within 15 min than the standard 500-U dose of the drug that works in 30–45 min. Moreover, approximately 30% of the laryngeal attacks treated with 500-U plasma-derived C1-inh need a second dose while patients with laryngeal edema treated with a 20-U/kg dose do not require an additional dose. Therefore, a 20-U/kg-dosing regimen induces a quicker and more effective response [42].

5.3. Icatibant

Icatibant is a potent bradykinin B2 receptor antagonist. After application, symptoms begin to resolve within 30–45 min, an improvement of symptoms occurs in an average of 1.16 h, and 7–14% of patients with laryngeal edema need a second dose of the drug [42, 43]. It has some advantages including its subcutaneous application, its ready form, and preservation in room temperature. Therefore, it can be easily carried and taken by the patient. Disadvantages include side effects like pain at the injection site and a short half-life, which can lead to rebound attacks [9].

5.4. Ecallantide

Ecallantide is a recombinant protein and a potent kallikrein inhibitor [44]. It effectively improves acute angioedema attacks and is used subcutaneously like icatibant, but it is a frozen product and has a short half-life. Ecallantide was licensed for patients 16 years old and older at first but recently was approved for those 12 years and older [45]. It leads to an improvement in symptoms within approximately 93 min and 10% of the patients treated with laryngeal edema need a second dose [46]. Although ecallantide is generally well tolerated, anaphylaxis was observed in 4% of the patients, so it is not approved for self-administration and has a warning sign on its box [47].

5.5. Long-term prophylaxis

Determining if patients are in need of long-term prophylaxis can be a compelling problem for physicians. The decision depends on the frequency, severity, and location of the episodes, the presence of comorbidity, access to emergency medical attention, and the patient's preference. According to a previous consensus report, patients who have attacks more than once a month, who have attacks more than 5 days in a month, and those with a history of obstruction of the respiratory airways should take a long-term prophylaxis [20]. In the years that followed with the approval for self-administration of icatibant, the human C1-inhibitors in some countries provided appropriate control of attacks and less need for long-term prophylaxis [48].

Anabolic steroids (17α-alkylated androgens), antifibrinolytics, and C1-inh concentrates can be utilized for this purpose (**Table 3**).

17α-alkylated androgens leading to an increase in the serum level of C1-inh decrease the severity and frequency of episodes in most patients, but they have adverse effects [49, 50]. Both adverse effects and the efficacy of 17α-alkylated androgens are dose-dependent; therefore, adjustment of the minimum dose, which is both protective against severe attacks and

Drug	Recommended dosage for adults (usual, range)	Recommended dosage for children (usual, range)	FDA approved/HAE indication	Adverse effects
17-α alkylated androgens				Common: weight gain, virilization, acne, altered libido, muscle pains, and cramps, headaches, depression, fatigue, nausea, constipation, menstrual abnormalities, and increase in liver enzymes, hypertension, alterations in lipid profile Unusual: decreased growth rate in children, masculinization of the female fetus, cholestatic jaundice, peliosis hepatis, and hepatocellular adenoma
Danazol	Minimal effective dose does not exceed 200 mg/day	Not recommended; if absolutely necessary do not exceed 2.5 mg/kg/day (50 mg/week to 200 mg/day)	Yes/yes	
Stanozolol	Minimal effective dose does not exceed 2 mg/day	0.5 mg/day (0.5 mg/week to 2 mg/day)	Yes/yes	
Oxandrolone	Minimal effective dose does not exceed 10 mg/day	0.1 mg/kg/day (2.5 mg/week to 7.5 mg/day)	Yes/no	
Antifibrinolytics				
ε-Aminocaproic acid	2 g three times daily (1 g twice daily to 4 g three times daily)	0.05 g/kg twice daily (0.02 g/kg twice daily to 0.1 g/kg twice daily)	Yes/no	Common: nausea, vertigo, diarrhea, postural hypotension, fatigue, muscle cramps with increased muscle enzymes Unusual: enhanced thrombosis
Tranexamic acid	1 g twice daily (0.25 g twice daily to 1.5 g twice daily)	20 mg/kg twice daily (10 mg/kg twice daily to 25 mg/kg three times daily)	Yes/no	

[a]Registration and availability of these drugs differ from country to country. FDA, Food and Drug Administration; HAE, hereditary angioedema [34]. http://dx.doi.org/10.1016/j.anai.2012.10.008

Table 3. Drugs used for long-term prophylaxis in HAE[a] [34].

cause fewer side effects, is crucial and varies from patient to patient [21]. Treatment with 17α-alkylated androgens can be started with a high dose that can be reduced to reach the most effective but least harmful dose. The most frequent adverse effects of the 17α-alkylated androgens are menstrual irregularities, changes in libido, hirsutism, acne, changes in mood, weight gain, myalgia, erythrocytosis, increased blood pressure, and abnormalities in lipid profiles [51, 52]. Less commonly, these drugs can lead to hepatotoxicity involving hepatic adenomas and hepatic carcinoma [53, 54]. Because of these adverse effects, patients should be periodically monitored by blood count, liver enzyme, lipid profiles, and liver ultrasound [14]. Moreover, the attenuated androgens lead to the closure of epiphyseal cartilage prematurely [55]. Stanozolol is used more commonly in some European countries since it was observed to cause fewer side effects and is more effective as well as it is approved for children's use in the US [10, 56]. 17α-alkylated androgens are relatively contraindicated in patients with prostate or breast cancer, known hepatic dysfunction, children, and pregnant women [57, 58]. Because of these side effects, they are no longer authorized in German-speaking European countries [48].

Antifibrinolytics including ε-aminocaproic acid and tranexamic acid are helpful in treating HAE by inhibiting the production of plasmin from plasminogen [55]. Although they have few side effects involving most commonly nausea, vomiting, and diarrhea, which are dose-dependent, they are not as effective as androgens. In some earlier studies, antifibrinolytics were observed to decrease the frequency of attacks; however, in a recently published study, no differences were detected between groups with and without antifibrinolytics [59–61]. As a consequence, they suggested antifibrinolytics for long-term prophylaxis where plasma-derived C1-inh is not accessible and androgens are not suitable for use [55].

In recent guidelines, the importance of quality-of-life scores of the patients is more emphasized than the number of attack days for making the decision of long-term prophylaxis [48]. Cinryze® was approved in 2011 in Europe and in 2008 in the US for the use of long-term prophylaxis and its recommended dose for adolescents and adults is 1000 U every 3–4 days [48]. Recombinant human C1-inh, which is used in the treatment of attacks, was shown to be effective for long-term prophylaxis in preliminary data [62]. A possible side effect of long-term and high dose of C1-inh therapy is the undesirable immunization with this protein [48].

5.6. Short-term prophylaxis

Short-term prophylactic therapy protects patients with HAE from acute attacks caused by a known triggering factor such as dental, minor, or major surgical interventions [21]. For this purpose, various prophylactic regimens are used. C1-inh concentrates between 1000 and 2000 U for adults and 20 U/kg for children or two units of fresh-frozen plasma for adults and 10 ml/kg for children can be administered before procedures [10]. Another regimen includes a high dose of 17α-alkylated androgens starting with 6–10 mg/kg/day in divided doses, such as danazol 200 mg three times a day for 5–10 days before and 2 days after the procedure. No studies comparing the efficacy of these prophylactic modalities have been published. Therefore, it must be individualized according to the cost, benefit-harm ratio, and the patient's preferences. In pregnant patients, C1-inh administration is preferred [21]. In children, if plasma-derived C1-inh is not available, danazol can be used for a short duration [55].

6. HAE in pregnancy

The influence of pregnancy on the course of the HAE is variable. Some patients can experience fewer attacks while others experience them more frequently [9]. There are a few case series about pregnancy and delivery in HAE, which include few patients. Therefore, the approach and management of pregnancies is debated. In a recently published study, 125 pregnancies in 61 patients were analyzed and 59.2% of the patients reported a mild increase in HAE symptoms, 14% reported no symptoms, and the symptoms of 40% of the patients were sustained in a similar severity and frequency throughout the pregnancy. A HAE diagnosis was known before gestation in 30.7% of the pregnancies. Long-term prophylaxis was used in nine pregnancies including one with epsilon-amino-caproic acid, two with tranexamic acid, two with anabolic steroids (temporary usage for 8 and 12 weeks in two male-confirmed fetuses), and four with plasma-derived C1-inh concentrates. None of the babies experienced side effects from these drugs. Most of the deliveries were vaginal (88%) with cesarean sections required in 15 patients. Ten patients did not receive prophylaxis and one of them experienced mild symptoms during delivery and was treated with a plasma-derived C1-inh concentrate. After vaginal delivery without prophylaxis, a few patients developed mild local edema [63]. Similar observations were also reported by other authors [64, 65]. In another study, none of the patients who received prophylactic treatment before cesarean sections experienced any symptoms [66].

In conclusion, the course of HAE varies from patient to patient in pregnancy. Although the frequency and severity of episodes can increase in some patients, others may not have any symptoms. Patients who have had severe or more frequent episodes during this pregnancy or a previous pregnancy or have additional risk factors are recommended to have a vaginal delivery with a prophylactic plasma-derived C1-inh concentrate before delivery [63]. In addition, plasma-derived C1-inh should be accessible during delivery and hospitalization [63].

7. HAE in childhood

Episodes of angioedema and abdominal pain can begin in childhood; however, an accurate diagnosis is often delayed leading to the administration of inadequate or incorrect therapies and even to death [55, 67]. Moreover, life-threatening laryngeal edema can be the first clinical presentation [67, 68]. Therefore, it is crucial to scan the entire family, including children, in a newly diagnosed patient. In this way, the disease can be detected and serious angioedema attacks can be prevented through prophylactic or therapeutic modalities [55].

A consensus of treatment strategies in pediatric patients with HAE was reported in 2007 [69]. Afterwards, a German group covered the treatment options in pediatric patients and addressed the problem that previous consensus reports could not meet the needs of individual countries because of different approved drugs. Therefore, they suggested treatment strategies for German-speaking countries and pointed out that in every country physicians should consider the approved treatment options in their country before choosing an off-label drug approved in other countries [55].

For long-term prophylaxis, the only choice is plasma-derived C1-inh. Androgens should be avoided for long-term usage. If plasma-derived C1-inh is not available, danazol can be substituted for short-term prophylaxis [55]. Although the effectiveness of tranexamic acid is lower than the androgens, in children tranexamic acid can be used for long-term prophylaxis [55].

The drugs used in the management of HAE in children are shown in **Tables 2** and **3** [34].

8. Future promising interventions

Preventing angioedema episodes in HAE patients is still an important problem since there are limited options comprising oral-attenuated androgens, which have various side effects leading to dose limitations and plasma-derived C1-inh, which is administered intravenously and therefore not practical [70, 71]. Additionally, on-demand treatment of acute episodes has the risk of laryngeal angioedema and leads to a reduction in the quality of life since the angioedema attacks continue to occur [72–74]. Given these problems, new practical safe and effective treatment options to prevent acute episodes are necessary.

Avoralstat is a newly developed oral plasma kallikrein inhibitor for which studies are ongoing. In the recently published first in-human study, the authors observed that the amount of the drug sufficient to inhibit the plasma kallikrein (400 mg every 8 h) was well tolerated [75].

There is no curative treatment for HAE. Amerantunga et al. argued that HAE can be considered a metabolic liver disease and as in other metabolic liver disorders liver transplantation and hepatocyte transformation can be curative options [76, 77]. However, these treatments have surgical risks and need long-term immunosuppression [77]. They also asserted that although liver-based gene therapies are not practical, they can be the alternative curative options where a recombinant virus as a vector can infect the hepatocytes leading to the production of the targeted protein [77].

Another future concern is to prevent the development of HAE with prenatal genetic diagnosis before implantation occurs [78]. Although it seems to be reasonable, the strategy has some limitations. First of all, in some parents, the mutations causing the disease cannot be determined, and in one quarter of the patients, the disease is caused by de novo mutations. Furthermore, because of the hormonal stimulation during in vitro fertilization, it can possibly lead to angioedema attacks. Lastly, there is a risk of having mild influenced offspring [78]. Therefore, patients need intensive genetic counseling before such a therapy.

9. Conclusion

In summary, HAE is a rare life-threatening disease with highly variable clinical presentations. Physicians and the public are not familiar with the disease. There are still unknown features of the disease and delay in diagnosis or misdiagnosis leading to inaccurate treatment. It is, however, crucial to recognize the disease to prevent mortality and morbidity. Therefore, more comprehensive studies are needed to describe the disease, and social work is essential to increase the awareness.

Author details

Asli Gelincik* and Semra Demir

*Address all correspondence to: gelincik@istanbul.edu.tr

Department of Internal Medicine, Division of Immunology and Allergy, Istanbul Faculty of Medicine, Istanbul University, Istanbul, Turkey

References

[1] Longhurst H, Cicardi M. Hereditary angio-edema. Lancet 2012;379:474–81. DOI: 10.1016/S0140-6736(11)60935-5.

[2] Osler W. Hereditary angio-neurotic oedema. Am J Med Sci 1888;95:362–7.

[3] Donaldson VH, Evans RR. A biochemical abnormality in hereditary angioedema: absence of serum inhibitor of C1-esterase. Am J Med 1963;35:37–44.

[4] Rosen FS, Charache P, Pensky J, Donaldson VH. Hereditary angioneurotic edema: two genetic variants. Science 1965;148:957–8.

[5] Davis AE III. C1 inhibitor and hereditary angioneurotic edema. Annu Rev Immunol 1988;6:595–628.

[6] Binkley KE, Davis A, 3rd. Clinical, biochemical and genetic characterization of a novel estrogen-dependent inherited form of angioedema. J Allergy Clin Immunol 2000;106:546–50.

[7] Bork K, Barnstedt SE, Koch P, Traupe H. Hereditary angioedema with normal C1-inhibitor activity in women. Lancet 2000;356:213–7.

[8] Serrano C, Guilarte M, Tella R, et al. Oestrogen dependent hereditary angio-edema with normal C1 inhibitor: description of six new cases and review of pathogenic mechanisms and treatment. Allergy 2008;63:735–41.

[9] Gulbahar O, Gokmen NM. Hereditary angioedema. In: Buyukozturk S, editor. Allerjik Hastalıklara Pratik Yaklasım. 1st ed. Selen; 2014. pp. 201–217. ISBN: 978-605-64466-3-4.

[10] Zuraw BL, Christiansen SC. Hereditary Angioedema and Bradykinin-mediated Angioedema. In: Adkinson NF, Jr, Bochner BS, Burks AW, Busse WW, Holgate ST, Lemanske RF, Jr, O'Hehir RE, editors. Middleton's Allergy Principles and Practice. 8th ed. Elsevier; 2014. pp. 588–601. ISBN: 9780323085939.

[11] Zuraw BL. Hereditary angioedema: a current state-of-the art review, IV: short- and long-term treatment of hereditary angioedema: out with the old and in with the new? Ann Allergy Asthma Immunol 2008;100(Suppl 2):S13–12.

[12] Moore GP, Hurley WT, and Pace SA. Hereditary angioedema. Ann Emerg Med 1988; 17:1082–1086.

[13] Bork K, Hardt J, Witzke G. Fatal laryngeal attacks and mortality in hereditary angioedema due to C1-INH deficiency. J Allergy Clin Immunol 2012; 30:692–697. DOI: 10.1016/j.jaci.2012.05.055.

[14] Zuraw BL. Clinical practice. Hereditary angioedema. N Engl J Med 2008;359:1027–1036. DOI:10.1056/NEJMcp0803977.

[15] Bork K, Meng G, Staubach P, et al. Hereditary angioedema: new findings concerning symptoms, affected organs, and course. Am J Med 2006;119:267–274.

[16] Frank MM. Hereditary angioedema: the clinical syndrome and its management in the United States. Immunol Allergy Clin North Am 2006;26:653–668.

[17] Agastoni A, Cicardi M. Hereditary and acquired C1-inhibitor deficiency: biological and clinical characteristics in 235 patients. Medicine (Baltimore) 1992;71:206–215.

[18] Farkas MM, Varga L, Szeplaki G, et al. Management of hereditary in paediatric patients. Pediatrics 2007;120:713–722.

[19] Bork K, Staubach P, Eckardt AJ, et al. Symptoms, course, and complications of abdominal attacks in hereditary angioedema due to C1 inhibitor deficiency. Am J Gastroenterol 2006;101:619–627.

[20] Bowen T, Cicardi M, Bork K, et al. Hereditary angioedema: a current state-of-the art review, VII: Canadian Hungarian 2007 International consensus Algorithm for the diagnosis, therapy and management of Hereditary angioedema. Ann Allergy Asthma Immunol 2008;100(Suppl 2):S30–40.

[21] Zuraw BL, Bernstein JA, Lang DM, et al. A focused parameter update: Hereditary angioedema, acquired C1 inhibitor deficiency, and angiotensin-converting enzyme inhibitor-associated angioedema. J Allergy Clin Immunol 2013;131:1491–3. DOI:10.1016/j.jaci.2013.03.034.

[22] Agostoni A, Cicardi M, Cugno M, et al. Angioedema due to angiotensin-converting enzyme inhibitors. Immunopharmacology 1999;44:21–25.

[23] Frank MM. Effect of sex hormones on the complement related clinical disorder of hereditary angioedema. Arthritis Rheum 1979;22:1295–1299.

[24] Prematta MJ, Kemp JG, Gibbs JG, Mende C, Rhoads C, Craig TJ. Frequency, timing, and type of prodromal symptoms associated with hereditary angioedema attacks. Allergy Asthma Proc 2009;30:506–11. DOI: 10.2500/aap.2009.30.3279

[25] Davis AE III. New treatments addressing the pathophysiology of hereditary angioedema. Clin Mol Allergy 2008;6:2. DOI:10.1186/1476-7961-6-2.

[26] Kesim B, Uyguner ZO, Gelincik A, et al. The Turkish Hereditary Angioedema Pilot Study (TURHAPS): the first Turkish series of hereditary angioedema. Int Arch Allergy Immunol 2011;156(4):443–50. DOI: 10.1159/000323915.

[27] Kalmár L, Hegedüs T, Farkas H, Nagy M, Tordai A. HAEdb: a novel interactive, locus-specific mutation database for the C1 inhibitor gene. Hum Mutat 2005;25:1–5.

[28] Cichon S, Martin L, Hennies HC, et al. Increased activity of coagulation factor XII (Hageman factor) causes hereditary angioedema type III. Am J Hum Genet 2006; 79:1098–104.

[29] Bork K, Kleist R, Hardt J, Witzke G. Kallikrein-kinin system and fibrinolysis in hereditary angioedema due to factor XII gene mutation Thr309Lys. Blood Coagul Fibrinolysis 2009;20:325–32. DOI:10.1097/MBC.0b013e32832811f8.

[30] Bork K, Fischer B, Dewald G. Recurrent episodes of skin angioedema and severe attacks of abdominal pain induced by oral contraceptives or hormone replacement therapy. Am J Med 2003;114:294–298.

[31] Bygum A. Hereditary angioedema in Denmark: a nationwide survey. Br J Dermatol 2009;161:1153–1158. DOI: 10.1111/j.1365-2133.2009.09366.x

[32] Zanichelli A, Magerl M, Longhurst H, Fabian V, Maurer M. Hereditary angioedema with C1 inhibitor deficiency: delay in diagnosis in Europe. Allergy Asthma Clin Immunol 2013;9:29. DOI: 10.1186/1710-1492-9-29.

[33] Bork K. Hereditary angioedema with normal C1 inhibitor activity including hereditary angioedema with coagulation factor XII gene mutations. Immunol Allergy Clin North Am 2006;26:709–724.

[34] Lang DM, Aberer W, Bernstein JA, Chng HH, Sevciovic Grumach A, Hide M, et al. International consensus on hereditary and acquired angioedema. Ann Allergy Asthma Immunol 2012;109:395–402. DOI: 10.1016/j.anai.2012.10.008.

[35] Gulbahar O, Gelincik A, Sin A, Gulec M, Yılmaz M, Mete Gokmen N, et al. The working group of hereditary angioedema (TNSACI). Herediter anjiyoödem. Asthma Allergy Immunol 2010;8:125–138.

[36] Gompels MM, Lock RJ, Abinun M, et al: C1 inhibitor deficiency: consensus document. Clin Exp Immunol 2005;139:379–394.

[37] Xu YY, Buyantseva LV, Agarwal NS, et al. Update on treatment of hereditary angioedema. Clin Exp Allergy 2013;43(4):395–405. DOI: 10.1111/cea.12080.

[38] Zuraw B, Cicardi M, Levy RJ, et al. Recombinant human C1-inhibitor for the treatment of acute angioedema attacks in patients with hereditary angioedema. J Allergy Clin Immunol 2010;126(4):821–7. DOI:10.1016/j.jaci.2010.07.021

[39] Riedl MA, Levy RJ, Suez D, et al. Efficacy and safety of recombinant C1-inhibitor for the treatment of hereditary angioedema attacks: a North American open-label study. Ann Allergy Asthma Immunol 2013;110(4):295–9. DOI: 10.1016/j.anai.2013.02.007

[40] Moldovan D, Reshef A, Fabiani J, et al. Efficacy and safety of recombinant human C1-inhibitor for the treatment of attacks of hereditary angioedema: European open-label extension study. Clin Exp Allergy 2012;42(6):929–35. DOI: 10.1111/j.1365-2222.2012.03984.x.

[41] Riedl MA, Bernstein JA, Li H, et al. Recombinant human C1-esterase inhibitor relieves symptoms of hereditary angioedema attacks: phase 3, randomized, placebo-controlled trial. Ann Allergy Asthma Immunol 2014;112(2):163–9. DOI: 10.1016/j.anai.2013.12.004.

[42] Bork K, Bernstein JA, Machnig T, Craig TJ. Efficacy of different medical therapies for the treatment of acute laryngeal attacks of hereditary angioedema due to C1-esterase inhibitor deficiency. J Emerg Med 2016;50(4):567–80.e1. DOI: 10.1016/j.jemermed.2015.11.008.

[43] Bork K. Hereditary angioedema with normal C1 inhibitor activity including hereditary angioedema with coagulation factor XII gene mutations. Immunol Allergy Clin North Am 2006;26:709–724.

[44] Farkas H, Varga L. Ecallantide is a novel treatment for attacks of hereditary angioedema due to C1 inhibitor deficiency Clin Cosmet Investig Dermatol 2011;4:61–68. DOI: 10.2147/CCID.S10322.

[45] Duffey H, Firszt R. Management of acute attacks of hereditary angioedema: role of ecallantide. J Blood Med 2015;6:115–123. DOI:10.2147/JBM.S66825.

[46] Sheffer AL, MacGinnitie AJ, Campion M, et al. Outcomes after ecallantide treatment of laryngeal hereditary angioedema attacks. Ann Allergy Asthma Immunol 2013;110:184–188. DOI: 10.1016/j.anai.2012.12.007

[47] KALBITOR® (Ecallantide) Injection, for Subcutaneous Use [Prescribing Information] [Internet] Cambridge, MA: Dyax Corp; 2014. Available from:http://www.kalbitor.com/hcp/rems/pdf/KalbitorFullPrescribing-Information.pdf. [Accessed October 18, 2014].

[48] Greve J, Strassen U, Gorczyza M, Dominas N, Frahm UM, Mühlberg H, Wiednig M, Zampeli V, Magerl M. Prophylaxis in hereditary angioedema (HAE) with C1 inhibitor deficiency. J Deutsch Dermatol Ges 2016;14(3):266–75. DOI: 10.1111/ddg.12856.

[49] Gelfand JA, Sherins RJ, Alling DW, Frank MM. Treatment of hereditary angioedema with danazol. Reversal of clinical and biochemical abnormalities. N Engl J Med 1976;295:1444–8.

[50] Bork K, Bygum A, Hardt J. Benefits and risks of danazol in hereditary angioedema: a long term survey of 118 patients. Ann Allergy Asthma Immunol 2008;100:153–61. DOI: 10.1016/S1081-1206(10)60424-3.

[51] Cicardi M, Castelli R, Zingale LC, Agostoni A. Side effects of long-term prophylaxis with attenuated androgens in hereditary angioedema: comparison of treated and untreated patients. J Allergy Clin Immunol 1997;99:164–6.

[52] Szeplaki G, Varga L, Valentin S, et al. Adverse effects of danazol prophylaxis on the lipid profiles of patients with hereditary angioedema. J Allergy Clin Immunol 2005;115:864–9.

[53] Bork K, Pitton M, Harten P, Koch P. Hepatocellular adenomas in patients taking danazol for hereditary angioedema. Lancet 1990;353:1066–7.

[54] Farkas H, Varga L, Szeplaki G, Visy B, Harmat G, Bowen T. Management of hereditary angioedema in pediatric patients. Pediatrics 2007;120:e713–22.

[55] Wahn V, Aberer W, Eberl W, et al. Hereditary angioedema (HAE) in children and adolescents—a consensus on therapeutic strategies. Eur J Pediatr 2012;171(9):1339–48. DOI: 10.1007/s00431-012-1726-4.

[56] Cicardi M, Castelli R, Zingale LC, Agostoni A. Side effects of long term prophylaxis with attenuated androgens in hereditary angioedema: comparison of treated and untreated patients. J Allergy Clin Immunol 1997;99:194–6.

[57] Bowen T, Cicardi M, Farkas H, et al. 2010 international consensus algorithm for the diagnosis, therapy and management of hereditary angioedema. Allergy Asthma Clin Immunol 2010;6:24. DOI: 10.1186/1710-1492-6-24.

[58] Frank MM, Sergent JS, Kane MA, Alling DW. Epsilon aminocaproic acid therapy of hereditary angioneurotic edema. A double-blind study. N Engl J Med 1972;286:808–812.

[59] Sheffer AL, Austen KF, Rosen FS. Tranexamic acid therapy in hereditary angioneurotic edema. N Engl J Med 1972;287:452–454.

[60] Zanichelli A, Vachini R, Badini M, Penna V, Cicardi M. Standard care impact on angioedema because of hereditary C1 inhibitor deficiency: a 21-month prospective study in a cohort of 103 patients. Allergy 2011;66:192–196. DOI:10.1111/j.1398-9995.2010.02433.x.

[61] Reshef A, Moldovan D, Obtulowicz K, et al. Recombinant human C1 inhibitor for the prophylaxis of hereditary angioedema attacks: a pilot study. Allergy 2013;68(1):118–24. DOI:10.1111/all.12060.

[62] Gonzalez-Quevedo T, Larco JI, Marcos C, et al. Management of pregnancy and delivery in patients with hereditary due to C1 inhibitor deficiency. J Investig Allergol Clin Immunol 2016;26(3):161–167. DOI: 10.18176/jiaci.0037.

[63] Czaller I, Visy B, Csuka D, Füst G, Toth F, Farkas H. The natural history of hereditary angioedema and the impact of treatment with C1 inhibitor concentrate during pregnancy: a long term survey. Eur J Obstet Gynecol Reprod Biol 2010;152(1):44–9. DOI: 10.1016/j.ejogrb.2010.05.008.

[64] Chinniah N, Katelaris CH. Hereditary angioedema and pregnancy. Austr N Z J Obstet Gynaecol 2009;49(1):2–5. DOI:10.1111/j.1479-828X.2008.00945.x.

[65] Martinez-Saguer I, Rusicke E, Aygören-Pürsün E, Heller C, Klingebiel T, Kreuz W. Characterization of acute hereditary angioedema attacks during pregnancy and breast-feeding and their treatment with C1 inhibitor concentrate. Am J Obstet Gynecol 2010;203(2):131.e1–7. DOI:10.1016/j.ajog.2010.03.003.

[66] Bork K, Siedlecki K, Bosch S, et al. Asphyxiation by laryngeal edema in patients with hereditary angioedema. Mayo Clin Proc 2000;75:349–354.

[67] Bork K, Hardt J, Schicketanz KH, Ressel N. Clinical studies of sudden upper airway obstruction in patients with hereditary angioedema due to C1 esterase inhibitor deficiency. Arch Intern Med 2003;163:1229–1235.

[68] Boyle RJ, Nikpour M, Tang MLK. Hereditary angioedema in children: a management guideline. Pediatr Allergy Immunol 2005;16:288–294.

[69] Zuraw BL, Banerji A, Bernstein JA, et al. US Hereditary Angioedema Association Medical Advisory Board 2013 recommendations for the management of hereditary angioedema due to C1 inhibitor deficiency. J Allergy Clin Immunol Pract 2013;1:458–467. DOI: 10 1016/j.jaip.2013.07.002.

[70] Maurer M, Magerl M. Long-term prophylaxis of hereditary angioedema with androgen derivates: a critical appraisal and potential alternatives. J Dtsch Dermatol Ges 2011;9:99–107. DOI: 10.1111/j.1610-0387.2010.07546.x.

[71] Lumry WR, Castaldo AJ, Vernon MK, Blaustein MB, Wilson DA, Horn PT. The humanistic burden of hereditary angioedema: impact on health-related quality of life, productivity, and depression. Allergy Asthma Proc 2010;31:407–414. DOI:10.2500/aap.2010.31.3394.

[72] Caballero T, Aygoren-Pursun E, Bygum A, et al. The humanistic burden of hereditary angioedema: results from the Burden of Illness Study in Europe. Allergy Asthma Proc 2014;35:47–53. DOI: 10.2500/aap.2013.34.3685.

[73] Nordenfelt P, Dawson S, Wahlgren CF, Lindfors A, Mallbris L, Bjorkander J. Quantifying the burden of disease and perceived health state in patients with hereditary angioedema in Sweden. Allergy Asthma Proc 2014;35:185–190. DOI:10.2500/aap.2014.35.3738.

[74] Bork K, Hardt J, Witzke G. Fatal laryngeal attacks and mortality in hereditary angioedema due to C1-INH deficiency. J Allergy Clin Immunol 2012;130:692–69772. DOI: 10.1016/j.jaci.2012.05.055.

[75] Cornpropst M, Collis P, Collier J, et al. Safety, pharmacokinetics, and pharmacodynamics of avoralstat, an oral plasma kallikrein inhibitor: phase 1 study. Allergy 2016;71:1676–1683. DOI:10.1111/all.12930.

[76] Ameratunga R, Bartlett A, McCall J, Steele R, Woon ST, Katelaris CH. Hereditary angioedema as a metabolic liver disorder: novel therapeutic options and prospects for cure. Front Immunol. 2016 Nov 30;7:547. DOI:10.3389/fimmu.2016.00547

[77] Zarrinpar A, Busuttil R. Liver transplantation: past, present and future. Nat Rev Gastroenterol Hepatol 2013;10(7):434–40. DOI:10.1038/nrgastro.2013.88.

[78] Bautista-Llacer R, Alberola TM, Vendrell X, Fernandez E, Perez-Alonso M. Case report: first successful application of preimplantation genetic diagnosis for hereditary angioedema. Reprod Biomed Online 2010;21(5):658–62. DOI: 10.1016/j.rbmo.2010.05.016.

Chapter 12

Pathophysiology of Bradykinin-Mediated Angioedema: The Role of the Complement System

Jesús Jurado-Palomo and Teresa Caballero

Additional information is available at the end of the chapter

http://dx.doi.org/10.5772/67704

Abstract

The "complement system" is one of the effector pathways of the immune system against microorganisms and tumor cells. The complement system can be activated through three major pathways: classical, lectin, and alternative. The sequential activation through the generation of complex enzymes from inactive zymogens produces a cascade in which a capable enzyme generates a large number of active downstream molecules.

C1 inhibitor (C1-INH) is a serine protease inhibitor (serpin) that regulates the following closely interrelated proteolytic pathways: complement system, coagulation system, contact system, and fibrinolysis system. The absence or malfunction of C1-INH results in the presence of attacks of angioedema (AE) due to uncontrolled activation of the contact system, with the generation of bradykinin (BK), a vasoactive peptide released from high-molecular-weight kininogen (HMWK). Some drugs that inhibit the catabolism of BK have been implicated in the development of AE. These include angiotensin-converting enzyme inhibitors (ACEIs), dipeptidyl peptidase IV (DPP-IV) inhibitors, aminopeptidase P (APP) inhibitors, and neutral endopeptidase (NEP) inhibitors.

We describe in this chapter the biochemistry pathways implicated in the pathophysiology of bradykininergic angioedema (BK-AE) and the role of the complement system in the prototype of BK-AE, in hereditary angioedema with C1-INH deficiency (C1-INH-HAE), and also in acquired angioedema with C1-INH deficiency (C1-INH-AAE).

Keywords: acquired angioedema, aminopeptidase P, angioedema, angiotensin-converting enzyme, bradykinin, C1 inhibitor, carboxypeptidase, complement system, contact system, dipeptidyl peptidase-IV, endothelin-converting enzyme-1, factor XII, fibrinolysis system, hereditary angioedema, neutral endopeptidase

1. Introduction: definition of angioedema and differentiation between histaminergic and bradykininergic angioedema

The term "angioedema" (AE) is defined as localized and transient subcutaneous and/or submucosal swelling (which may affect the gastrointestinal, respiratory, or genitourinary tract) [1, 2]. It occurs when there is vasodilation with consequent increase in capillary permeability and extravasation of fluid into the interstitial space [2, 3].

A variety of inflammatory mediators have been described that can lead to this process, such as histamine, prostaglandins, leukotrienes, and bradykinin [4]. The most frequent type of AE is produced by histamine release, as a consequence of mast cell activation, and is called "histaminergic angioedema."

It includes allergic reactions, but also idiopathic AE in the context of chronic spontaneous urticaria [5]. Histaminergic AE can be associated to urticaria [6], is usually erythematous, warm, and pruritic, and is responsive to treatment with antihistamines [7]. The clinical expression of urticarial lesions is mainly a consequence of inflammation and edema of the upper dermis, whereas swellings are located in the deep dermis and even in the subcutaneous tissue.

Another important type of AE is produced by an increase in bradykinin (BK). This AE type is non-erythematous, non-pruritic, cold, non-responsive to antihistamines and urticaria is not associated [7]. This subgroup is known as bradykininergic angioedema (BK-AE).

2. Classification of bradykinin-mediated angioedema (BK-AE)

BK-AE comprises several entities (**Table 1**). In recent years, there has been a dramatic increase in knowledge about this condition, particularly on the role of BK as the "final common mediator." The Spanish Study Group for Angioedema due to C1-inhibitor deficiency was established in 2007 within the Committee of Immunology of the Spanish Society of Allergology and Clinical Immunology (SEAIC). However, such was the progress in the understanding of the pathophysiology of different types of BK-AE that this group's name quickly changed to "Spanish Study Group on Bradykinin-Induced Angioedema" (SGBA).

BK-AE is mainly classified into two subtypes depending on whether or not there is a functional deficiency of C1 esterase inhibitor, better known as C1 inhibitor (C1-INH) (**Table 1**) [8]. Another common way to classify BK-AE is hereditary angioedema (HAE) and acquired angioedema (AAE) [8]. There are two forms of AE with C1-INH deficiency, a hereditary form (C1-INH-HAE) and an acquired form (C1-INH-AAE).

Among the forms of AE with no functionally active C1-INH deficiency are hereditary angioedema with normal C1-INH (nC1-INH-HAE), with/without mutation in the *F12* gene that encodes coagulation factor XII (FXII-HAE/U-HAE) or acquired AE associated with drugs that inhibit the metabolic pathways of BK, angiotensin-converting enzyme inhibitors (ACEi-AAE).

http://dx.doi.org/10.5772/67704

Other drugs that inhibit the catabolism of BK have been implicated in the development of AE. These include dipeptidyl peptidase IV (DPP-IV) inhibitors, aminopeptidase P (APP) inhibitors, neutral endopeptidase (NEP) inhibitors, and others.

Along with progress in biochemical-molecular knowledge, much has been learned about the different pathophysiological mechanisms of the different types of AE. For example, the initial term "HAE type III or oestrogen-induced" has evolved into the term FXII-HAE due to the description in some of these patients of mutations in the *F12* gene. Another example would be the recognition of antihypertensives belonging to the group of ACE inhibitors (ACEIs) as producers of AE by increased BK, secondary to the inhibition of its catabolism. This has led to classifications over time by different groups. In order to agree on a common name for all types of AE "without papules" described so far, the HAE International Working Group (HAWK), under the sponsorship of the European Academy of Allergy and Clinical Immunology (EAACI), proposed a classification of AE without wheals as seen in **Figure 1** [7], with four types of AAE and three types of HAE.

Bradykinin (BK)-mediated angioedema (AE)	With verified C1-inhibitor protein deficiency	Hereditary (C1-INH-HAE)	Type I (C1-INH-HAE type I)
			Type II (C1-INH-HAE type II)
		Acquired (C1-INH-AAE)	
	No verified C1 inhibitor protein deficiency	Hereditary (related to estrogen) (HAE type III)	With known mutation of *F12* gene (FXII-HAE)
			Without known mutation of *F12* gene (U-HAE: HAE unknown)
		Acquired associated with angiotensin-converting enzyme (ACE) inhibitors (ACEis) (AAE-ACEi)	

Table 1. Classification of different types of bradykinin-mediated AE (modified from SGBA Consensus) [9].

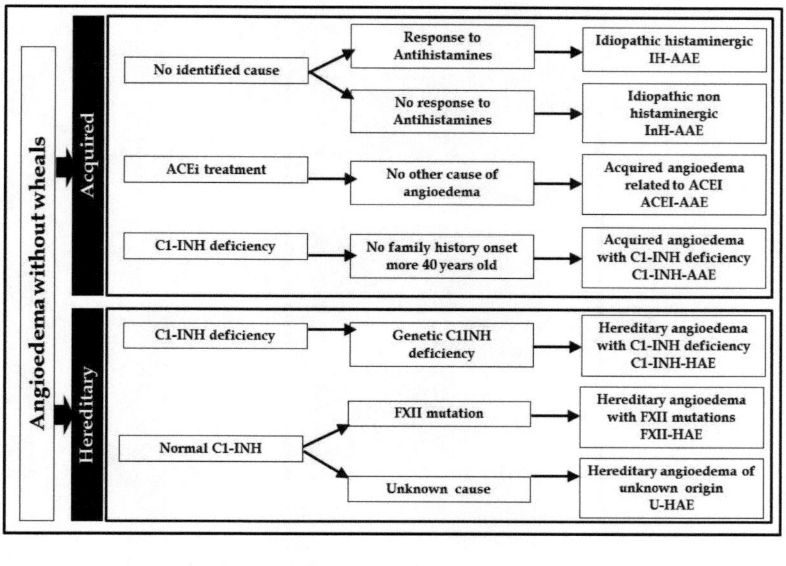

Figure 1. Classification of angioedema without wheals [7].

However, this classification has some limitations such as the noninclusion of AE caused by non-steroidal anti-inflammatory drugs (NSAIDs), which often occurs without associated urticaria [10]. These drugs act by inhibiting the enzyme cyclooxygenase in the metabolic pathways of arachidonic acid and increasing leukotrienes.

A classification of AE according to endotypes was proposed later [11]. In this classification, three subtypes of AE were included: (1) mast cell and basophil-driven AE, (2) bradykininergic AE, and (3) idiopathic AE [11]. It has the advantage that NSAIDs induced or exacerbated AE and allergic AE are both included within the mast cell and basophil-driven AE.

3. C1-inhibitor deficiency

C1-INH is a serine protease inhibitor (serpin) that regulates the following closely interrelated proteolytic pathways: complement system, coagulation system, contact system, and fibrinolysis system [12, 13] (**Figure 2**). It is also known as SERPING1, belongs to the SERPIN superfamily, and is mainly synthesized in hepatocytes [9].

First, C1-INH inhibits C1r, C1s, and mannose-binding-lectin-associated serine proteases (MASP1, MASP2) in the complement system. The inhibition of C1r and C1s is the function that gives name to this protein, "C1 inhibitor." The C1 fraction of complement, also known as C1 esterase, is the first protein of the complement system, and circulates in an inactive form. C1 esterase is activated during immunological processes, initiating the complement cascade and splitting off proteins from the classical pathway (C4 and C2) [9]. In patients with C1-INH deficiency, an increase in C1 esterase functioning produces decreased C2, C4 levels, the natural substrates of the complement C1s fraction, which diminish much more during AE attacks [9]. C3, the protein that follows C2 in the classical complement cascade, is usually normal in patients with C1-INH-HAE, since it is not controlled by C1-INH [9].

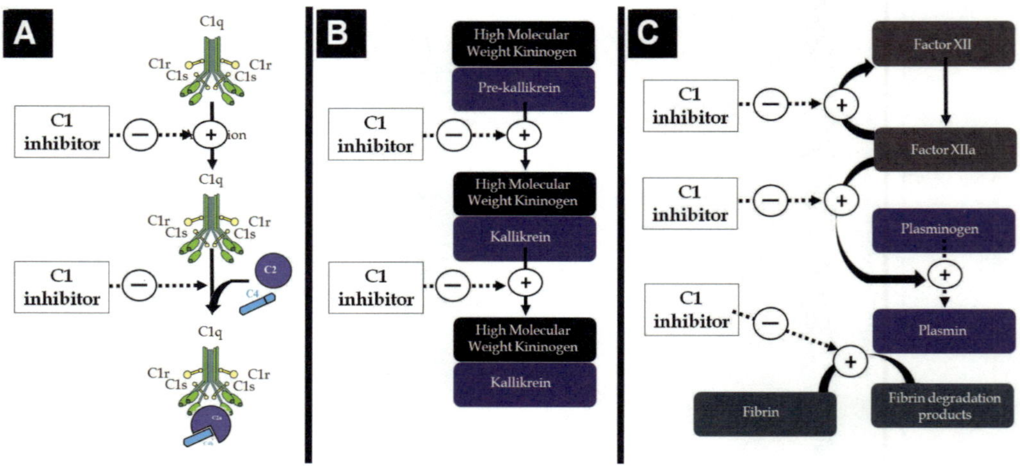

Figure 2. C1-INH regulates different pathways: (A) complement system, (B) contact system, and (C) fibrinolysis system.

Besides, C1-INH inhibits factor XI and thrombin in the coagulation system and tissue plasminogen activator and plasmin in the fibrinolytic system [9].

Finally, C1-INH also inhibits factor XII and kallikrein in the contact system, being the main inhibitor of the contact system and of BK formation [9]. This is the crucial action involved in AE development when C1-INH is lacking.

C1-INH deficiency can produce an activation of the four described cascades, with a final increase in BK. BK produces vascular hyperpermeability and edema formation [9].

C1-INH is the most potent inhibitor of the contact system and thus low C1-INH function can activate this system, with uncontrolled activation of FXII and increased formation of kallikrein. Kallikrein releases BK from high-molecular-weight kininogen (HMWK). The lack of C1-INH also produces an increase in plasmin through the activation of the fibrinolytic system. The split of BK from HMWK induced by kallikrein is facilitated by the presence of plasmin [9].

C1-INH is a glycoprotein with 478 amino acids. It is heavily glycosylated (approximately 30% by weight). Its apparent molecular weight on sodium dodecyl sulfate polyacrylamide gel electrophoresis (SDS-PAGE) is 104 kilodalton (kDa), but its calculated molecular weight is 76 kDa. It is formed by an N-terminal domain of 113 amino acids and a serpin domain of 365 amino acids [14].

The genetic study of *SERPING1* gene, which codes C1-INH, has identified more than 300 different mutations causing C1-INH-HAE [7].

There are classically two main types of AE due to C1-INH deficiency: hereditary (C1-INH-HAE) and acquired (C1-INH-AAE). In turn, two types of C1-INH-HAE [9] have been described; in patients with type I (85%) there is decreased antigenic C1-INH (consequently resulting in decreased functional activity); type II (15%) is characterized by normal C1-INH levels with decreased functional C1-INH (the molecule being dysfunctional) [9]. The acquired subtype is characterized by low levels of either antigenic and/or functional C1-INH, associated in most cases with B-cell lymphoproliferative disorders.

Hereditary or acquired deficiency of C1-INH is characterized by recurrent episodes of circumscribed, non-itchy AE in submucosal or subcutaneous locations. AE attacks can be triggered by estrogens, trauma, infection, or stress.

4. What is the complement system?

The "Complement System" is one of the effector pathways of the immune system against microorganisms and tumor cells, consisting of about 30 molecules, part of the complement factors enhance "inflammation" and "phagocytosis," producing lysis of cells and microorganisms. The sequential activation through the generation of complex enzymes from inactive zymogens produces a cascade in which a capable enzyme generates a large number of active downstream molecules. Very strict regulation of downstream activation processes can be expected to restrict such activation to the foci where it started, thereby preventing possible tissue damage [15, 16]. This set of molecules, those involved in the activation and the regulators (distinguishing between "triggers"—those able to bypass control systems—and "nontriggers"), is called the "complement system." The need for both "amplification" and "regulation" with strict control gives an idea of the complexity of the "Complement System."

5. Description of the complement system:

5.1. Alternative pathway of the "complement system"

We begin with the description of this pathway, which although referred to as "alternative" is phylogenetically older than the "classical pathway." It does not require the presence of antibodies (Abs) for activation, thus constituting an important defense in the early stages of infection, when there are no significant amounts of Ab synthesized. Continuously "at rest," it operates at a low level, and it is amplified in the presence of certain factors. So we can differentiate as follows:

(a) Alternative pathway "resting," "idle," or "pacemaker"

(1) In normal plasma conditions (absence of infection), the internal thioester bond of the C3 fraction is spontaneously hydrolyzed in a low ratio with a water molecule (H_2O) forming the complex C3(H_2O), also referred to as "C3i" ("tick-over" or "idle" activation) **(Figure 3)**.

(2) C3(H_2O) or "C3i": It binds to factor B, forming the C3(H_2O)B complex, also referred to as "C3iB." Factor B is equivalent to the C2 factor of the classical pathway detailed later.

(3) The D factor acting on the C3(H_2O)B complex, breaking fraction B and generating subproducts B1 and C3iBb.

(4) The C3iBb complex acts as a "C3 convertase" in fluid phase cleaving C3 into C3a and C3b*.

(5) The "C3b*" in fluid phase is hydrolyzed by water inactivating it. However, if by some chance the "C3b*" bonds covalently to an external surface ("recognition of the strange"), the "amplification of the alternative pathway" would occur. It is said that "C3b *"does not start this amplification within the body due to regulatory proteins that prevent it, such as the following:

a. Factor H binds to C3b*, attaching to the cytoplasmic membranes.

b. Factor I breaks the C3, displacing Factor H that returns intact to serum (would be ready to start its action again).

c. Factor I inactivates the free C3b bound to the cytoplasmic membrane itself (iC3b).

d. Factor I cleaves iC3b into C3c (small fragment in solution) and C3dg (inactive larger fragment bound to membrane).

http://dx.doi.org/10.5772/67704

(b) "Amplification" of the alternative pathway ("positive feedback loop")

(1) The "C3b*" binds covalently to an external surface ("recognition of the strange") that amplifies in such a way that many C3b molecules anchor **(Figure 3)**.

(2) The membrane-bound C3b binds to Factor B, forming the C3bB complex.

(3) Factor D (with serine protease activity) acts on C3bB, breaking the bound "B," releasing Ba and forming the active C3bBb complex.

(4) The C3bBb complex (with C3 convertase activity in Bb) is quickly dissociated, unless it is stabilized by binding to the host Factor P (also called "properdin"), forming the stable complex C3bBbP (the C3 convertase bound to alternative pathway membrane).

(5) The C3bBb complex produces rupture of numerous C3 molecules, whose C3b fragments bind near the same membrane-bound convertase.

(6) Such "feedback loop" is also activated by the C4b2a complex (C3 convertase) of the classical complement pathway.

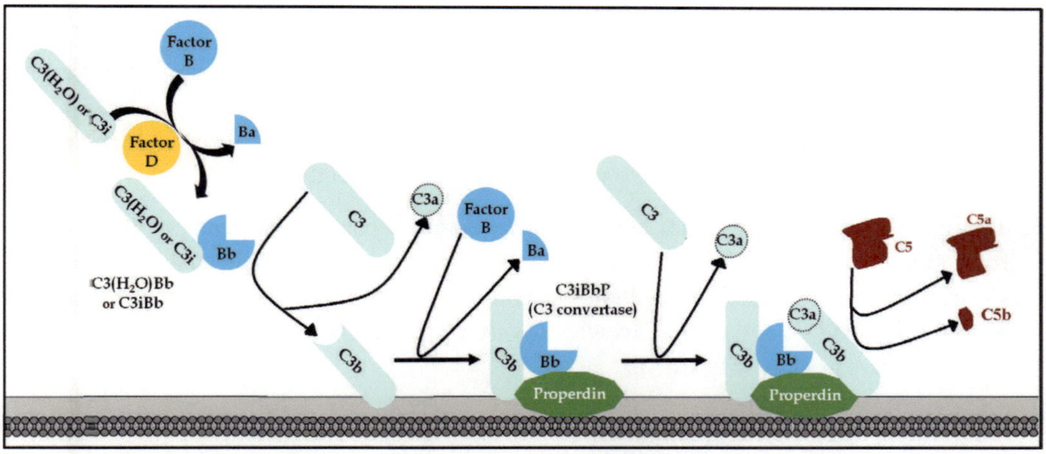

Figure 3. Alternative pathway activation of the complement system.

5.2. Classical pathway of the "complement system"

1. Activation of the complement system via the classical pathway requires the formation of the antigen-antibody complex (Ag-Ab), being the Ab of the subisotypes IgM, IgG1, IgG2 or IgG3. This interaction gives rise to conformational changes in the Fc fragment of immunoglobulin (Ig) generating an attachment site for the C1 fraction in the Cγ2 domain (constant part "2" of the IgG heavy chain) or the Cμ3 domain (constant part "3" of the IgM heavy chain).

2. The C1 fraction of the complement system is composed of five subunits: a "C1q" subunit (stem with six helical arms, three copies of a fundamental unit in a "Y," which in turn consists of two groups of three chains each together form a triple helix), two C1r subunits (arranged resting on the two arms of C1q), and two C1s subunits (arranged resting on the two arms of C1q, whose catalytic domains are arranged toward the center), stabilized by the Ca^{++} cation.

3. The C1q fraction is capable of binding to the Fc region of immunoglobulins provided they form part of immunocomplexes, such that

   a. It can bind to two or more IgG molecules through the Cγ2 domain when bound to the same Ag molecule (several IgG molecules are part of the same immunocomplex). IgG has only one binding site per molecule, so at least two IgG molecules are necessary to activate the complement system.

   b. It can bind to two or more Cμ3 domains of different pentametric IgM subunits. The free pentametric IgM is "flat" but on binding to Ag, the Fab arms adopt angles with the Fc portions (in the "staple" configuration), and then C1q can bind to different monomers of the same pentametric IgM. The IgM exposes more adhesion sites when it is in "staple" configuration, explaining why the IgM is more likely to activate the complement system.

4. Binding of multiple domains of the same C1 complex induces a conformational change that activates a "C1r" molecule by autocatalysis, which in turn activates the other "C1r" molecule. Once activated, the two "C1r" molecules exert hydrolysis of both C1s molecules to be activated, which is when they possess serine esterase activity.

5. The binding of several globular domains of the same C1 complex appears to induce a conformational change in this, which involves the activation of a C1r molecule by autocatalysis; in turn, this activated C1r activates the other C1r molecule. The two active molecules exert C1r hydrolysis of the two C1s, whereby they are activated: the two active C1s possess serine esterase activity (**Figure 4**).

6. C1s has two substrates: C2 and C4. Note at this point the regulatory role of the C1 inhibitor (C1-INH) molecule. A deficiency in this would result in uncontrolled activation of C1s acting on C2 and C4, with the consequent decrease in the levels of these two complement fractions that is apparent in patients with C1-INH-HAE:

   a. C1s bind to C4, producing two fragments: C4a (small fragment that diffuses into the plasma) and C4b (large fragment that binds to the membrane of the "target cell"). The C4a fraction is an "anaphylotoxin" that has importance later in this chain.

   b. C1 finds a binding site on C4b, and like everything around C1s is cleaved into two fragments: C2a (large fragment attached to C4b) and C2b (small fragment that diffuses into the plasma).

7. The C4bC2a complex (formed by the C2a and C4b bond) is called "C3 convertase" since it activates C3 in fragments C3a and C3b (**Figure 5**):

a. The intact C3 fraction has a very stable internal thioester bond between a cysteine and a glutamine (product of posttranslational modification) whose half-life is close to 600 h.

b. The C4bC2a complex catalyzes the proteolytic cleavage of C3 near the amino terminus of the α chain, with generation of the C3a and C3b fraction*.

c. The unstable C3b* component has the very unstable thioester bond, whose half-life is only 60 μs because it is susceptible to nucleophilic attack (this is due to the negative charge of sulfur (—S), while carbon remains as carbonyl group (—C⁺=O)).

d. A nearby nucleophilic group belonging to protein or cell surface carbohydrate reacts with the electrophilic C3b* carbonyl group, resulting in covalent bond (by —CO—O—) between the C3b and the cell surface.

e. The C3a fraction is an "anaphylotoxin" that will be important later in this chain.

f. Note that it is able to generate "tens" of C3b fragments, which is why this step is considered an "amplifier." However, not all "C3b" generated participate in the complement pathway since a portion diffuses into the plasma functioning as an "opsonizing agent."

8. The C3b fraction binds to C4bC2a, forming the C4b2aC3b complex, called "C5 convertase," as the portion of the C3b fraction of this complex binds to C5, hydrolyzing it into C5a and C5b. The C5a fraction is an "anaphylotoxin" that will be important later in this chain. The C5b fraction is a key element for the formation of the membrane "attack complex" (**Figure 3**). This step is already part of the "final common lytic pathway" between the "classical pathway" and "lectin pathway."

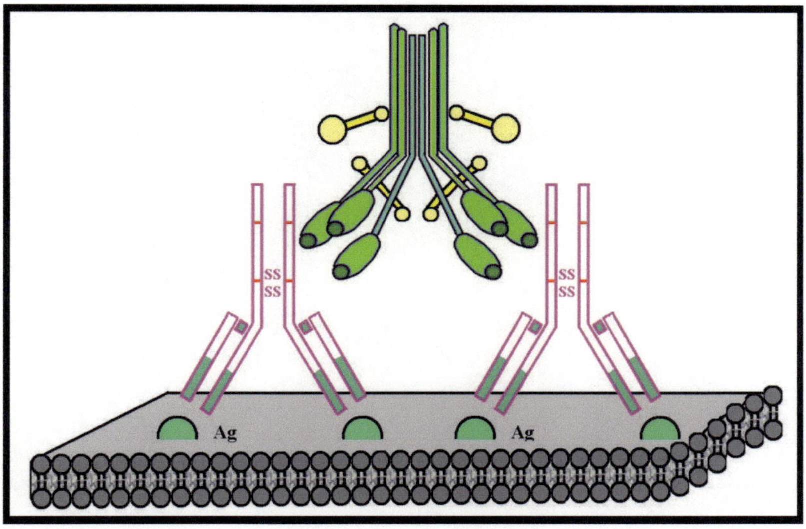

Figure 4. Classical pathway activation of the complement system, showing the binding of the C1q subunit to the Ig Fc, which is bound in turn to the cell membrane.

5.3. Lectin pathway of the "complement system"

The lectin pathway is a third way of complement system pathway activation different from the classical activation of C2 and C4 fractions (**Figure 6**). It starts with the action of the "mannan-binding protein" (MBP), which is structurally very similar to the C1q fraction (hexamers with 18 identical polypeptide chains coiled in groups of 3) and can bind two C1r subunits and two C1s subunits. However, it brings its own serine protease (called MASP) with 40% homology to C1r or C1s. MBP binds preferentially to the ends of mannose, fucose, and glucosamine of glycoproteins or polysaccharides present in the bacterial membrane. In a similar manner as described in the "classical pathway" with C1q2r2s complex, when MBP binds to carbohydrates it undergoes a conformational change, which in turn activates the serine protease (MASP). Activated MASP acts sequentially on C2 and C4 fractions to produce the "C3 convertase of the classical pathway."

MASP-1 has been recently shown to cleave bradykinin from HMWK [17] and its levels, together with the complex MASP1-C1-INH, have been related to disease severity in C1-INH-HAE [18].

5.4. Common final pathway of the "complement system"

The three activation pathways of the complement system (the classical pathway, the alternative pathway, and the lectin pathway) converge in a common final lytic pathway. The C5b, C6, C7, C8, and C9 fractions participate in the final lytic complement pathway and form a molecular structure known as "membrane attack complex" (MAC) (**Figure 7**).

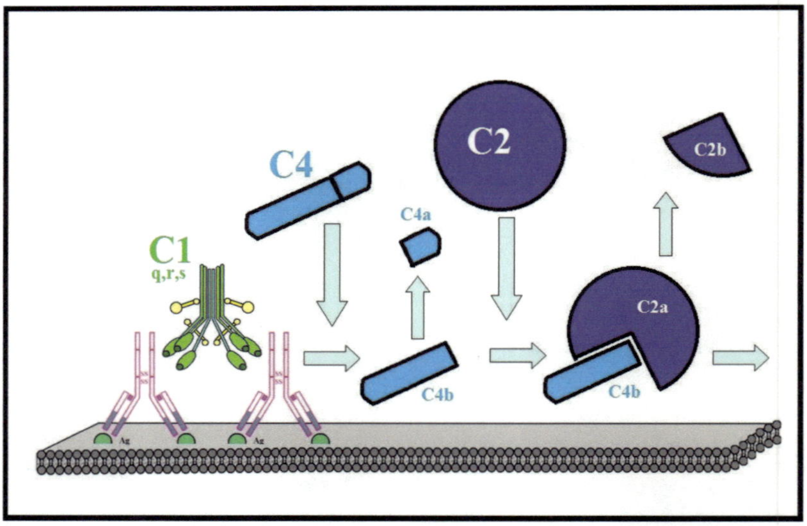

Figure 5. Classical pathway for the activation of the complement system, where the formation of the C1qrs complex until the formation of the C3b molecule can be observed.

http://dx.doi.org/10.5772/67704

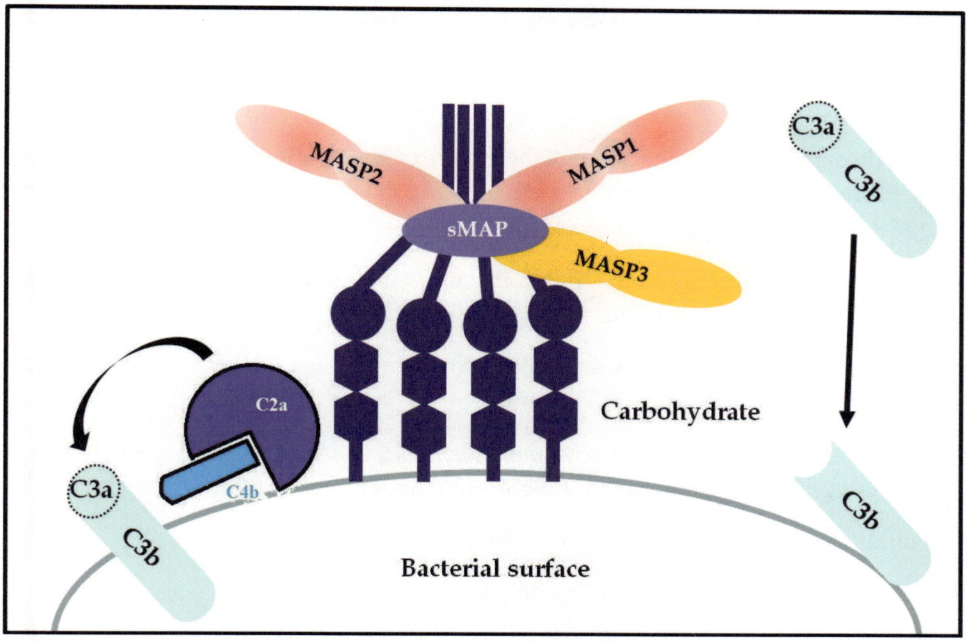

Figure 6. Lectin pathway for the activation of the complement system.

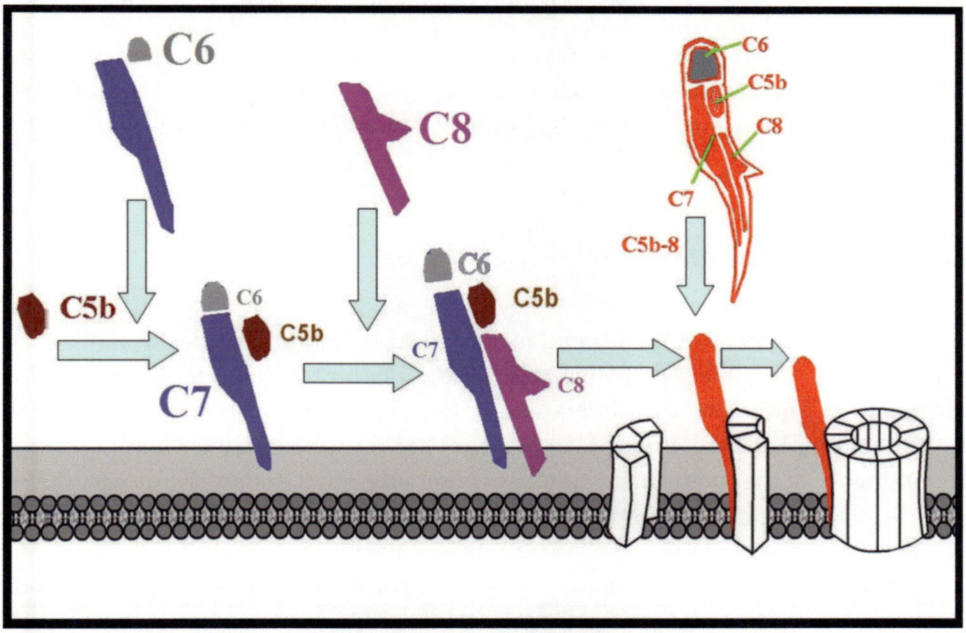

Figure 7. Major events in the lytic pathway cell membrane leading to the C9 polymerization and pore formation in the cell membrane.

MAC insertion into the cytoplasmic membrane causes an intercellular-extracellular communication pore with consequent ion exchange leading to cell death. The sequential steps are as follows:

1. As already mentioned, the final stage of the three activation pathways is common and consists in the formation of the "C5 convertase" that breaks the C5 fraction and triggers the appearance of the "membrane attack complex" (MAC). The steps at every pathway are as follows:
   a. The "classical pathway": the C4b2aC3b complex catalyzes the cleavage of C5 into C5a and C5b.
   b. The "lectin pathway": the C4b2aC3b complex catalyzes the cleavage of C5 into C5a and C5b.
   c. The "alternative pathway": a covalent attachment of a "new" C3b that forms part of the "C3 convertase," forming the C3bBb3b complex.
2. C5b binds to the cytoplasmic membrane hydrophilic region.
3. C5b binds to C6, forming the C5bC6 complex.
4. C5bC6 binds to C7, forming C5bC6-7 complex, which has already hydrophobic regions that are capable of penetrating into the inner section of the lipid bilayer.
5. C5bC6-7 binds to C8, forming C5bC6-7-8 complex, which is capable of forming a 10 Armstrong pore capable of destroying erythrocytes but not able to destroy nucleated cells.
6. C5bC6-7-8 binds to about 14 C9 units to form the C5b-C6-7-8-poli9 complex (or MAC), which is capable of forming a 70–100 Armstrong pore by contacting the intracellular with the extracellular medium with the subsequent ion and water exchange, leading to cell death.

6. Complement disorders

Complement disorders have been traditionally linked to immunodeficiency and associated with severe or frequent infections. More recently, complement has been recognized for its role in inflammation, autoimmune disorders, and vision loss [19]. The identification of hereditary and acquired complement deficiencies in humans has led to a better understanding of the biologic importance of the complement system in immunity and autoimmune disease (**Table 2**).

Complement protein	Gene (chromosome)	Effects of deficiency (commonly associated infections)
C1q	1p36.12 (A, B, and C chains)	Immune-complex disease Meningitis, pneumonia, sepsis (*Streptococcus pneumoniae, Neisseria meningitidis*)
C1r	12p13.31	Meningitis, pneumonia, sepsis (encapsulated bacteria)

Complement protein	Gene (chromosome)	Effects of deficiency (commonly associated infections)
C1s	12p13.31	Meningitis, pneumonia, sepsis (encapsulated bacteria)
C1-INH	11q11-q13.1	C1-INH-HAE
C2	6p21.33	Immune-complex disease Meningitis, osteomyelitis, pneumonia, sepsis (*Staphylococcus aureus, Streptococcus pneumoniae, Neisseria meningitidis*)
C3	19p13.3	Respiratory tract infections (*Haemophilus influenzae, Streptococcus pneumoniae, Streptococcus pyogenes, Neisseria meningitidis*)
C4	6p21.33 (Rodgers blood group and Chido blood group)	Immune-complex disease Meningitis, pneumonia, sepsis (encapsulated bacteria)
C5	9q33.2	SLE-like symptoms Meningitis, sepsis (*Neisseria meningitidis*)
C6	5p13.1	SLE-like symptoms MPGN Meningitis, sepsis (*Neisseria meningitidis*)
C7	5p13.1	Scleroderma, rheumatoid arthritis, and an SLE-like syndrome Meningitis, sepsis (*Neisseria meningitidis*)
C8	1p32.2 (alpha chain) 1p32.2 (beta chain) 9q34.3 (gamma chain)	Meningitis, sepsis (*Neisseria meningitidis*)
C9	5p13.1	Meningitis, sepsis (*Neisseria meningitidis*)
Factor D	19p13.3	Meningitis (*Neisseria meningitidis*)
Factor H	1q31.3	Recurrent pyogenic infections (*Haemophilus influenzae, Streptococcus pneumoniae, Neisseria meningitidis*)
Factor I	4q25	Recurrent pyogenic infections (*Haemophilus influenzae, Streptococcus pneumoniae, Neisseria meningitidis*)
Factor P (properdin)	Xp11.23	Meningitis (*Neisseria meningitidis*)
MBL (or MBP)	10q11.2-q21	Respiratory tract infections
MASP2	1p36.22	Respiratory tract infections
CD59 (or MAC-IP, MAC-IP, protectin)	11p13	Autoimmune-like conditions including paroxysmal nocturnal hemoglobinuria
DAF (or CD55)	1q32.2	Autoimmune-like conditions including paroxysmal nocturnal hemoglobinuria

C1-INH-HAE = hereditary angioedema with C1 inhibitor deficiency; CD59 = cluster of differentiation 59; MAC-inhibitory protein (MAC-IP), membrane inhibitor of reactive lysis (MIRL) or protectin; DAF = complement decay-accelerating factor; MASP2 = manna-binding lectin serine protease 2 (also called mannan-binding protein-associated serine protease 2); MBL = mannose-binding lectin (also called mannose-binding protein or mannan-binding protein (MBP); MPGN = membranoproliferative glomerulonephropathy; SLE = systemic lupus erythematous.

Table 2. Clinical significance of complement deficiencies [20–24].

7. Classification of angioedema due to functionally active C1 esterase inhibitor protein (C1 inhibitor) deficiency

Functionally active C1-INH deficiency can be hereditary or acquired. The hereditary form is a primary immunodeficiency [25] and is the most common genetic defect of the complement system [26]. The absence or malfunction of C1-INH results in the presence of attacks of AE (subcutaneous or mucosal swelling) due to uncontrolled activation of the contact system, with the generation of bradykinin, a vasoactive peptide released from HMWK [9].

7.1. Hereditary angioedema

C1-INH-HAE is a genetic autosomal dominant disease characterized by a deficiency of the functionally active C1 esterase inhibitor (C1 inhibitor) protein. Initially, it was believed that it affected one individual per 10,000–150,000 people, but being a rare disease it makes an estimate of prevalence difficult to pinpoint [27]. It could affect around 2000–3000 people in the USA [28]. There is a register of patients in Spain where the minimum prevalence is 1.09 per 100,000 inhabitants [29], while another register in Denmark describes a prevalence rate of 1.41 per 100,000 inhabitants [30]. The highest published prevalence is in Norway with 1.75 per 100,000 inhabitants [31]. Delays in diagnosis (an average of 13.1 years in the Spanish study) [29] along with the possibility of misdiagnosis and lack of recognition of the disease may mean that the true prevalence may be higher than estimates suggest. To date, no studies have shown differences in prevalence between ethnic groups.

Two phenotypic variants were described [32, 33]. *Type I* (HAE-I) is the most common (85%), characterized by a quantitative decrease of C1-INH, which results in a decrease in functional activity; *type II* (HAE-II) (15%) is characterized by normal or elevated levels of dysfunctional C1-INH. In both cases, the defect is transmitted as an autosomal dominant form, although with different genetic alterations. There is another estrogen-dependent hereditary AE variant in which both levels and function of C1-INH are normal and which has been called HAE *type III* [34, 35].

7.2. Acquired angioedema

C1-INH-AAE is biochemically characterized by low C1-INH concentrations and/or functions and no evidence of heredity. It is mainly associated with B cell lymphoproliferative disorders and occasionally with autoimmune, neoplastic, or infectious diseases [14]. Initially, it was classified into two types: type I, with most patients having an associated B cell line malignancy; type II, there were anti-C1-INH autoantibodies that interfered with C1-INH functional activity [36]. C1-INH production is normal or slightly increased. In many patients with type I, the paraproteinemia or M component actually behaves as an anti-C1-INH autoantibody, so some authors such as Cicardi suggest that the distinction between types I and II may be artificial [37].

Acquired C1-INH deficiency is characterized by the activation of the classical complement pathway and accelerated catabolism of C1-INH and the activation of the contact system [9]. This results in low C4 and C2 levels and normal C3 levels in plasma. C1q levels are frequently very low in C1-INH-AAE and this feature is frequently used to differentiate the acquired from the hereditary form of C1-INH deficiency [14].

8. Bradykinin as common final mediator of "bradykininergic" angioedema

8.1. Formation of bradykinin

BK is a linear nonapeptide (with sequence Arg1-Pro2-Pro3-Gly4-Phe5-Ser6-Pro7-Phe8-Arg9) produced endogenously in humans and other mammals as a result of the proteolytic activity of kallikrein on kininogens [38, 39].

Kallikreins belong to serine proteases and fall into two groups: tissue and plasma kallikreins. Within the tissue kallikreins, a family of 15 proteins is true kallikrein (hk1) and prostate-specific antigen (PSA or hk3) [39–41]. Plasma kallikrein is involved in processes that initiate coagulation especially during the activation phase due to contact with negatively charged surfaces. The plasma and tissue kallikreins release vasoactive peptides known as kinins implicated in biological processes such as the relaxation of vascular smooth muscle (hypotension), increased vascular permeability, smooth muscle contraction of the bronchial tree, and pain [39–41]. This peptide family produces BK release due to plasma kallikrein action on the HMWK, while it also releases Lys-bradykinin (Lys-BK) by the action of tissue kallikrein hk1 on low-molecular-weight kininogen (LMWK) [39–41] (**Figure 8**).

8.2. Other forms of angioedema with activation of the contact system

HAE *type III*, described in 2000 by two independent research groups [35, 42], has been also named as hereditary angioedema with normal C1-INH (nC1-INH-HAE) [7]. A subgroup of patients with nC1-INH-HAE (approximately 30%) has a mutation in exon 9 of *F12* gene [7] and this type of AE is known as FXII-HAE [7]. The rest have not known mutation and are known as unknown-HAE (U-HAE) [7].

FXII is a protease involved in the activation of the coagulation and contact systems and these mutations found in *F12* gene in patients with FXII-HAE have been shown to produce hyperactivability of coagulation factor FXII, with the consequent activation of the contact system [43].

8.3. Inhibition of bradykinin-metabolizing enzymes

Once produced, kinins are rapidly metabolized by metallopeptidases: neutral endopeptidase (NEP), angiotensin-converting enzyme (ACE), dipeptidyl peptidase-IV (DPP-IV), aminopeptidase P (APP), carboxypeptidases (CPN, CPM), and endothelin-converting enzyme-1 (ECE-1). Dendorfer et al. [44] described the metabolic pathways of BK degradation in murine models. In human plasma, BK is cleaved on the Pro7-Phe8 and Phe8-Arg9 bonds by the action of the two largest kininases: ACE and CPN [45]. Besides, in the 1960s it was reported that carboxypeptidase A cleaved the Pro7-Phe8 bond [46], while carboxypeptidase B cleaved the

Phe8-Arg9 bond [46]. Generally, carboxypeptidases remove Arg9 (carboxyl terminus) from the kinin molecule. Although NEP plays an important role in the kidney and epithelium, unlike ACE it barely exerts its action in plasma. APP cleaves BK in the Arg1-Pro2 bond [47]. NEP and ACE cleave BK at the Pro7-Phe8 bond (releasing the dipeptide Phe8-Arg9) [48]; NEP further cleaves the Gly4-Phe5 bond and ACE in the Phe5-Ser6 bond [48].

The following drug classes can cause acute AE by inhibition of the BK-metabolizing pathway (**Figure 8**):

- ACE (EC 3.4.15.1) inhibitors: lisinopril, captopril, enalapril, and ramipril.
- DPP-IV (EC 3.4.14.5) inhibitors: sitagliptin, vildagliptin, saxagliptin, alogliptin, and linagliptin.
- APP (EC 3.4.11.9) inhibitors: apstatin [49].
- CPN and CPM inhibitors.
- NEP, also known as neprilysin (EC 3.4.24.11) inhibitor: SQ29072 [50], SCH39370 [51], candoxatrilat [52], phosphoramidon [53], BP102 [54], and ecadotril [55].
- ECE-1 (EC 3.4.24.71) inhibitor: CGS35066 [56].
- Dual inhibitor of NEP and ACE: omapatrilat [57], fasidotril [58], sampatrilat [59], and mixanpril [60].
- Dual inhibitor of NEP and ECE-1: SLV-306 [61], S-17162 [62], CGS 26303 [63, 64], CGS 26393 [65], CGS 31447 [66], WS 75624B [67], B-90063 [68], CGS 34226 [69], and CGS 34043 [70].
- Triple inhibitor of ECE-1, NEP, and ACE: CGS 35601 [71–73] and CGS 37808 [74].

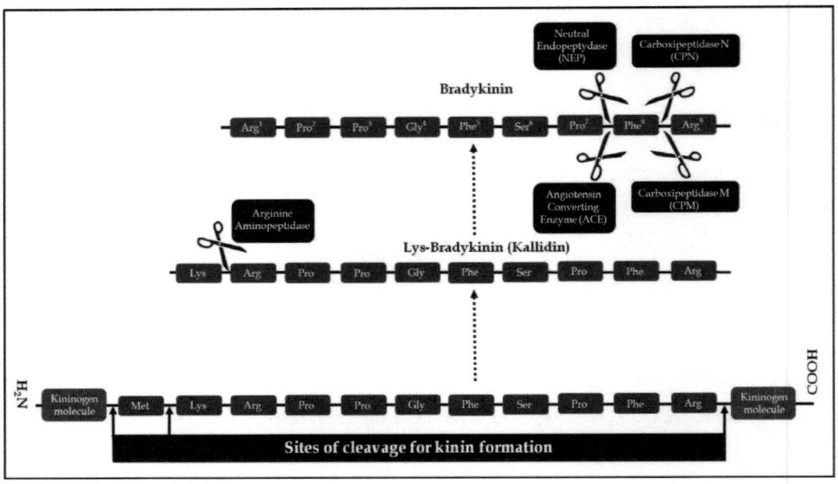

Figure 8. Formation of kinins in plasma and tissues. Each kinin is formed from kininogen by the action of a different enzyme.

http://dx.doi.org/10.5772/67704

8.4. Bradykinin receptor ligands

The biological effects of kinins involve the activation of specific receptors on the surface of the target cell. At least two different kinin receptors are known [75, 76]: BK receptor B1 (bradykinin receptor B1, also known as BDKRB1, B1R, BKR1, B1BKR, BKB1R, and BRADYB1) [77], which is coded in region 14q32.1-q32.2, and BK receptor B2 (bradykinin receptor B2, also known as BDKRB2, B2R, BK2, BK-2, BKR2, and BRB2) [78], which is coded in region 14q32.1-q32.2.

BKR1 binds and is activated by des-[Arg9]-bradykinin (DBK) and des-[Arg9]-Lys-bradykinin (Lys-BK), formed by the action of carboxypeptidases on Lys-BK and BK, respectively [79].

BKR1 is expressed in low amounts on normal physiological conditions in smooth muscle of blood vessels being regulated additively by inflammation [75, 79]. During stressful situations (trauma, tissue pressure, or inflammation with increase of IL1β or TNFα) [80, 81], the effects on BKR1 can predominate.

On the contrary, BKR2 binds selectively with BK and kallidin, mediating most of the effects of the contact system activation in the absence of inflammation.

Antagonists have been developed for both types of receptors, such as des-[Arg9]-bradykinin-Leu8 for BKR1 and HOE140 (icatibant acetate) for BKR2 [82]. Icatibant acetate has been shown to be effective for the treatment of acute AE attacks in C1-INH-HAE [7, 8, 83].

In summary, most of the biological effects of kinins are mediated by BKR2 and under conditions of inflammation or tissue damage there is induction of BKR1 [84] (**Figure 9**).

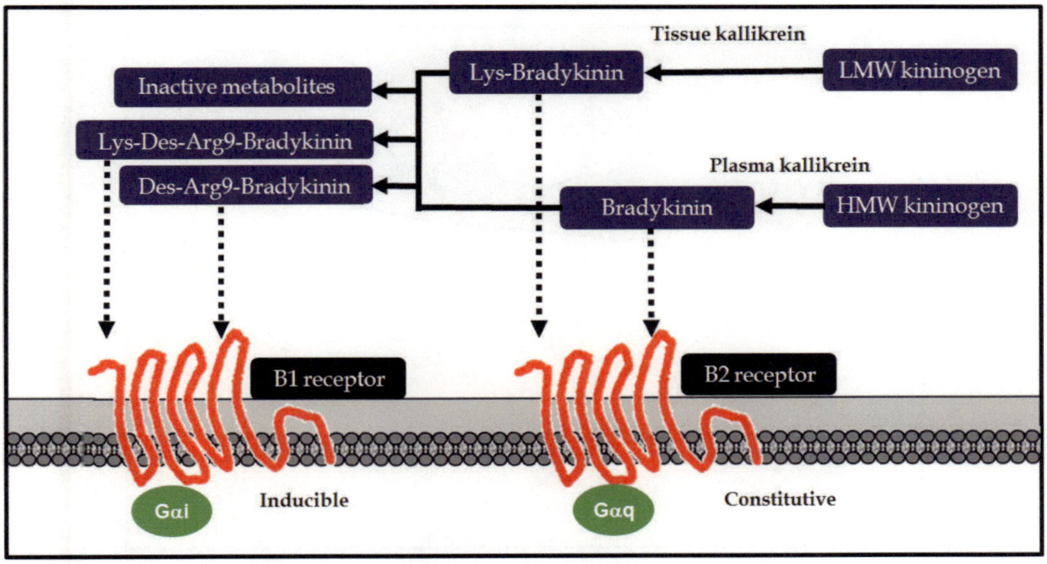

Figure 9. Bradykinin receptor ligands.

Both receptors belong to the superfamily of receptors that have seven transmembrane domains coupled to G proteins, differing both in primary structure, expression, and regulation of their tissue distribution [85, 86].

Two types of G protein-coupled receptors have been found that bind to BK mediating its response in pathophysiological conditions. To summarize, there are stimulatory G proteins (Gs and Gq) and inhibitory G proteins (Gi). Gs binds to GTP and activates adenylate cyclase, increasing the amount of intracellular cAMP. Gi binds to GTP and inactivates adenylate cyclase, indirectly reducing the amount of intracellular cAMP. Gq binds to GTP and activates PLC, increasing the amount of DAG, IP, and intracellular Ca^{++}. Transduction pathways stimulated by kinins have been extensively investigated in endothelial cells, where BKR1 interacts with Gq and Gi proteins, using the same signaling pathways as BKR2 (**Figure 10**).

BKR2 binds to G proteins and activates phospholipases A_2 and C. The kinin-induced increase in phospholipase C (PLC) causes it to act on their specific substrate, phosphatidylinositol biphosphate (PIP2), hydrolyzing it generating the two metabolites: inositol triphosphate (IP_3) and diacylglycerol (DAG). IP3 binds to a specific receptor (IP3R) in the endoplasmic reticulum facilitating the release of intracellular Ca^{++}. IP3, possibly together with its metabolite, IP4, can regulate calcium channels of the plasma membrane allowing the entry of extracellular calcium into the cell [87, 88]. The other metabolite of PIP2 hydrolysis, DAG, is responsible for the activation of protein kinase C (PKC) [89, 90]. PKC consists of one polypeptide chain with two functional domains: (a) a hydrophobic domain for binding to the cell membrane and (b) a hydrophilic domain, which possesses catalytic function. PKC at cellular rest is found in an inactive form in the cytosol, but once stimulated by DAG together with Ca^{++} ions it translocates to the cell membrane to exert its function of protein kinase in serine and threonine

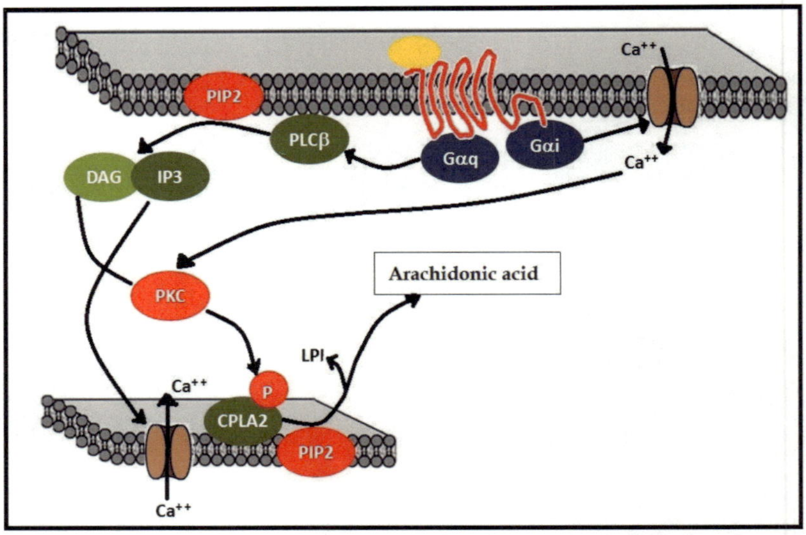

Figure 10. Bradykinin receptors and G-protein–coupled receptor-signaling pathway.

amino acids. BK has been shown to activate a Ca^{++}-dependent PKC and PKC not dependent on this ion, as well as atypical isoforms [91]. The stimulation of phospholipase A_2 (PLA_2) releases arachidonic acid from membrane phospholipids [92], which can be metabolized in the form of powerful inflammatory mediators.

In addition, BKR2 transitorily promotes phosphorylation of tyrosine from tyrosine kinases such as MAP kinase ("mitogen-activated protein kinase"), as well as the activation of the JAK/STAT pathway. Activated BKR2 interacts directly with nitric oxide synthase (NOS) resulting in nitric oxide (NO) [93].

9. Conclusions

C1-INH-HAE is a rare inherited disorder, characterized by recurrent AE attacks in various regions of the body. C1-INH-AAE is an acquired disease usually due to the presence of anti-C1-INH autoantibodies. The lack of C1-INH leads to inappropriate activation of the kallikrein-kinin system and release of BK, a vasoactive mediator.

nC1-INH-HAE is another inherited form of AE, with no C1-INH deficiency, but a probable increase in BK formation due to mutation in exon 9 of *F12* gene with subsequent hyper-activability.

BK (common final mediator of BK-AE) is a linear nonapeptide (with sequence Arg1-Pro2-Pro3-Gly4-Phe5-Ser6-Pro7-Phe8-Arg9) produced endogenously in humans and other mammals as a result of the proteolytic activity of kallikrein on kininogens.

Some drugs that inhibit the catabolism of BK have been implicated in the development of AE. These include ACEIs, DPP-IV inhibitors, APP inhibitors, and NEP inhibitors.

Author details

Jesús Jurado-Palomo[1,2]* and Teresa Caballero[2,3,4]

*Address all correspondence to: h72jupaj@yahoo.es

1 Department of Allergology, Nuestra Señora del Prado University General Hospital, Talavera de la Reina, Spain

2 Spanish Study Group on Bradykinin-Induced Angioedema (SGBA), Spanish Society of Allergology and Clinical Immunology (SEAIC), Madrid, Spain

3 Department of Allergology, Hospital La Paz Health Research Institute (IdiPAZ), Madrid, Spain

4 Biomedical Research Network on Rare Diseases, CIBERER (U754), Madrid, Spain

References

[1] Jaiganesh T, Wiese M, Hollingsworth J, Hughan C, Kamara M, Wood P, et al. Acute angioedema: recognition and management in the emergency department. Eur J Emerg Med. 2013;20:10–7.

[2] Grigoriadou S, Longhurst HJ. Clinical immunology review series: an approach to the patient with angio-oedema. Clin Exp Immunol. 2009;155:367–77.

[3] Bork K. Angioedema. Immunol Allergy Clin N Am. 2014;34:23–31.

[4] Kaplan AP, Greaves MW. Angioedema. J Am Acad Dermatol. 2005;53:373–88.

[5] Powell RJ, Leech SC, Till S, Huber PA, Nasser SM, Clark AT; British Society for Allergy and Clinical Immunology. BSACI guideline for the management of chronic urticaria and angioedema. Clin Exp Allergy. 2015;45:547–65.

[6] Kaplan AP. Clinical practice. Chronic urticaria and angioedema. N Engl J Med. 2002;346:175–9.

[7] Cicardi M, Aberer W, Banerji A, Bas M, Bernstein JA, Bork K, et al. Classification, diagnosis, and approach to treatment for angioedema: consensus report from the Hereditary Angioedema International Working Group. Allergy. 2014;69:602–16.

[8] Caballero T, Baeza ML, Cabañas R, Campos A, Cimbollek S, Gómez-Traseira C, et al. Consensus statement on the diagnosis, management, and treatment of angioedema mediated by bradykinin. Part II. Treatment, follow-up, and special situations. J Investig Allergol Clin Immunol. 2011;21:422–41; quiz 442–3. Review. Erratum in: J Investig Allergol Clin Immunol. 2012;22:3 p following 153.

[9] Caballero T, Baeza ML, Cabañas R, Campos A, Cimbollek S, Gómez-Traseira C, et al. Consensus statement on the diagnosis, management, and treatment of angioedema mediated by bradykinin. Part I. Classification, epidemiology, pathophysiology, genetics, clinical symptoms, and diagnosis. J Investig Allergol Clin Immunol. 2011;21(5):333–47; quiz follow 347. Review. Erratum in: J Investig Allergol Clin Immunol. 2012;22(2):3 p following 153.

[10] Prieto-García A, Marcos C, Caballero T; Spanish Group for Study of Bradykinin-Mediated Angioedema. Classification of angioedema without wheals. Ann Allergy Asthma Immunol. 2016;116:177.

[11] Giavina-Bianchi P, Aun MV, Motta AA, Kalil J, Castells M. Classification of angioedema by endotypes. Clin Exp Allergy. 2015;45:1142–43.

[12] Cugno M, Zanichelli A, Foieni F, Caccia S, Cicardi M. C1-inhibitor deficiency and angio-edema: molecular mechanisms and clinical progress. Trends Mol Med. 2009;15:69–78.

[13] Kaplan AP, Ghebrehiwet B. The plasma bradykinin forming pathways and its interrelationships with complement. Mol Immunol. 2010;47:2161–9.

[14] Agostoni A, Aygören-Pürsün E, Binkley KE, Blanch A, Bork K, Bouillet L, et al. Hereditary and acquired angioedema: Problems and progress: Proceedings of the third C1 esterase Inhibitor deficiency workshop and beyond. J Allergy Clin Immunol. 2004;114:S51–131.

[15] Peña J. Immune system. Chapter 1. Immunology (3rd edition, ISBN: 84-368-1213-1). Ed. Jose Peña. Ed Pirámide (Grupo Anaya). 1998. pp. 33–46.

[16] García-Olivares E, Alonso A, Peña J. Complement system. Chapter 13. Immunology (3rd edition, ISBN: 84-368-1213-1). Ed. Jose Peña. Ed Pirámide (Grupo Anaya). 1998.pp. 225–38.

[17] Dobó J, Major B, Kékesi KA, Szabó I, Megyeri M, Hajela K, Juhász G, Závodszky P, Gál P. Cleavage of kininogen and subsequent bradykinin release by the complement component: mannose-binding lectin-associated serine protease (MASP)-1. PLoS One 2011;6:e20036.

[18] Hansen CB, Csuka D, Munthe-Fog L, Varga L, Farkas H, Hansen KM, Koch C, Skjødt K, Garred P, Skjoedt MO. The levels of the lectin pathway serine protease MASP-1 and its complex formation with C1 inhibitor are linked to the severity of hereditary angioedema. J Immunol. 2015;195:3596–604.

[19] Frazer-Abel A, Sepiashvili L, Mbughuni MM, Willrich MA. Overview of laboratory testing and clinical presentations of complement deficiencies and dysregulation. Adv Clin Chem. 2016;77:1–75.

[20] Pettigrew HD, Teuber SS, Gershwin ME. Clinical significance of complement deficiencies. Ann N Y Acad Sci. 2009;1173; 108–23.

[21] Nesargikar PN, Spiller B, Chavez R. The complement system: history, pathways, cascade and inhibitors. Eur J Microbiol Immunol (Bp). 2012;2:103–111.

[22] Prohászka Z, Nilsson B, Frazer-Abel A, Kirschfink M. Complement analysis 2016: Clinical indications, laboratory diagnostics and quality control. Immunobiology. 2016;221:1247–51.

[23] Audemard-Verger A, Descloux E, Ponard D, Deroux A, Fantin B, Fieschi C, et al. Infections revealing complement deficiency in adults. Medicine. 2016;95:e3548.

[24] Gene Family: Complement system. URL disponible en: http://www.genenames.org/cgi-bin/genefamilies/set/492

[25] Notarangelo L, Casanova JL, Fischer A, Puck J, Rosen F, Seger R, et al. Primary immunodeficiency diseases: An update. J Allergy Clin Immunol. 2004; 114: 677–87.

[26] Carreer FMJ. The C1 inhibitor deficiency. A review. Eur J Clin Chem Clin Biochem. 1992; 30: 793–807.

[27] Lunn ML, Santos CB, Craig TJ. Is there a need for clinical guidelines in the United States for the diagnosis of hereditary angioedema and the screening of family members of affected patients? Ann Allergy Asthma Immunol. 2010;104:211–4.

[28] Zuraw BL. Hereditary angioedema: a current state-of-the art review, IV: short- and long-term treatment of hereditary angioedema: out with the old and in with the new? Ann Allergy Asthma Immunol. 2008;100(Suppl 2):S13–8.

[29] Roche O, Blanch A, Caballero T, Sastre N, Callejo D, López-Trascasa M. Hereditary angioedema due to C1 inhibitor deficiency: patient registry and approach to the prevalence in Spain. Ann Allergy Asthma Immunol. 2005;94:498–503.

[30] Bygum A. Hereditary angio-oedema in Denmark. A nationwide survey. Br J Dermatol. 2009;161:1153–8,

[31] Stray-Pedersen A, Abrahamsen TG, Frøland SS. Primary immunodeficiency diseases in Norway. J Clin Immunol. 2000;20:477–85.

[32] Rosen FS, Charche P, Pensky J, Donaldson V. Hereditary angioneurotic edema. Two genetic variants. Science. 1965; 148: 957–8.

[33] Rosen FS, Alper CA, Pensky J, Klemperer MR, Donaldson VH. Genetically determined heterogeneity of the C1 esterase inhibitor in patients with hereditary angioneurotic edema. J Clin Invest. 1971; 50: 2143–9.

[34] Bork K, Barnstedt SE, Koch P, Traupe H. Hereditary angioedema with normal C1 inhibitor activity in women. Lancet. 2000; 356;213–7.

[35] Binkley K, Davis A 3rd. Clinical, biochemical and genetic characterization of a novel estrogen-dependent inherited form of angioedema. J Allergy Clin Immunol. 2000; 106: 546–50.

[36] Orfan NA, Kolski GB. Angioedema and C1 inhibitor deficiency. Ann Allergy. 1992; 69: 167–74.

[37] Cicardi M, Beretta A, Colombo M, Gioffré D, Cugno M, Agostoni A. Relevance of lymphoproliferative disorders and of anti-C1 inhibitor autoantibodies in acquired angiooedema. Clin Exp Immunol. 1996; 106: 475–80.

[38] Elliot DF. Structure of bradykinin. Biochem Pharmacol. 1962;10:25–8.

[39] Bhoola KD, Figueroa CD, Worthy K. Bioregulation of kinins: kallikreins, kininogens, and kininases. Pharmacol Rev. 1992;44:1–80.

[40] Blais C, Mareau F, Rouleau J-L, Adam A. The kallikrein-kininogen-kinin system: lessons from the quantification of endogenous kinins. Peptides. 2000;21:1903–40.

[41] Leeb-Lundberg FML, Marceu F, Müller-Esterl W, Pettibone DJ, Zuraw BL. Classification of the kinin receptor family: from molecular mechanism to pathophysiological consequences. Pharmacol Rev. 2005;57:27–77.

[42] Bork K, Barnstedt SE, Koch P, Traupe H. Hereditary angioedema with normal C1 inhibitor activity in women. Lancet. 2000; 356;213–7.

[43] de Maat S, Björkqvist J, Suffritti C, Wiesenekker CP, Nagtegaal W, Koekman A, et al. Plasmin is a natural trigger for bradykinin production in patients with hereditary angioedema with factor XII mutations. J Allergy Clin Immunol. 2016;138:1414–1423.e9.

[44] Dendorfer A, Wolfrum S, Wagemann M, Qadri F, Dominiak P. Pathways of bradykinin degradation in blood and plasma of normotensive and hypertensive rats. Am J Physiol Heart Circ Physiol. 2001;280:H2182–8.

[45] Sheikh IA, Kaplan AP. Mechanism of digestion of bradykinin and lysyl bradykinin (kallidin) in human serum. Role of carboxypeptidase, angiotensin-converting enzyme and determination of final degradation products. Biochem Pharmacol. 1989;38:993–1000.

[46] Greenbaum LM, Yamafuji K. The in vitro inactivation and formation of plasma kinins by spleen cathepsins. Br J Pharmacol Chemother. 1966;27:230–8.

[47] Sidorowicz W, Szechiński J, Canizaro PC, Běhal FJ. Cleavage of the Arg1-Pro2 bond of bradykinin by a human lung peptidase: isolation, characterization, and inhibition by several beta-lactam antibiotics. Proc Soc Exp Biol Med. 1984;175:503–9.

[48] Gafford JT, Skidgel RA, Erdos EG, Hersh LB. Human kidney "enkephalinase" a neutral metalloendopeptidase that cleaves active peptides. Biochemistry. 1983;22:3265–71.

[49] Prechel MM, Orawski AT, Maggiora LL, Simmons WH. Effect of a new aminopeptidase P inhibitor, apstatin, on bradykinin degradation in the rat lung. J Pharmacol Exp Ther. 1995;275:1136–42.

[50] Seymour AA, Norman JA, Asaad MM, Fennell SA, Swerdel JN, Little DK, Dorso CR. Renal and depressor effects of SQ 29,072, a neutral endopeptidase inhibitor, in conscious hypertensive rats. J Cardiovasc Pharmacol. 1990;16:163–72.

[51] Charles CJ, Espiner EA, Richards AM, Sybertz EJ. Endopeptidase inhibition in angiotensin-induced hypertension. Effect of SCH 39370 in sheep. Hypertension. 1995;26:89–94.

[52] McDowell G, Nicholls DP. The endopeptidase inhibitor, candoxatril, and its therapeutic potential in the treatment of chronic cardiac failure in man. Expert Opin Investig Drugs. 1999;8:79–84.

[53] Oefner C, D'Arcy A, Hennig M, Winkler FK, Dale GE. Structure of human neutral endopeptidase (Neprilysin) complexed with phosphoramidon. J Mol Biol. 200018;296:341–9.

[54] Nakajima S, Majima M, Ito H, Hayashi I, Yajima Y, Katori M. Effects of a neutral endopeptidase inhibitor, BP102, on the development of deoxycorticosterone acetate-salt hypertension in kininogen-deficient Brown Norway Katholiek rats. Int J Tissue React. 1998;20:45–56.

[55] Nawarskas J, Rajan V, Frishman WH. Vasopeptidase inhibitors, neutral endopeptidase inhibitors, and dual inhibitors of angiotensin-converting enzyme and neutral endopeptidase. Heart Disease. 2001;3: 378–85.

[56] Trapani AJ, Beil ME, Bruseo CW, De Lombaert S, Jeng AY. Pharmacological properties of CGS 35066, a potent and selective endothelin-converting enzyme inhibitor, in conscious rats. J Cardiovasc Pharmacol. 2000;36(5 Suppl 1):S40–3.

[57] Zanchi A, Maillard M, Burnier M. Recent clinical trials with omapatrilat: new developments. Curr Hypertens Rep. 2003;5:346–52.

[58] Laurent S, Boutouyrie P, Azizi M, Marie C, Gros C, Schwartz JC, Lecomte JM, Bralet J. Antihypertensive effects of fasidotril, a dual inhibitor of neprilysin and angiotensin-converting enzyme, in rats and humans. Hypertension. 2000;35:1148–53.

[59] Maki T, Nasa Y, Tanonaka K, Takahashi M, Takeo S. Beneficial effects of sampatrilat, a novel vasopeptidase inhibitor, on cardiac remodeling and function of rats with chronic heart failure following left coronary artery ligation. J Pharmacol Exp Ther. 2003;305:97–105.

[60] Fournié-Zaluski MC, Gonzalez W, Turcaud S, Pham I, Roques BP, Michel JB. Dual inhibition of angiotensin-converting enzyme and neutral endopeptidase by the orally active inhibitor mixanpril: a potential therapeutic approach in hypertension. Proc Natl Acad Sci U S A. 1994;91:4072–6.

[61] Thöne-Reinke C, Simon K, Richter CM, Godes M, Neumayer HH, Thormählen D, et al. Inhibition of both neutral endopeptidase and endothelin-converting enzyme by SLV306 reduces proteinuria and urinary albumin excretion in diabetic rats. J Cardiovasc Pharmacol. 2004;44(Suppl.1):S76–9.

[62] Descombes JJ, Mennecier P, Versluys D, Barou V, de Nanteuil G, Laubie M, et al. S 17162 is a novel selective inhibitor of big ET-1 responses in the rat. J Cardiovasc Pharmacol. 1995;26(Suppl.3):S61–4.

[63] Sorokin A, Kohan DE. Physiology and pathology of endothelin-1 in renal mesangium. Am J Physiol Renal Physiol. 2003;285:F579–F589.

[64] Feldman DL, Mogelesky TC, Chou M, Jeng AY. Attenuation of puromycin aminonucleoside-induced glomerular lesions in rats by CGS 26303, a dual neutral endopeptidase/endothelin-converting enzyme inhibitor. J Cardiovasc Pharmacol. 2000;36:S342–S345.

[65] Pelletier S, Battistini B, Jeng AY, Sirois P. Effects of dual endothelin-converting enzyme/neutral endopeptidase inhibitors, CGS 26303 and CGS 26393, on lipopolysaccharide or interleukin-1 beta-stimulated release of endothelin from guinea pig tracheal epithelial cells. J Cardiovasc Pharmacol. 1998;31(Suppl.1):S10–2.

[66] Shetty SS, Savage P, DelGrande D, De Lombaert S, Jeng AY. Characterization of CGS 31447, a potent and nonpeptidic endothelin-converting enzyme inhibitor. J Cardiovasc Pharmacol. 1998;31(Suppl.1):S68–70.

[67] Tsurumi Y, Ueda H, Hayashi K, Takase S, Nishikawa M, Kiyoto S, et al. WS75624 A and B, new endothelin converting enzyme inhibitors isolated from Saccharothrix sp. No. 75624. I. Taxonomy, fermentation, isolation, physico-chemical properties and biological activities. J Antibiot (Tokyo). 1995;48:1066–72.

[68] Takaishi S, Tuchiya N, Sato A, Negishi T, Takamatsu Y, Matsushita Y, et al. B-90063, a novel endothelin converting enzyme inhibitor isolated from a new marine bacterium, Blastobacter sp. SANK 71894. J Antibiot (Tokyo). 1998;51:805–15.

[69] Jeng AY, Savage P, Beil ME, Bruseo CW, Hoyer D, Fink CA, et al. CGS 34226, a thiol-based dual inhibitor of endothelin converting enzyme-1 and neutral endopeptidase 24.11. Clin Sci (Lond). 2002;103(Suppl.48):98S–101S.

[70] Trapani AJ, De Lombaert S, Beil ME, Bruseo CW, Savage P, Chou M, et al. CGS 34043: a non-peptidic, potent and long-acting dual inhibitor of endothelin converting enzyme-1 and neutral endopeptidase 24.11. Life Sci. 2000;67:1025–33.

[71] Inguimbert N, Poras H, Teffo F, Beslot F, Selkti M, Tomas A, et al. N-[2-(indan-1-yl)-3-mercapto-propionyl] amino acids as highly potent inhibitors of the three vasopeptidases (NEP, ACE, ECE): in vitro and in vivo activities. Bioorg Med Chem Lett. 2002;12:2001–5.

[72] Daull P, Blouin A, Beaudoin M, Gadbois S, Belleville K, Cayer J, et al. The hemodynamic and metabolic profiles of Zucker diabetic fatty rats treated with a single molecule triple vasopeptidase inhibitor, CGS 35601. Exp Biol Med (Maywood). 2006;231:824–9.

[73] Battistini B, Daull P, Jeng AY. CGS 35601, a triple inhibitor of angiotensin converting enzyme, neutral endopeptidase and endothelin converting enzyme. Cardiovasc Drug Rev. 2005;23:317–30.

[74] Trapani AJ, Beil ME, Bruseo CW, Savage P, Firooznia F, Jeng AY. CGS 35601 and its orally active prodrug CGS 37808 as triple inhibitors of endothelin-converting enzyme-1, neutral endopeptidase 24.11, and angiotensin-converting enzyme. J Cardiovasc Pharmacol. 2004;44:S211–S215.

[75] Regoli D, Barabé J. Pharmacology of bradykinin and related kinins. Pharmacol Rev. 1980,32:1–46.

[76] Regoli D, Rhaleb NE, Drapeau G, Dion S. Kinin receptor subtypes. J Cardiovasc Pharmacol. 1990;15Suppl 6:S30–8.

[77] Menke JG, Borkowski JA, Bierilo KK, MacNeil T, Derrick AW, Schneck KA, et al. Expression cloning of a human B1 bradykinin receptor. J Biol Chem. 1994;269: 21583–6.

[78] Hess JF, Borkowski JA, Young GS, Strader CD, Ransom RW. Cloning and pharmacological characterization of a human bradykinin (BK-2) receptor. Biochem Biophys Res Commun. 1992;184:260–8.

[79] Dray A, Perkins M. Bradykinin and inflammatory pain. Trends Neurosci. 1993;16:99–104.

[80] Sardi SP, Ares VR, Errasti AE, Rothlin RP. Bradykinin B1 receptors in human umbilical vein: pharmacological evidence of up-regulation, and induction by interleukin-1 beta. Eur J Pharmacol. 1998; 358:221–7.

[81] Haddad EB, Fox AJ, Rousell J, Burgess G, McIntyre P, Barnes PJ et al. Post-transcriptional regulation of bradykinin B1 and B2 receptor gene expression in human lung fibroblasts by tumor necrosis factor-alpha: modulation by dexamethasone. Mol Pharmacol. 2000;57:1123–3.

[82] Wirth K, Hock FJ, Albus U, Linz W, Alpermann HG, Anagnostopoulos H et al. Hoe 140: a new potent and long acting bradykinin antagonist: in vivo studies. Br J Pharmacol. 1991;102:774–7.

[83] Cicardi M, Bork K, Caballero T, Craig T, Li HH, Longhurst H, et al. Evidence-based recommendations for the therapeutic management of angioedema owing to hereditary

C1 inhibitor deficiency: consensus report of an International Working Group. Allergy. 2012;67:147–57.

[84] Marceau F, Hess JF, Bachvarov DR. The B1 receptors for kinins. Pharmacol Rev. 1998;50:357–86.

[85] McEachern AE, Shelton ER, Bhakta S, Obernolte R, Bach C, Zuppan P, et al. Expression cloning of a rat B2 bradykinin receptor. Proc Natl Acad Sci USA. 1991;88:7724–8.

[86] Menke JG, Borkowski JA, Bierilo KK, MacNeil T, Derrick AW, Schneck KA et al. Expression cloning of a human B1 bradykinin receptor. J Biol Chem. 1994;269:21583–6.

[87] Allan D, Michell RH. Elevation of intracellular calcium ion concentration provokes production of 1,2-diacylglycerol and phosphatidate in human erythrocytes. Biochem Soc Trans. 1975;3:751–2.

[88] Allan D, Michell RH. A calcium-activated polyphosphoinositide phosphodiesterase in the plasma membrane of human and rabbit erythrocytes. Biochim Biophys Acta. 1978;508:277–86.

[89] Kuo JF, Shoji M, Girard PR, Mazzei GJ, Turner RS, Su HD. Phospholipid/calcium-dependent protein kinase (protein kinase C) system: a major site of bioregulation. Adv Enzyme Regul. 1986;25:387–400.

[90] Nelsestuen GL, Bazzi MD. Activation and regulation of protein kinase C enzymes. J Bioenerg Biomembr. 1991;23:43–61.

[91] Tippmer S, Quitterer U, Kolm V, Faussner A, Roscher A, Mosthaf L, Müller-Esterl W, Häring H. Bradykinin induces translocation of the protein kinase C isoforms alpha, epsilon, and zeta. Eur J Biochem. 1994 1;225:297–304.

[92] Schrör K. Role of prostaglandins in the cardiovascular effects of bradykinin and angiotensin-converting inhibitors. J Cardopvasc Pharmacol. 1992;20 Suppl.9:S68–73.

[93] Australian Public Assessment Report for icatibant. AusPAR Firazyr Icatibant Shire Australia Pty Ltd SM- 2009-00755-3-2. 07/06/2010. URL disponible en: http://www.tga.gov.au/pdf/auspar/auspar-firazyr.pdf (accessed on 13 December 2013)

Chapter 13

Short-Term Prophylaxis in Odontostomatological, Maxillofacial and ENT Procedures in Patients with Hereditary Angioedema Due to C1-Inhibitor Deficiency

Jesús Jurado-Palomo and Teresa Caballero

Additional information is available at the end of the chapter

http://dx.doi.org/10.5772/67713

Abstract

Oestrogens, trauma, infections or stress has been described as triggers for angioedema (AE) attacks in patients with hereditary angioedema due to C1-inhibitor deficiency (C1-INH-HAE). Microtrauma can precipitate the onset of acute AE attacks, and thus, dental-oral procedures carry a high risk of triggering them and also an increased risk of death from asphyxiation due to the AE location. In the past, without proper specific treatment, the overall mortality after dental surgery in patients with C1-INH-HAE was up to 30–40%. Some dental-oral, medical and/or surgical procedures are susceptible to receive "short-term prophylaxis" (STP) in order to reduce the risk of AE. We describe the published case reports of dental-oral, maxillofacial and ear, nose and throat (ENT) procedures in patients with C1-INH-HAE. Different consensus algorithms and clinical guidelines have been published for managing dental-oral, maxillofacial and otolaryngological procedures (DOMFOPs) and will be reviewed below. Based on the clinical experience of the Department of Allergology of the University Hospital La Paz (Madrid) and the University General Hospital Nuestra Señora del Prado (Talavera de la Reina), these algorithms have been updated and modified. We advise to classify procedures according to the risk of producing AE as minor, intermediate and major risks.

Keywords: algorithm, angioedema, antifibrinolytic agents, attenuated androgens, bradykinin, C1 inhibitor, dental-oral procedures, dental surgery, ecallantide, hereditary angioedema, icatibant acetate, recombinant human C1 inhibitor, plasma-derived human C1-inhibitor concentrate, short-term prophylaxis, solvent/detergent-treated plasma, treatment

1. Introduction

Hereditary angioedema due to C1-inhibitor deficiency (C1-INH-HAE) is a genetic autosomal dominant disease characterized by a deficiency of the functionally active C1 esterase inhibitor (C1-INH) protein [1]. This deficiency results in an excess of bradykinin (BK), which increases vascular permeability and produces angioedema (AE) [1].

The minimum prevalence of C1-INH-HAE is 1.09 per 100,000 inhabitants in Spain [2], 1.41 per 100,000 inhabitants in Denmark [3], 1.54 per 100,000 inhabitants in Italy [4] and 1.75 per 100,000 inhabitants in Norway [5].

Other forms of BK-mediated AE are: acquired angioedema due to C1-INH deficiency (C1-INH-AAE), hereditary angioedema with normal C1-INH (C1-INH-nC1-INH), with/without mutation in the F12 gene that encodes Factor XII coagulation (HAE-FXII/HAE-D) and acquired angioedema associated with angiotensin converting enzyme inhibitors (ACEi) (AAE-ACEi). ACEis are drugs that inhibit the metabolic pathways of BK and thus produce an increase in BK. Other drugs that inhibit BK catabolism have been implicated in the development of AE. These include dipeptidyl peptidase IV (DPPIV) inhibitors, aminopeptidase P (APP) inhibitors, neutral endopeptidase (NEP) inhibitors and others. In this chapter, we will focus on C1-INH-HAE.

2. The importance of cervicofacial anatomical location in C1-INH-HAE angioedema attacks

Oestrogens, trauma, infections or stress has been described as triggers for AE attacks in 21 patients with C1-INH-HAE [6]. Microtrauma can precipitate the onset of acute AE attacks, and thus, dental-oral procedures carry a high risk of triggering them and also an increased risk of death from asphyxiation due to the AE location [7]. Treatment with adrenaline, antihistamines or glucocorticoids is not effective in this type of BK-mediated AE [8].

In the past, without proper specific treatment, overall mortality after dental surgery in patients with C1-INH-HAE was up to 30–40% [9–12]. Some dental-oral, medical and/or surgical procedures are susceptible to receive "short-term prophylaxis" (STP) (also called "pre-procedural prophylaxis") [8, 13–15] in order to reduce the risk of AE. Such prophylaxis in patients with C1-INH-HAE usually consists of introducing oral antifibrinolytics or attenuated androgens (AAs) or administering intravenous pdhC1INH before the procedure [8, 13]. There are currently two brands of pdhC1INH available: Berinert® (CSL-Behring, Marburg, Germany) and Cinryze® (Shire-HGT, Zug, Switzerland). Since upper airway AE can cause death from asphyxiation [13, 16], adequate monitoring of upper airway permeability is imperative, so that appropriate emergency treatment (endotracheal intubation and/or tracheotomy) is performed if the upper airway is threatened despite medical treatment [8, 17]. Nevertheless, the availability of specific drugs for the treatment of acute AE attacks and of plasma-derived human C1-inhibitor concentrates (pdhC1INH) (Berinert®, CSL Behring, Marburg, Germany and Cinryze®, Shire HGT, Zug, Switzerland) for STP, together with the increased awareness of

http://dx.doi.org/10.5772/67713

pre-procedural prophylaxis, has reduced the prevalence of upper airway respiratory AE and death from asphyxiation after dental procedures [15, 18].

3. Management of dental-oral, maxillofacial and ENT procedures (DOMFOPs) in patients with C1-INH-HAE

A review of published case reports of dental-oral, maxillofacial and ear, nose and throat (ENT) procedures in patients with C1-INH-HAE is shown in **Table 1**.

Case report (gender/age)	STP			AE type	AE development	Reference
	pdhC1INH	FFP	Icatibant acetate			
One male and five females aged between 18 and 64 y.o.	N.AD	2 Units	N.AD	C1-INH-HAE type I	None	Jaffe et al. [19]
Three males aged between 41 and 56 y.o.	N.AD	N.AD	N.AD	C1-INH-HAE	None	Heft and Flynn [20]
One female of 28 y.o.	N.AD	N.AD	N.AD	C1-INH-HAE	None	
One female of 45 y.o.	N.AD	1 Unit	N.AD	C1-INH-HAE type I	None	Delfino et al. [21]
One female of 22 y.o.	N.AD	2 Units	N.AD	C1-INH-HAE type I	None	Allbright and Taylor [22]
One male of 20 y.o.	N.AD	N.AD	N.AD	C1-INH-HAE	None	Sturdy et al. [23]
One female of 32 y.o.	N.AD	2 Units	N.AD	C1-INH-HAE type I	None	Mauro et al. [24]
One male of 37 y.o.	N.AD	2 Units	N.AD	Unknown	None	Malmstrom et al. [25]
One female of 40 y.o.	N.AD	4 Units	N.AD	C1-INH-AAE type II	Laryngeal oedema	Degroote et al. [26]
One male of 32 y.o.	N.AD	6 Units	N.AD	C1-INH-HAE type I	None	Phillips et al. [27]
One female of 18 y.o.	2000 IU	N.AD	N.AD	C1-INH-HAE type I	None	Leimgruber et al. [28]
	N.AD	N.AD	N.AD		Laryngeal oedema	
One male and two females aged between 34 and 49 y.o.	N.AD	4 Units	N.AD	C1-INH-HAE type I	None	Peled et al. [29]
	N.AD	4 Units	N.AD	C1-INH-HAE type I	None	
One female of 10 y.o.	N.AD	2 Units	N.AD	C1-INH-HAE type I	None	Karlis et al. [30]

Case report (gender/age)	STP			AE type	AE development	Reference
	pdhC1INH	FFP	Icatibant acetate			
Six males and six females aged between 21 and 50 y.o.	N.AD	N.AD	N.AD	C1-INH-HAE type I	None	Farkas et al. [31]
One male of 4 y.o.	N.AD	Used	N.AD	Unknown	None	Webb et al. [32]
One female of 6 y.o.	N.AD	N.AD	N.AD	HAE	None	
One female of 54 y.o.	500 IU	N.AD	N.AD	C1-INH-HAE type I	None	Maeda et al. [33]
Three females aged between of 27 and 32 y.o.	N.AD	N.AD	N.AD	C1-INH-HAE type I	Laryngeal oedema	Börk and Barnstedt [18]
One male of 46 y.o.	N.AD	N.AD	N.AD	C1-INH-HAE type I	Laryngeal oedema	
One female of 28 y.o.	N.AD	N.AD	N.AD	C1-INH-HAE type I	Laryngeal oedema	Rice et al. [34]
One female of 49 y.o.	N.AD	N.AD	N.AD	C1-INH-HAE type I + AAE-ACEi	Laryngeal oedema	Van Sickels et al. [35]
One female of 33 y.o.	N.AD	N.AD	N.AD	C1-INH-HAE type I	None (danazol)	
One female of 8 y.o.	Used	N.AD	N.AD	C1-INH-HAE	None (danazol)	Moraes et al. [36]
One male of 36 y.o.	N.AD	N.AD	N.AD	C1-INH-HAE type II	Laryngeal oedema	Baccioglu Kavut [37]
	1000 IU	N.AD	N.AD		None	
One female of 28 y.o.	N.AD	N.AD	SC 30 mg	C1-INH-HAE type I	None	Senaratne et al. [38]
One female of 45 y.o.	N.AD	N.AD	SC 30 mg	C1-INH-HAE	None	Angeletti et al. [39]
One female of 6 y.o.	500 IU	N.AD	N.AD	C1-INH-HAE type II	None	Narayanan et al. [40]
Two males aged between 19 and 57 y.o. and one female of 20 y.o.	N.AD	N.AD	N.AD	C1-INH-HAE type I	Minimal pharyngeal oedema	Jurado-Palomo et al. [15]
One female of 26 y.o.	1000 IU	N.AD	N.AD	C1-INH-HAE type I	None	Sanuki et al. [41]
One female of 50 y.o.	N.AD	N.AD	N.AD	C1-INH-HAE	Laryngeal oedema	Forrest et al. [42]

FFP = fresh frozen plasma, IU = International Unit, N.AD = not administered, pdhC1INH = plasma-derived human C1 esterase inhibitor, SC = subcutaneous, STP = short-term prophylaxis and y.o. = years old.

Table 1. Literature review of dental-oral, maxillofacial and ENT procedures in patients with C1-INH-HAE.

http://dx.doi.org/10.5772/67713

4. The development of diagnostic-therapeutic algorithms for dental-oral, maxillofacial and otolaryngological procedures (DOMFOPs) according to the risk of triggering angioedema attacks

In the last 12 years, different consensus algorithms and clinical guidelines have been published for managing DOMFOP STP and will be reviewed below.

4.1. The 2003 Hungarian-Canadian consensus algorithm

The 2003 Hungarian-Canadian consensus was the first consensus document on the management of C1-INH-HAE [43]. It attempted to establish a separation between minor and major DOMFOPs but did not go deeper in differentiating clearly which procedures were considered minor or major (**Figure 1**) [43].

According to the 2003 Hungarian-Canadian consensus, the STP in DOMFOPs should be as follows:

1. If only a minimum dental manipulation was going to be performed and pdhC1INH was available for the treatment of acute AE attacks, no pre-procedural prophylaxis was indicated. However, if pdhC1INH was not available, STP with danazol or tranexamic acid was recommended. Local injection of local anaesthetic was recognized as being able to precipitate an AE attack [43].

2. For a manipulation that was not considered minor, danazol was recommended (even in children and pregnant women in the last trimester). Tranexamic acid was considered as an

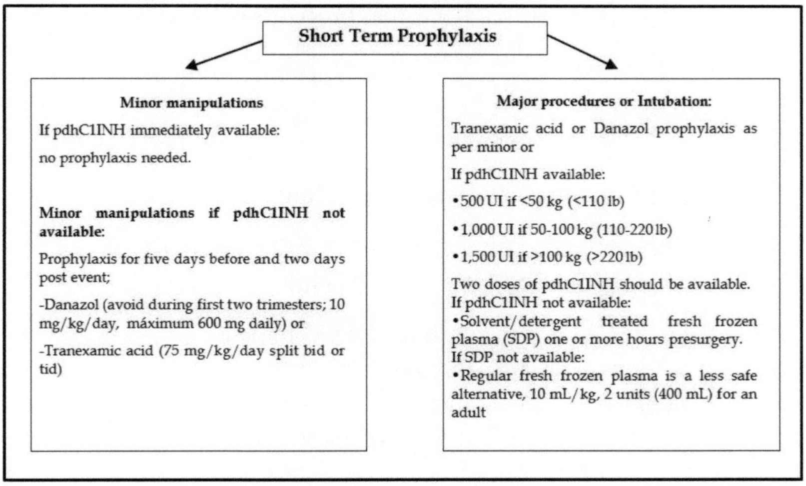

Figure 1 Short-term prophylaxis algorithm for C1-inhibitor deficiency according to the 2003 Hungarian-Canadian consensus [43].

alternative to danazol. pdhC1INH should be available for immediate administration if an AE attack developed [43]. In case of a major surgical procedure or if the patient was being intubated, intravenous pdhC1INH had to be administered 1 hour before surgery. A second pdhC1INH dose should be administered during surgery and even repeated daily or as much as needed until there was no risk of developing AE. If pdhC1INH was not available, STP with danazol or tranexamic acid was recommended. Solvent/detergent-treated fresh frozen plasma (SD-FFP) 1 or more hours before procedure could be another alternative if pdhC1INH was not available; regular FFP would be a fourth option, although less safe than SD-FFP [43].

The algorithm summarizing the recommendations for surgical risk of the Hungarian-Canadian consensus 2003 can be seen in **Figure 1** [43].

4.2. The 2005 British consensus algorithm

According to the 2005 British consensus [16], STP was not only indicated before risky procedures or surgeries but also during periods of physiological or psychological stress (also called intermittent long-term prophylaxis). It was the first time that the term "intermittent long-term prophylaxis" was used. The proposed STP scheme was as follows:

- pdhC1INH (500–1500 U, generally 1000 U) up to 24 hours before. Additional doses may be required later, basically if postoperative infection occurs. It was the treatment of choice in major dental procedures such as tooth extractions.
- Tranexamic acid from 2 to 5 days before procedure until 2 days after procedure

  – 4 g/day (1 g 4 times/day)
- Attenuated androgens from 2 to 5 days before procedure to 2 days after procedure

  – Danazol: 100–600 mg/day

  – Stanozolol: 2–6 mg/day

4.3. The 2007 Hungarian-Canadian consensus algorithm

The 2007 Hungarian-Canadian consensus (published in 2008) continued the distinction between minor or major procedures and intubation (**Figure 2**) [44].

Unlike the 2003 Hungarian-Canadian algorithm, the recommendation of the use of tranexamic acid in minor manipulations with available pdhC1INH was removed. In addition, in major procedures or intubation, the recommendation of the use of danazol or tranexamic acid was also removed, and recommendations differed according to the availability or non-availability of pdhC1INH.

4.4. The 2010 international consensus algorithm

The International consensus published in Allergy, Asthma and Clinical Immunology (official publication of the Canadian Society of Allergy and Clinical Immunology) in 2010 updated the STP recommendations (**Figure 3**) [13].

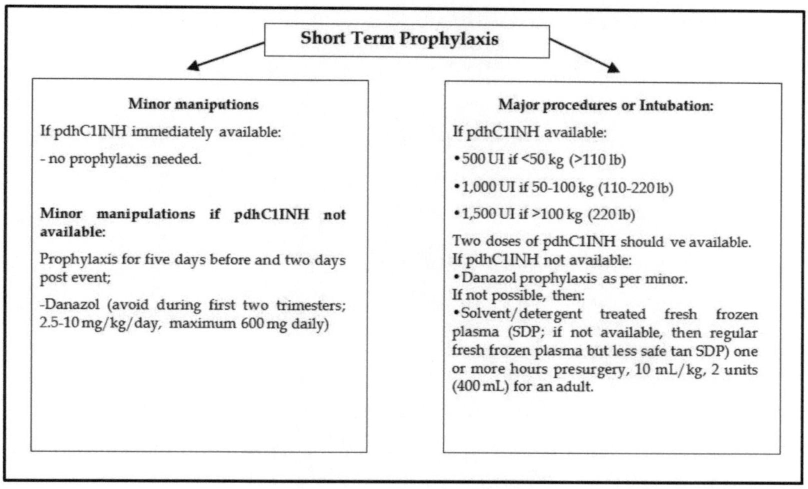

Figure 2. Prophylaxis algorithm in C1-inhibitor deficiency of the 2007 Hungarian-Canadian consensus [44].

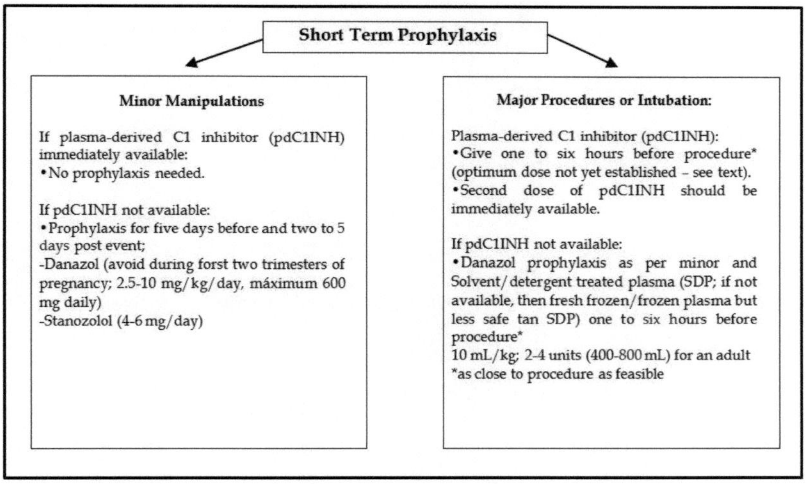

Figure 3. Prophylaxis algorithm in C1-inhibitor deficiency in the 2010 international consensus [44].

A distinctive feature is that the time period for STP with oral drugs for minor risk procedures was increased from 5 days before the procedure to 2–5 days after the completion of the procedure [13]. It also emphasizes the non-use of danazol during the first two trimesters of pregnancy because of the obvious risks of AAs. Antifibrinolytics are still not recommended for STP in this type of procedures.

In procedures involving a higher AE risk or endotracheal intubation, pdhC1INH should be administered from 1 to 6 hours before the procedure, if available. As in previous consensus documents, it only distinguishes between DOMFOPs of minor or major risk, not considering "intermediate risk".

4.5. The 2011 Spanish consensus algorithm

According to the Spanish consensus [8], STP was indicated in surgery or medical procedures that involve trauma in the cervicofacial region with the risk of laryngeal oedema development (e.g. dental manipulations, tonsillectomy, maxillofacial surgery, endoscopy, bronchoscopy or interventions requiring endotracheal intubation) and to prevent local oedema that could alter the surgeon's work area and may affect the surgical outcome.

Specific acute treatment (pdhC1INH or icatibant acetate) must be available with appropriate monitoring of the patient after surgery, including an action plan.

The recommendations were as follows:

- Intravenous pdhC1INH (500 U if the patient weighs less than 50 kg and 1000 U if he/she weighs more than 50 kg) administered from 1 to 4 hours prior to the procedure, with a required second dose (if available).
- Intravenous SD-FFP (if pdhC1INH is not available), two units administered 1 hour before the procedure.
- AAs from 5 to 7 days before to 2–3 days after the procedure (in case of postoperative complications such as infections, AAs should be continued for more than 5 days.)

  – Danazol: 400–600 mg/day

  – Stanozolol: 4–6 mg/day
- Antifibrinolytics

  – EACA

  – Tranexamic acid: 1–4 g/day or 75 mg/kg/day divided into 2–3 doses from 5 days before to 2 days after surgery

Drugs and doses for STP are summarized in **Table 2**.

Pharmacological group	Drug	Adults	Children
C1-INH replacement	pdhC1INH	500–1500 U, 1–4 hours before event	20 U/kg, 1 hour before event
	FFP	2 U (400 ml), 1 hour before procedure	10 mL/kg 1 hour before procedure
Attenuated androgens	Danazol	400–600 mg/24 hours for 5–7 days before and 2–3 days post-event	10 mg/kg/day for 5–7 days before to 2–3 days post-event
	Stanozolol	4–6 mg/24 hours for 5 days before and 3 days post-event	
Antifibrinolytics (seldom used)	Tranexamic acid	1 g/6 hours for 5 days before and 2 days post-event	500 mg/6 hours for 2 days before and 2 days post-event

Table 2. Short-term prophylaxis in the Spanish 2011 national consensus on C1-INH-HAE.

http://dx.doi.org/10.5772/67713

4.6. The 2012 management guidelines of the World Allergy Organization (WAO)

This was the first guideline on C1-INH-HAE and thus was the first time in which evidence levels were analysed and graded recommendations were given [45].

There was no evidence about the effectiveness of STP. The advice to administer STP was based on Expert Opinion. It was stated that even though STP was used, AE episodes could still occur and sometimes after minor procedures (case reports, series of patients). Nevertheless, several publications had reported a reduction in the incidence of AE with STP in both adults and children. In this guideline, the indications of STP varied according to:

- The patient's personal history: frequent episodes of AE, AE following a similar procedure (dental or oral surgery), need for intubation, more invasive procedures
- Probability of AE associated with such a procedure
- Periods of high risk of attacks (due to increased likelihood of AE attacks or increased consequences of AE attack): periods of stress, tests

STP administration had to be considered prior to surgery, especially in the case of dental/intraoral procedures, in which endotracheal intubation was required, when the airway or pharynx was manipulated and before bronchoscopy or endoscopy. This statement had a level of evidence D (adapted from previous consensus document or "statement" based on an expert opinion poll during a consensus conference) and a strength of recommendation A.

In DOMFOPs with minimal risk or if there was availability of safe drugs for on-demand treatment of "upper airway edema" (UAE) attacks, STP could be omitted. Two doses of pdhC1INH, ecallantide or icatibant had to be available for possible immediate administration. The patient had to know the risks and have a plan of action and treatment for AE attacks.

The recommendations were as follows:

- Intravenous pdhC1INH: 10–20 U/kg or 1000 U was recommended, administered from 1 to 6 hours before DOMFOP. Dosing studies were required, as AE attacks have even occurred with 1000 U doses
- SD-FFP (if pdhC1INH was not available)
- AAs from 5 days before to 5 days after the procedure (if the risk associated with the procedure or surgery was relatively low and no pdhC1INH was available). Its use was limited to elective surgery with a lower perceived effectiveness as compared to pdhC1INH, although there was no evidence. AAs have considerable side effects, being contraindicated during pregnancy (except in the last trimester of pregnancy) and during lactation

  – Danazol: 2.5–10 mg/kg/day, to a maximum dose of 600 mg/day

  – Stanozolol: 4–6 mg/day
- Antifibrinolytics

  – Tranexamic acid: 25 mg/kg/day divided into 2–3 doses

4.7. The 2013 guidelines for the management of HAE, C1-INH-AAE and ACEi-AAE

All HAE patients are candidates for STP when exposed to situations that could likely trigger an AE attack [46].

Two statements are particularly relevant in this field:

1. Summary statement 20: STP can be achieved by using FFP, pdhC1INH and high doses of AAs for short periods. Recommendation strength B (directly based on category II evidence or recommendation extrapolated from category I evidence).
2. Summary statement 25: New drugs for the treatment of C1-INH deficiency syndromes are costlier than the alternative treatment with AAs. Official studies of cost-utility and cost-effectiveness in helping healthcare providers in the management of patients with C1-INH deficiency syndromes are warranted. Strength of recommendation D.

The drugs and doses recommended are as follows:

- Intravenous pdhC1INH: 1000–2000 U
- Intravenous SD-FFP 2 U: several hours (up to 12 hours) before the procedure
- Oral 17-alpha-alkylated AAs, for 5–10 days before to 2 days after the procedure
  - Danazol: 6–10 mg/kg/day into divided doses; maximum 200 mg, 3 times per day or equivalent

There are no comparative studies between pdhC1INH and AAs. The decision on the drug to be prescribed should be based on an individualized assessment of damage/burden compared to the benefits, costs and patient preferences. In emergency procedures, pdhC1INH is the treatment of choice. Specific treatment for AE attacks (pdhC1INH, ecallantide or icatibant) should be available during and after any procedure.

4.8. The 2014 Canadian consensus

STP should be considered prior to the patient's specific known triggers and before any medical, surgical or dental procedures [47]. Evidence level is low, and the strength of the recommendation is strong.

Specific treatments for the acute attack of C1-INH-HAE should be available during and after the procedure. The level of evidence is low (our confidence in the estimated effect is limited: the true effect may be substantially different from the estimated effect). The strength of the recommendation is strong.

The drugs and doses recommended were as follows:

- pdhC1INH: pdhC1INH was recommended, although there were no data on the most appropriate dose. In Europe, it was marketed under the following brands:
  - Cinryze®: 1000 U up to 24 hours before, though there is not enough evidence that confirms that administering the drug more than 6 hours before the procedure is safe
  - Berinert®: 1000 U up to 6 hours before

- AAs from 5 days before to 2–3 days after the procedure (STP could be considered when the risk associated with surgery was low and there was no immediate availability of the specific treatments for acute attacks)

  – Danazol: 2.5–10 mg/kg/day, up to a maximum dose of 600 mg/day

- Antifibrinolytics

  – Tranexamic acid: 25 mg/kg/day (up to a maximum dose of 3000–6000 mg/day) divided into 2–3 doses from 5 days before to 2–5 days after the surgery or when a trigger was anticipated. Its effectiveness in preventing attacks was unknown, so it should only be used if other drugs were not available

4.9. The 2013 Spanish algorithm for short-term prophylaxis

A group of allergists along with clinical pharmacologists from different hospitals in Spain developed algorithms for the diagnosis, prophylaxis and treatment of C1-INH-HAE [48].

STP was not indicated in minor procedures with the availability of specific treatment for acute AE attacks. STP was indicated in all the procedures that involved trauma in the cervicofacial region because of the risk of developing AE in the upper airway and in any diagnostic or therapeutic procedure in order to avoid local edema in the working area so that the procedure result was not altered.

pdhC1INH was the election treatment for STP. Both Cinryze® 1000 U (1–24 horas pre-procedure) and Berinert® 10–20 U/kg (1–6 hours of pre-procedure) were available for their 20 use in adults.

In case pdhC1INH was not available, attenuated androgens (danazol, estanozolol) and antifibrinolytics (tranexamic acid, epsilon aminocaproic acid) were alternatives in programmed procedures and SD-FFP in case of emergency procedures.

- Danazol: 400–600 mg/day (divided into 2–3 doses/day—from 5 to 7 days pre-procedure to 2–3 days post-procedure)
- Stanozolol: 4–6 mg/day (divided into 2–3 doses/day—from 5 to 7 days pre-procedure to 3 days post-procedure)
- Tranexamic acid: 1,000 mg/6 hours (from 5 days pre-procedure to 2–3 days post-procedure (consider thrombotic risk)

It was advised that any patient receiving STP should be observed and the specific treatment for acute attacks should be available for 48 hours after the procedure, as the risk for AE is not totally cancelled with STP.

These authors specified STP for children. The election treatment was also intravenous—pdhC1INH (Berinert®: 10–20 U/kg, 1–6 hours pre-procedure or Cinryze® 1000 U).

In case pdhC1INH was not available, they advised to use attenuated androgens or tranexamic acid:

- Danazol: 10 mg/kg/day (divided into 2–3 doses/day—from 5 to 7 days pre-procedure to 2–3 days post-procedure)
- Tranexamic acid: 500 mg/6 hours (from 5 days pre-procedure to 2–3 days post-procedure)

4.10. International consensus for the management of children with C1-INH-HAE

According to the international consensus for the management of children [49] (**Figure 4**), indications for STP in paediatrics (as in adults) include patient-specific triggers, medical and dental procedures. For most "minor interventions", the recommendation is to choose an on-demand treatment if a swelling event is precipitated rather than prophylaxis, provided that a licensed on-demand medication is immediately available in the case of emergency (level III evidence).

4.11. US consensus for the management of children with C1-INH-HAE

Only Berinert® is approved for the treatment of children < 12 y.o. [50]. Berinert®, at 20 U/kg, has less risk of containing an infectious agent, is approved by the Food and Drug Administration (FDA) in children and is preferable when available [51–53].

FFP given empirically at 2 U per patient immediately before surgery has been reported to provide effective STP in adults and poses less risk [19]. It is critically important that effective on-demand treatment be available, whether the patient is given STP prophylaxis or not. Therapeutic approaches for C1-INH-HAE have been studied carefully in adults, but not all have not been investigated with the same level of care in children (**Table 3**).

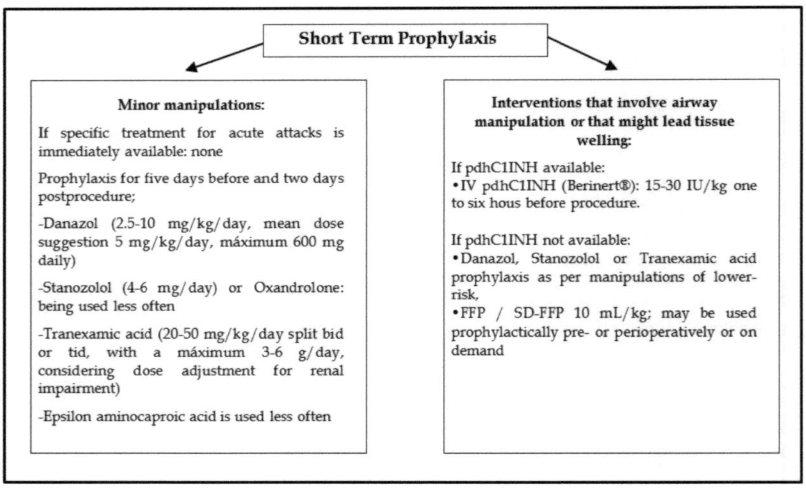

Figure 4. Prophylaxis algorithm in C1-inhibitor deficiency in the 2017 international consensus for the management of children [49].

http://dx.doi.org/10.5772/67713

Drugs	Type of evidence	Dosage	Use
Berinert®	I (adults) and II-3 (children)	20 IU/kg intravenous	On demand
Cinryze®	I (adults >18 y.o.) and II-3 (children)	1000 IU intravenous (adults)	Prophylaxis
Ruconest®	I (adults ≥ 18 y.o.)	50 IU/kg intravenous	On demand
Icatibant acetate	I (adults ≥ 18 y.o.) and II-3 (children)	30 mg subcutaneous	On demand
Ecallantide	I (adults, adolescents ≥ 12 y.o.) and II-3 (children)	30 mg subcutaneous	On demand
Danazol	I (adults) and II-3 (children, not recommended)	<200 mg oral	Prophylaxis
Tranexamic acid	II-3 (adults and children)	20–40 mg/kg up to 3 g/day oral	Prophylaxis
Fresh frozen plasma	II-3 (adults)	1–2 Units intravenous	On demand

Type of evidence I = randomized controlled trial and II-3 = dramatic results in uncontrolled trial.

Table 3. Drugs for prophylaxis and for the acute treatment of hereditary angioedema (modified Frank et al.) [50].

4.12. Available treatments for STP in C1-INH-HAE

4.12.1. Plasma-derived C1 esterase inhibitor concentrate (pdhC1INH)

pdhC1INH consists of a replacement therapy for the lacking C1-INH. There are currently several pdhC1INH pharmaceutical presentations: Berinert® (CSL-Behring GmbH, Marburg, Germany), Cebitor® (Sanquin, Amsterdam, The Netherlands) and Cinryze® (Shire HGT, Zug, Switzerland) (see **Table 4** for a comparison of the available drugs for short-term prophylaxis in C1-INH-HAE).

For nearly 25 years, Berinert-P (CSL-Behring GmbH) was available in Spain through the Foreign Medications office [8]. Afterwards, it was finally marketed in Spain as Berinert® in August 2009 [8]. Berinert® is a purified, pasteurized, nanofiltred pdhC1INH. It is presented in 500 U vials of a lyophilized product for intravenous administration, which has to be stored at 2–25°C [8], and when reconstituted, a 50 IU/mL solution is formed. It has an excellent safety post-launch record after more than 35 years of its availability [54–56].

Berinert® is currently approved by the FDA for the treatment of AE attacks in adults and adolescents, 12 years and older, with C1-INH-HAE, and by the European Medical Agencies (EMA) for the treatment of AE attacks and short-term prophylaxis in adults and children with C1-INH-HAE [56].

Cebitor® is only available in a few European countries.

Cinryze® comes in a package with two lyophilized 500 U C1 inhibitor (human) vials. After reconstitution, each vial contains a 100 U/ml solution. It has to be stored from 2 to 25°C.

The FDA approved Cinryze in October 2008 for long-term prophylaxis in adults (> 18 years) [8]. In 2010, the European Medicines Agency (EMA) approved the marketing of Cinryze® for long-term prophylaxis, short-term-prophylaxis and the treatment of acute attacks in adolescents and adults [57].

Drug	Trade name	Company	Drug description	Mechanism of action	Administration route	Indication for STP	Adverse events
Human plasma-derived C1-INH	Berinert®	CSL-Behring	Human plasma-derived C1-esterase inhibitor	C1-INH replacement[1]	Intravenous	- Adults: 1000 IU, 1–6 hours before procedure - Children: 15–30 IU/kg 1–6 hours before procedure	**Rare:** risk of anaphylaxis, thrombosis **Theoretical**: transmission of infectious agent
Human plasma-derived C1-INH	Cebitor®, Cinryze®	Sanquin, Shire HGT	Human plasma-derived C1-esterase inhibitor	C1-INH replacement	Intravenous	1000 U, 1–24 hours before procedure[2]	
Conestat-alfa (recombinant human C1-INH produced in transgenic rabbits)	Rhucin®/ Ruconest®[3]	Pharming NV	Recombinant human inhibitor of C1-esterase (produced in transgenic rabbits)	C1-INH replacement	Intravenous	No	**Rare:** risk of anaphylaxis (screening for IgE antibodies against rabbit dander is advised by EMA)
Icatibant acetate	Firazyr®	Shire HGT	Synthetic peptide (10 aa)	Blockage of B2R	Subcutaneous	No	**Common:** local swelling, pain and pruritus at injection site Attack can recur in the following 48 hours **Theoretical**: worsening of an ongoing acute coronary artery disease
Ecallantide	Kalbitor®	Shire HGT	Recombinant human protein (60 aa)	Selective inhibitor of plasma kallikrein	Subcutaneous	No	**Common:** prolonged PTT **Uncommon:** risk of anaphylaxis (must be administered by healthcare professionals)
Solvent/ detergent-treated plasma (SD-FFP)		Several	Plasma derivative	Replacement of deficient C1-INH protein	Intravenous	Adults: 2–4 U Children: 10 mL/kg 1–6 hours before procedure[4]	Transmission of infectious agents: only S/D treatment inactivates enveloped viruses but not non-enveloped ones Risk of hypervolaemia: large volumes can overload the circulatory system Allergenic potential: large

Drug	Trade name	Company	Drug description	Mechanism of action	Administration route	Indication for STP	Adverse events
							number of potentially allergenic constituents
Epsilon-amino-caproic acid (EACA)	Caproamin®, Amicar®	Rottapharm, Xanodyne Pharmaceuticals		Antifibrinolytic: antiplasmin and plasminogen activator inhibitor effect	Oral, intravenous		**Common:** nausea, vertigo, diarrhoea, postural hypotension, fatigue, muscle cramps with increased muscle enzymes **Uncommon:** thrombosis
Tranexamic acid	Amchafibrin®, Cyklokapron®	Pfizer, New York, NY	Cyclic derivative of epsilon amino-caproic acid		Oral, intravenous	500–3000 mg/day divided into 3–4 doses Adults: 1 g/6h Children: 500 mg/6h 2 days pre-procedure and 2 days post-procedure	
Stanozolol	Winstrol®	Winthrop, Barcelona, Spain	Attenuated androgen (17-alpha-alkylated androgens)	Increase in plasma C1-esterase inhibitor levels	Oral	2 mg/day or less 4–6 mg/day (divided into 2–3 doses), 5 days pre-procedure and 3–5 days post-procedure	**Common**: weight gain, virilization, acne, altered libido, muscle pain, headaches, depression, fatigue, nausea, constipation, menstrual abnormalities, increase in liver enzymes, hypertension, alterations in lipid profile **Uncommon**: decreased growth rate in children, masculinization of female foetus, cholestatic jaundice, peliosis hepatis, hepatocellular adenoma
Danazol	Danatrol, Danocrine, Danol	Sanofi-Aventis, Paris, France	Attenuated androgen (17-alpha-alkylated androgen)	Increase in plasma C1-esterase inhibitor levels; increase in plasma aminopeptidase P levels	Oral	200 mg/day or less, 5 days pre-procedure and 3–5 days post-procedure Adults: 400–600 mg/day (divided into 2–3 doses) Children: 10 mg/kg/day (divided into 2–3 doses)	
Oxandrolone	Oxandrin®	Savient Pharmaceu ticals, East Brunswick, NJ	Attenuated androgen (17-alpha-alkylated androgen)	Increase in plasma C1-esterase inhibitor levels	Oral	10 mg/day or less	

[1] Inhibits plasma kallikrein, factors XIIa and XIa, C1s, C1r, plasmin.
[2] Cinryze® SPC (Summary of Products Characteristics) indicates 1–24 hours, but the authors consider it should be administered as close as possible to the procedure and no longer than 6 hours prior to procedure.
[3] Conestat alfa is commercialized as Ruconest® in Europe and Rhucin® in other parts of the world.
[4] As close to procedure as possible.

Table 4. Drugs for the treatment of C1-INH-HAE with special focus on STP.

Both Berinert® and Cinryze® are currently authorized for intravenous self-administration by trained patients or their relatives.

The recommended doses for STP are 1000 U for adults both for Berinert® and Cinryze® and 15–30 IU/kg for children for Berinert®, 1–6 hours before procedure. Although the Cinryze® Summary of Products Characteristics (SPC) indicates 1–24 hours, most authors consider that it should be administered as close as possible to the procedure and no longer than 6 hours prior to procedure [58]. For long, complex surgeries and in the case of infection or other trigger factors, the pdhC1INH dose may have to be repeated.

At least one dose of a specific drug for the treatment of acute AE attacks (C1-INH concentrate, rhC1INH, ecallantide or icatibant) should be available for on-demand treatment in case it is needed.

4.12.2. Fresh frozen plasma

In countries where pdhC1INH is not available, fresh frozen plasma (FFP) is an alternative. FFP should be virally inactivated with solvents and detergents (SD-FFP) to be safer. FFP acts by supplying lacking C1-INH [8]. SD-FFP dosage for C1-INH-HAE has not been studied, and the generally used dose is the same than in coagulation disorders: 2 units of 200 mL each [8].

Among the possible FFP side effects are alloimmunization, anaphylactic or allergic reactions, transmission of infectious diseases (viruses, Creutzfeldt-Jakob disease) and excessive intravascular volume with the risk of hypervolemia and heart failure [8].

4.12.3. Attenuated androgens

Danazol and stanozolol are 17-α-alkylated synthetic derivatives, which are very effective and have fewer side effects than other androgens. Their mechanism of action in C1-INH-HAE is not well known. Several actions may contribute to their effectiveness. First, a significant increase in C1-INH plasma levels was reported with high AA doses. Second, an increase in the expression of C1-INH mRNA in mononuclear cells with the minimum effective dose was shown. Finally, an increase in the plasma levels of aminopeptidase P, one of the BK catabolizing enzymes, was published [8].

Danazol is a potent gonadotropic inhibitor with partial antigestagenic, anabolic and androgenic activity, whereas stanozolol is an anabolic steroid with certain anticoagulant properties [8].

Oxandrolone is another AA, which has been used in C1-INH-HAE to a lesser extent [8].

AAs have considerable side effects when used as long-term prophylaxis for long periods of time or at high doses [8]. The main secondary effects are disorders of libido, impotence, weight gain, menstrual irregularities, breast atrophy/hypotrophy, acne, voice changes, increased atherogenic index, polycythemia, hypertension, haematuria, transient increases in transaminases, hepatic necrosis, cholestatic hepatitis, hepatosplenic peliosis, transient increases in muscle enzymes (creatine phosphokinase and aldolase) and rhabdomyolysis. There have also been some cases of hepatic adenoma and adenocarcinoma. However, the data on increased risk of atherosclerosis are controversial. AAs used for short periods of time as STP are much better tolerated, and thus, they were advised as STP for children and pregnant women in the first consensus documents on C1-INH-HAE.

The effect of AAs takes approximately 5 days, and thus, AAs cannot be used in emergency situations that require STP. AA doses for STP can be seen in **Table 3**.

These drugs may have to be administered for more than 5 days after the procedure in the case of postoperative complications, especially infection [8].

4.12.4. *Antifibrinolytic agents*

The mechanism of action of antifibrinolytic agents in C1-INH-HAE is unknown.

4.12.4.1. *ε-Aminocaproic acid*

ε-Aminocaproic acid (EACA) (Amycar®, Rottapharm Madaus, Milan, Italy) is effective in preventing AE attacks in C1-INH-HAE if taken as long-term prophylaxis [8, 14]. There is a scarcity of data about its use as STP, although some consensus documents advise on its use [13, 44].

The most frequent side effect is a transient increase in creatine phosphokinase and aldolase associated with muscle pain, weakness and fatigue. Other side effects are thrombosis and extensive muscle necrosis [8].

4.12.4.2. *Tranexamic acid*

Tranexamic acid (Amchafibrin®, Rottapharm Madaus, Milan, Italy) is a cyclic derivative of EACA and has been proven efficacious in preventing AE attacks in patients with C1-INH-HAE [8, 14]. Tranexamic acid competitively inhibits the activation of plasminogen, which, under normal conditions, is inhibited by C1-INH, thus reducing the conversion of plasminogen to plasmin (fibrinolysis) [8].

Muscle cramps, nausea, diarrhoea, hypotension, dizziness and fatigue are among its described side effects.

The dose for STP is 1 g 4 times a day or 75 mg/kg/day divided into 2–3 doses from 5 days before to 2 days after the surgery or medical procedure.

Antifibrinolytics are seldom used in countries where other treatments are available. Antifibrinolytics should be discontinued before the surgery, as they may theoretically promote thromboembolic events [8].

4.12.5. *Icatibant acetate*

Icatibant acetate (Firazyr®, Shire HGT, Zug, Switzerland) is a synthetic decapeptide similar to BK and a highly specific, potent and competitive antagonist of the BK B2 receptor (B2R), inhibiting the vasodilation produced by BK [8]. Its effectiveness as the treatment for AE acute attacks in C1-INH-HAE has been shown in clinical trials and patient series [8] and in patient registries [59–61]. No serious adverse reactions have been reported, the only significant side effect being injection site reactions (in more than 95% of cases), consisting of self-limiting erythema, oedema, pruritus and pain [8]. The European Medicines Agency (EMA) approved icatibant acetate for the treatment of acute AE attacks in adult patients (≥ 18 y.o.) with C1-INH-HAE in July 2008, and it has been available in Spain since March 2009. It was approved by the

FDA in 2011. Icatibant acetate's self-administration was authorized by EMA in 2011. A registry on the use of icatibant acetate in real life has confirmed its safety [61].

Icatibant acetate is only approved for adults. A study on its safety and efficacy in children is currently going on. There is no information about its safety profile in women who are pregnant. Regarding breastfeeding, lactation should be avoided 12 hours after icatibant acetate's administration. According to prescribing information, icatibant acetate should not be used in patients with active ischemic heart disease or those who have had an ischemic stroke in the preceding 2 weeks [8].

Isolated cases of STP with off-label icatibant acetate prior to some medical, dental or surgical procedures in patients with C1-INH-HAE have been published [38, 62, 63]. First, a thyroid biopsy without later local oedema was published [62].

However, controlled studies are necessary. The short half-life (1–2 hours) of this agent and the fact that it blocks B2R but does not diminish the BK production may restrict its use in short-term prophylaxis, as there is a theoretical risk of late local oedema. The trauma may result in an increase in local BK through FXII activation. While B2R blockage continues, no oedema is produced, but when B2Rs are released (after icatibant is eliminated from the body), an oedema episode could develop 6–8 hours after the surgery if BK remains high [8]. Other authors do not support its use as short-term prophylaxis due to its short half-life [64].

4.12.6. Ecallantide (Kalbitor®, Shire HGT, Zug, Switzerland)

Ecallantide is a very potent, reversible and highly specific human plasma kallikrein inhibitor, whose half-life is 2.0 ± 0.5 hours [8]. Its effectiveness has been demonstrated in different clinical trials [8, 14, 58, 65].

The United States Food and Drug Administration approved its use in December 2009 for the treatment of acute AE episodes in patients aged 16 years and older with C1-INH-HAE. Later, its use was extended to adolescents.

Acute allergic reactions, as well as anaphylaxis, have been reported [8].

It is administered subcutaneously at 30 mg (divided into 3 doses) and should be stored refrigerated [8]. One isolated case of STP with a low dose of ecallantide (10 mg) plus FFP, which did not result in AE, was reported [66].

However, the short half-life of ecallantide (2.0 ± 0.5 hours) could restrict its use as short-term prophylaxis [8, 64]. It is necessary to carry out controlled studies or gain more experience in order to recommend its use in this indication.

4.12.7. Recombinant human C1 inhibitor

Recombinant human C1-INH (rhC1INH) (Ruconest®/Rhucin®, Pharming Group NV, Leiden, The Netherlands) is produced in transgenic female rabbits in which the human C1NH gene has been inserted. The resulting rhC1INH is excreted in the rabbit milk, from which it is obtained by purification. The active substance is also termed conestat alfa. rhC1INH is effective in the treatment of acute AE attacks. rhC1INH is a C1-INH replacement therapy but with

http://dx.doi.org/10.5772/67713

the advantages of the absence of the potential risk of transmitting blood-borne human infections and its suitability for large-scale production. It has a similar inhibitory potency and high structural analogy with phC1INH, although with a lower half-life (3 hours), due to differences in glycosylation. rhC1INH can be kept at room temperature (2–25°C). A 50 U/kg dose (maximum 4200 U) was approved by the EMA in October 2010 for the treatment of acute AE attacks in > 18 years with C1-INH-HAE, although it has not yet been marketed in Spain. In 2016, its approval was extended to adolescents.

FDA approved rhC1INH in 2014 for the treatment of acute AE attacks in adolescents and adult patients with C1-INH-HAE. The approved dose is 50 U/kg with a maximum dose of 4200 U administered intravenously.

A possible disadvantage of recombinant products is being potentially immunogenic and having the risk of producing neutralizing antibodies and/or allergic reactions. However, data on immunological safety are good, with no antibody production and no adverse immunological effects observed, except for an anaphylactic reaction in one patient with undisclosed rabbit allergy in a phase I clinical trial [8, 57].

rhC1INH is not recommended for short-term prophylactic management of C1-INH-HAE due to its short half-life [64].

Two consensus for the management of C1-INH-HAE in children have been published in 22 2016 [50, 65, 66].

Caballero et al. published a consensus document in which the management of STP in female patients was reviewed [67]. This information was updated later for HAE with and without C1-inhibitor deficiency [68].

The unavailability of STP should not delay an urgent procedure [69]. C1-INH-HAE should not be an obstacle for routine procedures [69].

In DOMFOP, it is advisable, provided that it is possible, to use regional anaesthesia to avoid the trauma that supposes oropharyngeal intubation [8, 13, 70].

It is impossible to predict which patients will develop angioedema after a determined medical/surgical procedure. Moreover, a single patient could present or not present AE after the same procedure [70–72]. There are no controlled studies that assess STP efficacy; current available data come from observational studies: The risk of perioperative AE without STP (not taking into account dental procedures) is 6–31% [73]. There is no increased risk related to the procedure location or surgical area size [73]. The prevalence of AE attacks after dental procedures performed without STP varies from 5 to 37% of patients [71–73]. Farkas et al. observed that 40% of the patients who had not performed STP developed AE post-procedures, when assessing all the interventions as a whole [74]. Most times, AE is local, but distant AE has also been described [72, 73]. AE can be triggered by minor procedures, such as local injection of a local anesthetic [43], suture of a hand cut or an aesthetic injection of hyaluronic acid in the lips [72]. In some patients, perioperative angioedema was the first manifestation of C1-INH-HAE [72].

The study of STP use in large patients' series has shown that STP with pdhC1INH or AAs reduced the number of patients who present AE attacks after medical/surgical procedures [15, 71, 73].

pdhC1INH reduced the AE risk more after invasive procedures than AAs and AAs more than tranexamic acid [73]. It is important to emphasize that the AE risk after surgical/medical procedures is not completely avoided with STP [71, 73] and is independent of C1-INH-HAE severity [15] and thus, at least one therapeutic dose of a specific treatment for acute AE attacks should be available during and after the procedure [8, 74]. If the procedure involves the ENT area, the patient should be informed about the possibility to develop a laryngeal oedema, not only in the 12 hours following the procedure but also later [72], and one should establish an action plan for the patient.

5. Conclusion: a proposal for STP algorithm

Based on the clinical experience of the Department of Allergology of the University Hospital La Paz (Madrid) and the University General Hospital Nuestra Señora del Prado (Talavera de la Reina), these algorithms have been updated and modified.

Most studies do not take into account the disease severity in order to plan STP and to study the STP efficacy.

Jurado-Palomo et al. [15] calculated retrospectively the C1-INH-HAE severity by using the Diagnostic, Therapeutic, and Management Algorithm for Hereditary Angioedema, from Agostoni et al. [70] (**Table 5**). They studied the efficacy of STP with AAs and/or pdhC1INH in patients with C1-INH-HAE and found that all the patients who suffered mild pharynx laryngeal AE curiously occurred in the group of patients with milder stages of C1-INH-HAE. Curiously, these patients had not received long- or short-term AA prophylaxis nor pre-procedural pdhC1INH [15].

Attack severity		Score
Mild attacks (discomfort noticed, but no disruption of normal daily activities)		0.5 for each 24 hours
Moderate attacks (discomfort sufficient to reduce or affect normal daily activities)		1 for each 24 hours
Severe attacks (inability to work or perform daily activity)		2 for each 24 hours
Need for treatment:		
- Emergency treatment: conservative, substitutive (C1-INH, FFP).		5 each
- Emergency treatment: invasive (intubation, tracheotomy).		25 each
- Long-term prophylaxis for more than 6 months.		25
- Long-term prophylaxis for 3–6 months.		12.5
Score	**Class**	**Degree**
>30	1	Severe
21–30	2	Moderate
11–20	3	Mild
1–10	4	Minimal
0	5	Asymptomatic

Table 5. Criteria for the evaluation of disease severity [70] (these parameters are determined over the period of 1 year. The sum of the scores defines the severity of the disease for that year).

We advise to classify procedures according to the risk of producing AE as minor, intermediate and major risks.

If we classified dental procedures according to the surgical risk, the injection of local anaesthetic would be of minor AE risk, but it has been identified to be able to precipitate an attack of AE [43]. In our series, even the placement of orthodontic appliances (lower risk according to our classification) showed triggering of mild palate oedema in the months after the placement [15]. Thus, it is important that patients have specific drugs, for the treatment of acute attacks, available.

We would recommend using danazol, stanozolol and tranexamic acid in minor risk manipulations and not using tranexamic acid for those procedures of intermediate or major AE risk and attenuated androgens if pdhC1INH is available.

Given this and in our experience, we would propose the following algorithms for the prophylaxis of DOMFOPs (**Figure 5**). To elaborate on this algorithm, three special mentions can be done:

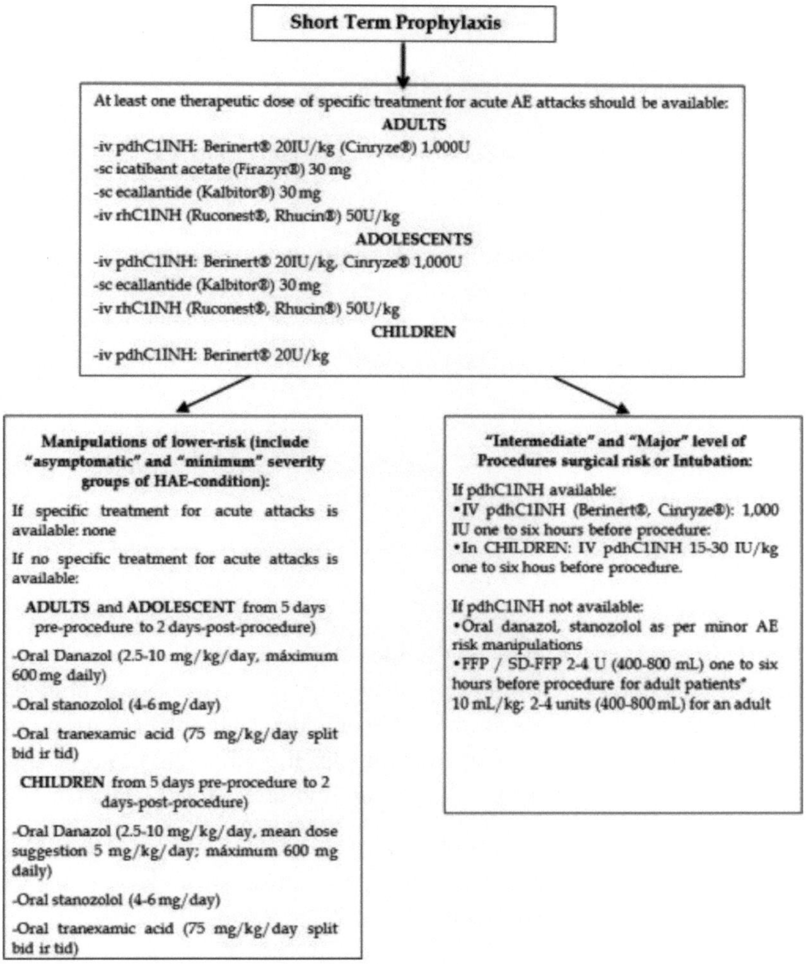

Figure 5. Proposed algorithm for short-term prophylaxis in C1-INH-HAE according to the authors' experience at University Hospital La Paz in Madrid and at University General Hospital Nuestra Señora del Prado in Talavera de la Reina.

1. In an "intermediate" level of procedures, surgical risk is included, although it includes the same prophylactic approach as greater surgical risk.
2. It is clearly specified that short-term prophylaxis to reduce AE risk after dental manipulations should be performed even in patients with asymptomatic activity or minimal disease.
3. Stanozolol is included as a recommendation in lower risk manipulations, at the same level as danazol or tranexamic acid.

Close coordination between different specialists is advisable to decide the attitude to follow pre-procedurally. Treatment for acute attacks should be available in the operating room, in the allergology department and even at patient's home.

Author details

Jesús Jurado-Palomo[1,2]* and Teresa Caballero[2,3,4]

*Address all correspondence to: h72jupaj@yahoo.es

1 Department of Allergology, Nuestra Señora del Prado University General Hospital, Talavera de la Reina, Spain

2 Spanish Study Group on Bradykinin-Induced Angioedema (SGBA), Spanish Society of Allergology and Clinical Immunology (SEAIC), Spain

3 Department of Allergology, Hospital La Paz Health Research Institute (IdiPAZ), Madrid, Spain

4 Biomedical Research Network on Rare Diseases, CIBERER (U754), Madrid, Spain

References

[1] Caballero T, Baeza ML, Cabañas R, Campos A, Cimbollek S, Gómez-Traseira C, et al. Consensus statement on the diagnosis, management, and treatment of angioedema mediated by bradykinin. Part I. Classification, epidemiology, pathophysiology, genetics, clinical symptoms, and diagnosis. J Investig Allergol Clin Immunol. 2011;21:333–47; quiz follow 347. Review. Erratum in: J Investig Allergol Clin Immunol. 2012;22:3 p following 153.

[2] Roche O, Blanch A, Caballero T, Sastre N, Callejo D, López-Trascasa M. Hereditary angioedema due to C1 inhibitor deficiency: patient registry and approach to the prevalence in Spain. Ann Allergy Asthma Immunol. 2005;94:498–503.

[3] Bygum A. Hereditary angio-oedema in Denmark. A nationwide survey. Br J Dermatol 2009;161:1153–8.

[4] Zanichelli A, Arcoleo F, Barca MP, Borrelli P, Bova M, Cancian M, et al. A nationwide survey of hereditary angioedema due to C1 inhibitor deficiency in Italy. Orphanet J Rare Dis. 2015;10:11.

[5] Stray-Pedersen A, Abrahamsen TG, Frøland SS. Primary immunodeficiency diseases in Norway. J Clin Immunol. 2000;20:477–85.

[6] Fay A, Abinun M. Current management of hereditary angioedema (C1 esterase inhibitor deficiency). J Clin Pathol 2002;55:266–70.

[7] Atkinson JC, Frank MM. Oral manifestations and dental management of patients with hereditary angioedema. J Oral Pathol Med. 1991;20:139–42.

[8] Caballero T, Baeza ML, Cabañas R, Campos A, Cimbollek S, Gómez-Traseira C, et al. Consensus statement on the diagnosis, management, and treatment of angioedema mediated by bradykinin. Part II. Treatment, follow-up, and special situations. J Investig Allergol Clin Immunol. 2011;21:422–41; quiz 442–3. Review. Erratum in: J Investig Allergol Clin Immunol. 2012;22:3 p following 153.

[9] Bork K, Barnstedt SE. Laryngeal edema and death from asphyxiation after tooth extraction in four patients with hereditary angioedema. J Am Dent Assoc. 2003;134:1088–94.

[10] Landerman NS. Hereditary angioneurotic edema. J Allergy Clin Immunol. 1962;33:316–29.

[11] Cicardi M, Bergamaschini L, Marasini B, Boccassini G, Tucci A, Agostoni A. Hereditary angioedema: an appraisal of 104 cases. Am J Med Sci. 1982;284:2–9.

[12] Bork K, Siedlecki K, Bosch S, Schopf RE, Kreuz W. Asphyxiation by laryngeal edema in patients with hereditary angioedema. Mayo Clin Proc. 2000;75:349–54.

[13] Bowen T, Cicardi M, Farkas H, Bork K, Longhurst HJ, Zuraw B, et al. International consensus algorithm for the diagnosis, therapy and management of hereditary angioedema. Allergy Asthma Clin Immunol. 2010;6:24-36.

[14] Cicardi M, Bork K, Caballero T, Craig T, Li HH, Longhurst H, et al. Evidence-based recommendations for the therapeutic management of angioedema owing to hereditary C1 inhibitor deficiency: consensus report of an International Working Group. Allergy. 2012;67:147–57.

[15] Jurado-Palomo J, Muñoz-Caro JM, López-Serrano MC, Prior N, Cabañas R, Pedrosa M et al. Management of dental-oral procedures in patients with hereditary angioedema due to C1 inhibitor deficiency. J Investig Allergol Clin Immunol. 2013;23:1–6.

[16] Gompels MM, Lock RJ, Abinun M, Bethune CA, Davies G, Grattan C, et al. C1 inhibitor deficiency: consensus document. Clin Exp Immunol. 2005;139:379–94.

[17] Wall RT, Frank M, Hahn M. A review of 25 patients with hereditary angioedema requiring surgery. Anesthesiology. 1989;71:309–11.

[18] Bork K, Barnstedt SE. Laryngeal edema and death from asphyxiation after tooth extraction in four patients with hereditary angioedema. J Am Dent Assoc. 2003;134:1088–94.

[19] Jaffe CJ, Atkinson JP, Gelfand JA, Frank MM. Hereditary angioedema: the use of fresh frozen plasma for prophylaxis in patients undergoing oral surgery. J Allergy Clin Immunol. 1975;55:386–93.

[20] Heft MW, Flynn PM. Hereditary angioedema: review of literature and dental treatment. J Am Dent Assoc. 1977;95:986–90.

[21] Delfino JJ, Sclaroff A, Giglio JA, Travis M. Management of a patient with hereditary angioneurotic edema. J Oral Surg. 1978;36:890–2.

[22] Albright BW, Taylor CG. Hereditary angioneurotic edema: report of case. J Oral Surg. 1979;37:888–90.

[23] Sturdy KA, Beastall RH, Grisius RJ, Oatis GW Jr. Hereditary angioedema controlled with danazol. Report of a case. Oral Surg Oral Med Oral Pathol. 1979;48:418–20.

[24] Mauro JV, Meyrowitz MR, Licari G, Jankowski R. Hereditary angioneurotic edema: clinical management and case report. J Am Dent Assoc. 1982;104:641–3.

[25] Malmstrom HS, Hock JM, Sandforf C. Dental management of patients with hereditary angioedema: report a case. J Am Dent Assoc. 1985;111:957–8.

[26] Degroote DF, Smith GL, Huttula GS. Acute airway obstruction following tooth extraction in hereditary angioedema. J Oral Maxillofac Surg. 1985;43:52–4.

[27] Phillips KM, Glock M, Cohen SG. Hereditary angioedema: report of case. Spec Care Dentist. 1989;9:23–6.

[28] Leimgruber A, Jacques WA, Spaeth PJ. Hereditary angioedema: uncomplicated maxillofacial surgery using short-term C1 inhibitor replacement therapy. Inn Arch Allergy Immunol. 1993;101:107–12.

[29] Peled M, Ardekian L, Schnarch A, Laufer D. Preoperative prophylaxis for C1 esterase-inhibitor deficiency in patients undergoing oral surgery: a report of three cases. Quintessence Int. 1977;28:169–71.

[30] Karlis V, Glickman RS, Stern R, Kinney L. Hereditary angioedema: case report and review of management. Oral Surg Oral Med Oral Pathol Oral Radiol Endod. 1997;83:462–4.

[31] Farkas H, Gyeney L, Gidofalvy E, Fust G, Varga L. The efficacy of short-term danazol prophylaxis in hereditary angioedema patients undergoing maxillofacial and dental procedures. J Oral Maxillofac Surg. 1999;57:404–8.

[32] Webb MD, Hakimeh S, Holly LK. Management of children with hereditary angioedema: a report of two cases. Pediatr Dent. 2000;22:141–3.

[33] Maeda S, Miyawaki T, Nombra S, Yagi T, Shimada M. Management of oral surgery in patients with hereditary or acquired angioedemas: review and case report. Oral Surg Oral Med Oral Pathol Oral Radiol Endod. 2003;96:540–3.

[34] Rice S, Cochrane TJ, Millwaters M, Ali NT. Emergency management of upper airway angio-oedema after routine dental extraction in a patient with C1 esterase deficiency. Br J Oral Maxillofac Surg. 2008;46:394–6.

[35] Van Sickels NJ, Hunsaker RB, Van Sickels JE. Hereditary angioedema: treatment, management, and precautions in patients presenting for dental care. Oral Surg Oral Med Oral Pathol Oral Radiol Endod. 2010;109:168–72.

[36] Moraes RS, Vieira AS, Primo LG. Management of a dentigerous cyst in a child with hereditary angioedema. J Dent Child (Chic). 2010;77:59–63.

[37] Baccioglu Kavut A. A case of hereditary angioedema type II diagnosed in adult age by his first and life-threatening attack. Allergy 2011;66(Suppl. 94):320–481 (p. 431).

[38] Senaratne KT, Cottrell AM, Prentice RI. Successful perioperative management of a patient with C1 esterase inhibitor deficiency with a novel bradykinin receptor B2 antagonist. Anaesth Intens Care. 2012;40:523–6.

[39] Angeletti C, Angeletti PM, Mastrobuono F, Pilotti L, Ciccozzi A, Guetti C. BradykininB2 receptor antagonist off label use in short-term prophylaxis in hereditary angioedema. Int J Immunopathol Pharmacol. 2014;27:653–9.

[40] Narayanan A, Date RR, Birur S, Bhakta P, Srinivasan S. Anaesthesia management of a patient with hereditary angioedema with prophylactic administration of C1 esterase inhibitor: case report and literature review. Sultan Qaboos Univ Med J. 2013;13:E467–71.

[41] Sanuki T Watanabe T, Kurata S, Ayuse T. Perioperative management of tooth extractions for a patient with hereditary angioedema. J Oral Maxillofac Surg. 2014;72:2421.e1–3.

[42] Forrest A, Milne N, Soon A. Hereditary angioedema: death after a dental extraction. Aust Dent J. 2016. doi:10.1111/adj.12447.

[43] Bowen T, Cicardi M, Farkas H, Bork K, Kreuz W, Zingale L, et al. Canadian 2003 international consensus algorithm for the diagnosis, therapy, and management of hereditary angioedema. J Allergy Clin Immunol. 2004;114:629–37.

[44] Bowen T, Cicardi M, Bork K, Zuraw B, Frank M, Ritchie B, et al. Hereditary angiodema: a current state-of-the-art review, VII: Canadian Hungarian 2007 international consensus algorithm for the diagnosis, therapy, and management of hereditary angioedema. Ann Allergy Asthma Immunol. 2008;100(1 Suppl 2):S30–40.

[45] Craig T, Aygören-Pürsün E, Bork K, Bowen T, Boysen H, Farkas H, et al. WAO guideline for the management of hereditary angioedema. World Allergy Organ J. 2012;5:182–99.

[46] Zuraw BL, Bernstein JA, Lang DM, Craig T, Dreyfus D, Hsieh F, et al. A focused parameter update: hereditary angioedema, acquired C1 inhibitor deficiency, and angiotensin-converting enzyme inhibitor-associated angioedema. J Allergy Clin Immunol. 2013;131:1491–3.

[47] Betschel S, Badiou J, Binkley K, Hébert J, Kanani A, Keith P, et al. Canadian hereditary angioedema guideline. Allergy Asthma Clin Immunol. 2014;10:50.

[48] Baeza ML, Caballero Molina T, Crespo Diz C, González-Quevedo, Guilarte Clavero M, Hernández Fernández de Rojas D, et al. Algorithm for diagnosis and treatment of hereditary angioedema as a tool for management. Farm Hosp. 2013;37:521–9. Erratum in: Farm Hosp. 2014;38:150.

[49] Farkas H, Martinez-Saguer I, Bork K, Bowen T, Craig T, Frank M, et al. International consensus on the diagnosis and management of pediatric patients with hereditary angioedema with C1 inhibitor deficiency. Allergy. 2017;72:300–313.

[50] Frank MM, Zuraw B, Banerji A, Bernstein JA, Craig T, Busse P, et al. Management of children with hereditary angioedema due to C1 Inhibitor deficiency. Pediatrics. 2016;138(5). pii: e20160575.

[51] Schneider L, Hurewitz D, Wasserman R, Obtulowicz K, Machnig T, Moldovan D, et al. C1-INH concentrate for treatment of acute hereditary angioedema: a pediatric cohort from the I.M.P.A.C.T. studies. Pediatr Allergy Immunol. 2013;24:54–60.

[52] Lumry W, Manning ME, Hurewitz DS, Davis-Lorton M, Fitts D, Kalfus IN, et al. Nanofiltered C1-esterase inhibitor for the acute management and prevention of hereditary angioedema attacks due to C1-inhibitor deficiency in children. J Pediatr. 2013;162:1017–22, e1–2.

[53] Frank MM. Update on preventive therapy (prophylaxis) of hereditary angioedema. Allergy Asthma Proc. 2011;32:17–21.

[54] De Serres J, Groner A, Lindner J. Safety and efficacy of pasteurized C1 inhibitor concentrate (Berinert P) in hereditary angioedema: a review. Transfus Apher Sci. 2003;29:247–54.

[55] Terpstra FG, Kleijn M, Koenderman AH, Over J, van Engelenburg FA, Schuitemaker H, van't Wout AB. Viral safety of C1-inhibitor NF. Biologicals. 2007;35:173–81.

[56] Riedl MA, Bygum A, Lumry W, Magerl M, Bernstein JA, Busse P, et al. Safety and usage of C1-inhibitor in hereditary angioedema: Berinert registry data. J Allergy Clin Immunol Pract. 2016;4:963–71.

[57] Caballero Molina T, Pedrosa Delgado M, Gómez Traseira C. Hereditary angioedema. Med Clin (Barc). 2015;145:356–65.

[58] Cicardi M, Aberer W, Banerji A, Bas M, Bernstein JA, Bork K, et al. Classification, diagnosis, and approach to treatment for angioedema: consensus report from the hereditary angioedema international working group. Allergy. 2014;69:602–16.

[59] Hernández Fernández de Rojas D, Ibañez E, Longhurst H, Maurer M, Fabien V, Aberer W, et al. Treatment of HAE attacks in the icatibant outcome survey: an analysis of icatibant self-administration versus administration by health care professionals. Int Arch Allergy Immunol. 2015;167:21–8.

[60] Longhurst HJ, Aberer W, Bouillet L, Caballero T, Fabien V, Zanichelli A, et al. Analysis of characteristics associated with reinjection of icatibant: results from the icatibant outcome survey. Allergy Asthma Proc. 2015;36:399–406. Erratum in: Allergy Asthma Proc. 2015;36:511.

[61] Zanichelli A, Maurer M, Aberer W, Caballero T, Longhurst H, Bouillet L, et al. Long-term safety of icatibant treatment of patients with angioedema in real-world clinical practice. Allergy. 2016. doi:10.1111/all.13103.

[62] Marqués L, Domingo D, Maravall FJ, Clotet J. Short-term prophylactic treatment of hereditary angioedema with icatibant. Allergy. 2010;65:137–8.

[63] Angeletti C, Angeletti PM, Mastrobuono F, Pilotti L, Ciccozzi A, Guetti C. Bradykinin B2 receptor antagonist off label use in short-term prophylaxis in hereditary angioedema. Int J Immunopathol Pharmacol. 2014;27:653–9.

[64] Bernstein JA. Managing hereditary angioedema patients undergoing otolaryngeal procedures. Am J Rhinol Allergy. 2013;27(6):522–7. doi:10.2500/ajra.2013.27.3964.

[65] Turner MD, Oughourli A, Heaney K, Selvaggi T. Use of recombinant plasma kallikrein inhibitor in hereditary angioedema: a case report and review of the management of the disorder. J Oral Maxillofac Surg. 2004;62:1553–6.

[66] Farkas H, Martinez-Saguer I, Bork K, Bowen T, Craig T, Frank M, et al. International consensus on the diagnosis and management of pediatric patients with hereditary angioedema with C1 inhibitor deficiency. Allergy. 2016. doi:10.1111/all.13001.

[67] Caballero T, Farkas H, Bouillet L, Bowen T, Gompel A, Fagerberg C, et al. International consensus and practical guidelines on the gynecologic and obstetric management of female patients with hereditary angioedema caused by C1 inhibitor deficiency. J Allergy Clin Immunol. 2012;129:308–20.

[68] Caballero T, Canabal J, Rivero-Paparoni D, Cabañas R. Management of hereditary angioedema in pregnant women: a review. Int J Womens Health. 2014;6:839–48.

[69] Longhurst H, Cicardi M. Hereditary angio-oedema. Lancet. 2012;379(9814):474–81.

[70] Agostoni A, Aygören-Pürsün E, Binkley KE, Blanch A, Bork K, Bouillet L, et al. Hereditary and acquired angioedema: problems and progress: proceedings of the third C1 esterase inhibitor deficiency workshop and beyond. J Allergy Clin Immunol. 2004;114: S51–131.

[71] Bork K, Hardt J, Staubach-Renz P, Witzke G. Risk of laryngeal edema and facial swellings after tooth extraction in patients with hereditary angioedema with and without prophylaxis with C1 inhibitor concentrate: a retrospective study. Oral Surg Oral Med Oral Pathol Oral Radiol Endod. 2011;112:58–64.

[72] Aygören-Pürsün E, Martinez Saguer I, Kreuz W, Klingebiel T, Schwabe D. Risk of angioedema following invasive or surgical procedures in HAE type I and II--the natural history. Allergy. 2013;68:1034–9.

[73] Farkas H, Zotter Z, Csuka D, Szabó E, Nébenfuhrer Z, Temesszentandrási G, et al. Short-term prophylaxis in hereditary angioedema due to deficiency of the C1-inhibitor--a long-term survey. Allergy 2012;67:1586–93.

[74] Zuraw B, Bersntein J, Lang D. A focused parameter update: hereditary angioedema, acquired C1 inhibitor deficiency, and angiotensin-converting enzyme inhibito-associated angioedema. J Allergy Clin Immunol. 2013;131:1491–3.

Chapter 14

Bradykinin-Mediated Angioedema Across the History

Jesús Jurado-Palomo, Irina Diana Bobolea,

Alexandru Daniel Vlagea and Teresa Caballero

Additional information is available at the end of the chapter

http://dx.doi.org/10.5772/67714

Abstract

The origins of the discovery of the "Complement System" date from the second half of the nineteenth century. The official paternity of the Complement System is attributed to Jules Bordet. The complement system can be activated through three major pathways. The classical pathway, the alternative pathway, and the lectin pathway converge in a common final lytic pathway. Hereditary angioedema (HAE) due to C1-inhibitor (C1-INH) deficiency (C1-INH-HAE) was first described by Robert Graves in his clinical lectures. The autosomal dominant pattern of HAE was recognized by Sir William Osler. The pathophysiologic basis of C1-INH-HAE as a deficiency of a plasma inhibitor was discovered in the early 1960s. In 1986, the C1NH gene was identified, which encodes the C1-INH protein. Although the possible relationship between angioedema and estrogens in women was described as early as 1986, it was not until the first decade of the twenty-first century when several series of patients with HAE were described with normal levels of the fractions of the complement system. In the last decade, several drugs have been approved and marketed in Europe, in the United States, and in other countries, contributing to the improved management of C1-INH-HAE and patient's quality of life.

Keywords: acquired angioedema, angioedema, bradykinin, c1 inhibitor, complement system, factor XII, hereditary angioedema, hereditary angioedema with mutation in *F12* gene, history, immunodeficiency

1. Introduction

The origins of the discovery of the "Complement System" date from the second half of the nineteenth century. The official paternity of the Complement System is attributed to Jules Bordet. The complement system can be activated through three major pathways. The classical pathway, the alternative pathway, and the lectin pathway converge in a common final lytic pathway. This chapter describes the historical discovery of biochemistry pathways implicated in the pathophysiology of bradykininergic angioedema (BK-AE).

2. Historical review of the Complement System

The origins of the discovery of the "Complement System" date from the second half of the nineteenth century. In that era, the works of Louis Pasteur (1822–1895), Robert Koch (1843–1910) [1], and Joseph Lister (1827–1912) [2] contributed to the knowledge needed to consider many microorganisms as producers of lethal effects in humans. It was obvious that the human body, despite being constantly exposed to microorganisms, successfully overcame their assaults, discovering that many of them were destroyed in the blood, one of whose effector systems of defense was the "complement system" [3] (**Figure 1**).

Taube and Gscheidlen made one of the first observations that the blood of various mammals possessed bactericidal activity [4]. These authors injected microorganisms in the bloodstream, sampling at 24 and 48 hours while preserving them aseptically. Even months after storage, bacterial multiplication was not observed. Wyssokowitsch [5] and von Fodor [6, 7] repeated the experiment, injecting microorganisms in the blood of mammals, noting that within minutes there were no viable organisms; they thought that they had been cleared by the blood cells. Metschnikoff [8] found phagocytes that engulfed and destroyed microorganisms, but soon discovered that blood cells were not solely responsible. Grohmann [9] was the first scientist who discovered that *in vitro* plasma (cell-free) was capable of lysing bacteria and fungi.

Nuttal [10], in experiments similar to those conducted previously by Wyssokowitsch [5] and von Fodor [6, 7], observed morphological changes in microorganisms (anthrax bacillus) that had escaped phagocytosis, concluding that they had been damaged by a noncellular process. After inoculating defibrinated sheep blood with bacteria, the bactericidal activity was preserved both *in vivo* and *in vitro*, but disappeared if the blood was heated to 45°C or was stored for several days at room temperature. A year later, Buchner [11, 12] reported that fresh serum was able to lyse bacteria, but if heated for 30 minutes at 55°C, this capacity was lost. He also found that the dialysis of fresh serum against water at 0°C for 18–36 hours abolished the lytic activity, but there was no loss when dialyzed against bicarbonate buffer containing 0.75–0.8% NaCl. He called fresh factor serum with bactericidal activity "alexina," concluding that it was due to proteins with enzymatic activity.

Pfeiffer and Issaeff [13] reported that the activity of alexina was due to the joint action of specific antibodies and specific serum factor. In their experiment, the blood of guinea pigs that recovered from cholera infection protected normal guinea pigs if they were injected alexina

http://dx.doi.org/10.5772/67714

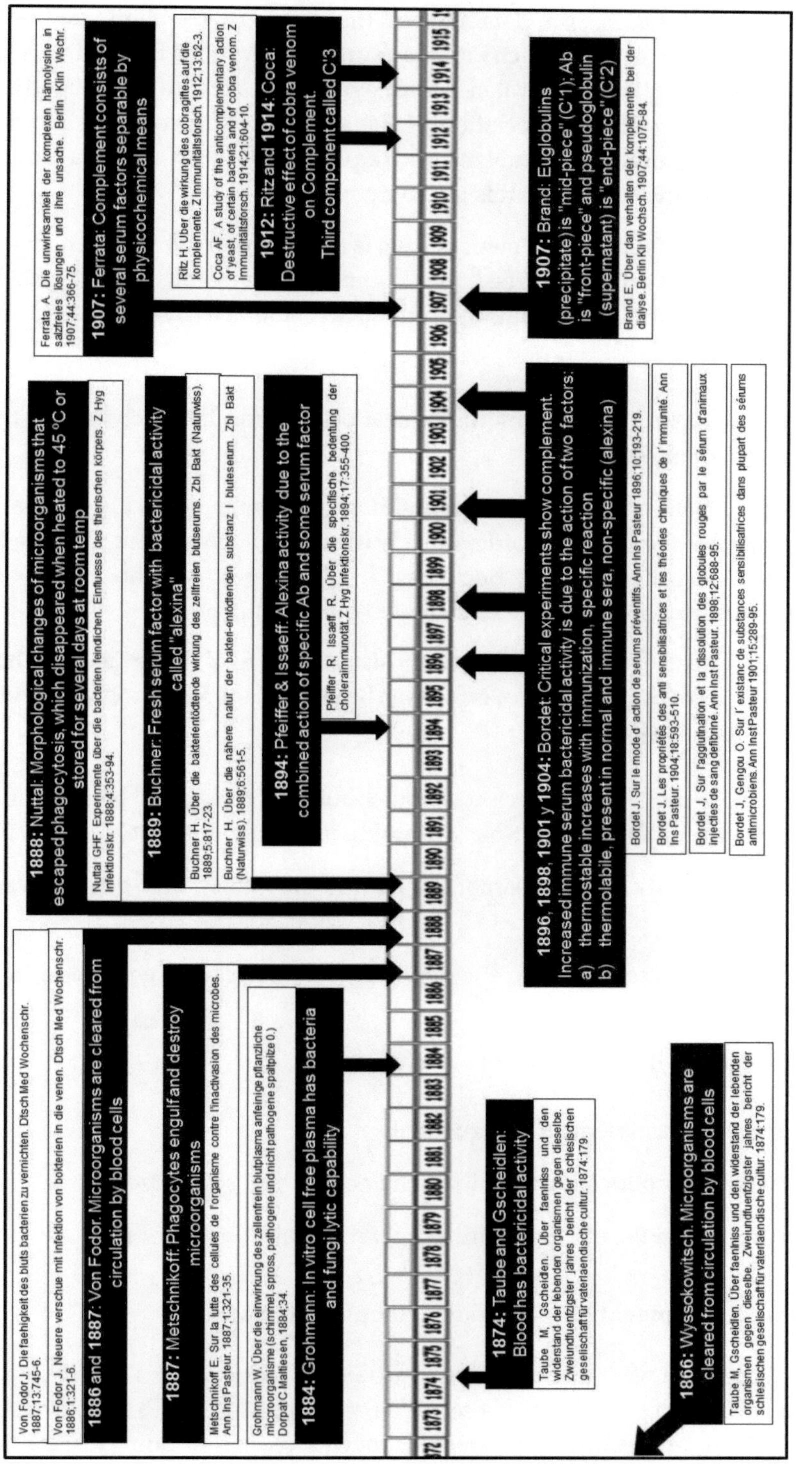

Figure 1. Historical review of the Complement System (from 1850 to 1930) [3].

mixed with live bacteria. *In vitro* data showed that vibrios were eliminated only by fresh immune serum, but not by heat-inactivated immune serum. Protection against cholera present during injections of heat-inactivated immune serum was due to the antibody. Therefore, bacterial lysis was due to the association of the antibody plus complement. Bacteriolytic ability of serum from animals immunized with a particular microorganism was higher than that of animals immunized against this microorganism.

The official paternity of the Complement System is attributed to Jules Bordet, who performed the critical experiments that identified the "complement system" in 1894 [14, 15]. Bordet [16, 17] showed that increased immune serum bactericidal activity was due to the action of two factors [3]:

(a) Thermostable factor increased by immunization, specifically reacting with the microorganism used to immunize.

(b) Thermolabile factor present in normal and immune sera, nonspecific (at least in the way the thermostable factor was). Bordet quickly identified such a factor with the bactericidal activity or alexina described by Buchner [11, 12]. He was also able to lyse erythrocytes sensitized with specific antibodies against erythrocyte antigens.

Ferrata [18] showed that the complement consisted of several serum factors that could be separated by physicochemical means, but it was Brand [19] the following year who best characterized both fractions [3]:

(a) He called the activity in the precipitate (euglobulins) "mid-piece" because he found that it acted after the antibody (front-piece) would bind to the cell (RBC).

(a) He called the activity in the supernatant (pseudo-globulins) "end-piece" because it acted only after the "mid-piece" had acted.

(b) Interaction of erythrocytes with the antibody, mid-piece, and end-piece, in that order, produced hemolysis.

Brand's works established a number of assumptions:

(a) The action of the complement is sequential.

(b) An intermediate product as a function of hemolysis was generated.

Both the mid-piece and the end-piece are temperature sensitive.

2.1. Historical development of the classical complement pathway

Ritz [20] and Coca [21] were the first to demonstrate the existence of a third component other than the mid- and end-piece following observation of the destructive effect of cobra venom on the complement [3] (**Figure 2**). Coca treated fresh serum with yeast, concluding that the third component was capable of combining with yeast and he called it C′3. Gordon et al. [22] showed a fourth component, which he called C′4 when observing that the ammonium destroyed a thermostable

http://dx.doi.org/10.5772/67714

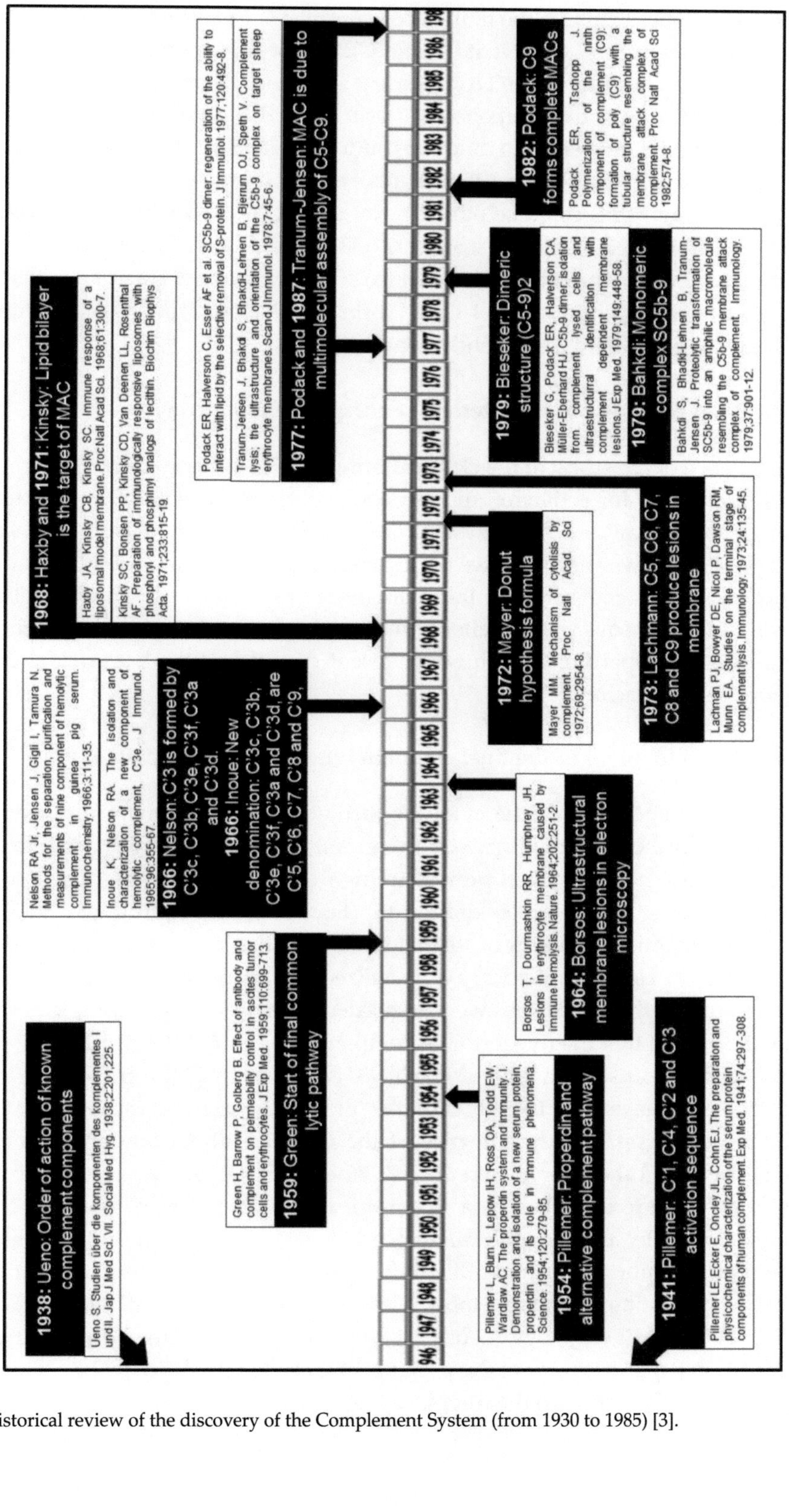

Figure 2. Historical review of the discovery of the Complement System (from 1930 to 1985) [3].

factor from serum other than C′3 (the mid-piece was called C′1 and the end-piece was renamed C′2). It should be noted at this point that C′1 and C′2 do not correspond to the current fractions C1 and C2, since both constitute the full complement including C′3 and C′4. Ueno [23] established the order of performance of the components known up to that time. Pillemer [24] managed to separate the four serum fractions into different components and set the activation sequence C′1, C′4, C′2, and C′3. It was not until the early 1960s, once chromatographic methods were developed, that the various components could be purified. Nelson [25, 26] showed that in reality the third component C′3 was formed by at least six factors (C′3c, C′3b, C′3e, C′3f, C′3a, and C′3d). Having established that these were proteins not related to C′3 acting at a later stage, he called them C′5, C′6, C′7, C′8, and C′9, respectively. As of 1968, World Health Organization (WHO) annulled the symbol "′" leaving it currently C1, C2, and so on.

2.2. Historical development of the alternative complement pathway

The heavy reliance of the study of the classical complement pathway using erythrocytes sensitized with antibodies for activation did not even consider the possibility of activation by other substances [3]. However, since the early twentieth century, there were data suggesting that it was possible to lyse erythrocytes with cobra venom without antibodies and with the participation of various components other than those of the classical pathway. Pillemer [27] was the father of the discovery of the alternative pathway upon describing a protein or a new component called "properdin," which when absent diminished the bactericidal potency of serum against certain bacteria.

2.3. Historical development of the final common lytic complement pathway

Green et al. [28] suggested that the cytolysis mediated by complement involved the production of pores in the cell membrane on the grounds that large molecules (dextrans and albumin) prevented cell lysis when present in high concentration in the reaction medium; on the contrary, but small molecules did not [3] (**Figure 2**). Cell rupture was thought to be due to a colloid-osmotic swelling process that finally finished by lysing the cell. Borsos et al. [29], with the use of electron microscopy, visualized ultrastructural lesions etched into cell membranes, showing that the lesions were associated with the cytolytic complement activity. Lachman [30] showed that the five terminal components C5, C6, C7, C8, and C9 were necessary and sufficient to cause such lesions. Haxby [31] and Kinsky [32] were the first to demonstrate that the lipid bilayer was the target of the "membrane attack complex" (MAC), noting that C5-C9 directly damaged the integrity of the bilayer without any enzymatic activity. Mayer [33] formulated the "donut hypothesis" where cell damage is achieved through the formation of a structure described as a donut, forming stable transmembrane pores. Lysis would be explained by the osmotic difference between the exterior and the interior cell through the transmembrane channel. Bhadki [34] and Podack [35] observed that the MAC was due to C5-C9 multimolecular assembly. Bieseker [36] initially postulated a dimeric structure (C5-9)2, but Bhakdi [37] suggested a monomeric complex with the same structure as the complex SC5b-9 ("S" was one of the proteins that control the MAC). The C9 alone forms complexes structurally similar to the full MAC [38].

http://dx.doi.org/10.5772/67714

3. Historical review (from C1 inhibitor to bradykinin)

Hereditary angioedema (HAE) due to C1-inhibitor (C1-INH) deficiency (C1-INH-HAE), also known as "non-allergic angioneurotic edema," "AE without urticaria," or "Osler's hereditary edema" is a potentially fatal clinical entity, which in recent years has become an example to be followed because of the great progress made from the union of researchers, physicians, and patient associations worldwide (**Figure 3**).

It was first described in 1843 by Robert Graves in his clinical lectures. In 1882, Heinrich Quincke documented some cases of acute, circumscribed edema, involving two generations of the same family and coined the term angioneurotic edema [39]. Subsequently, Sir William Osler in 1888 first described in detail an inherited form of angioedema (AE) [40], from which in 1917 the hereditary type was identified [41]. The disease was defined biochemically in 1963 by Donaldson and Evans [42], as an absence of serum inhibitor of the first component of the complement. Dating from 1972 is the first case of acquired angioedema due to C1 inhibitor deficiency (C1-INH-AAE) in lymphosarcoma [43].

The main symptom of C1-INH-HAE is the attack of AE, the laryngeal location being the most serious. Landerman [44] reviewed all the medical literature published between 1888 and 1962 and found 28 publications of more than one case of death from fatal laryngeal attacks in more than one family with C1-INH-HAE. The total number of deaths due to C1-INH-HAE was 92.

In 1960, Spaulding demonstrated the efficacy of methyl testosterone in the treatment of C1-INH-HAE in a family [45]. In 1976, a double-blind placebo-controlled trial demonstrated the efficacy of danazol for the treatment of C1-INH-HAE [46]. It was then when stanozolol, another attenuated androgen, started to be used [47].

In 1968, the first case of C1-INH-HAE successfully treated with epsilon-aminocaproic acid (EACA) was published [48], although it was not until 1972 when the efficacy of anti-fibrinolytic agents (AFs), EACA, and tranexamic acid was demonstrated in double-blind clinical trials [49, 50]. AFs are reserved for those patients who cannot tolerate attenuated androgens or present contraindications for their administration.

An article published in 1973 described for the first time the administration of concentrated C1-INH (pdC1INH), partially purified from a mixture of human plasma, in two patients [51]. Previously, replacement therapy in patients with C1-INH-HAE in the attack phase had been attempted with fresh-frozen plasma [52], which was abandoned later because of the risk of viral transmission, although it was still used in case of pdC1INH being unavailable [53].

In the USA, two double-blind placebo-controlled clinical trials had been conducted with pdC1INH, which had proven its efficacy and safety [54]; however, the Food and Drug Administration (FDA) had not yet approved its use in the 2000s. At that time, Berinert-P® (Behring, Marburg, Germany) was commercialized in Germany and a few European countries [55] and was available in Spain, where it was imported through the Foreign Medicines service [56].

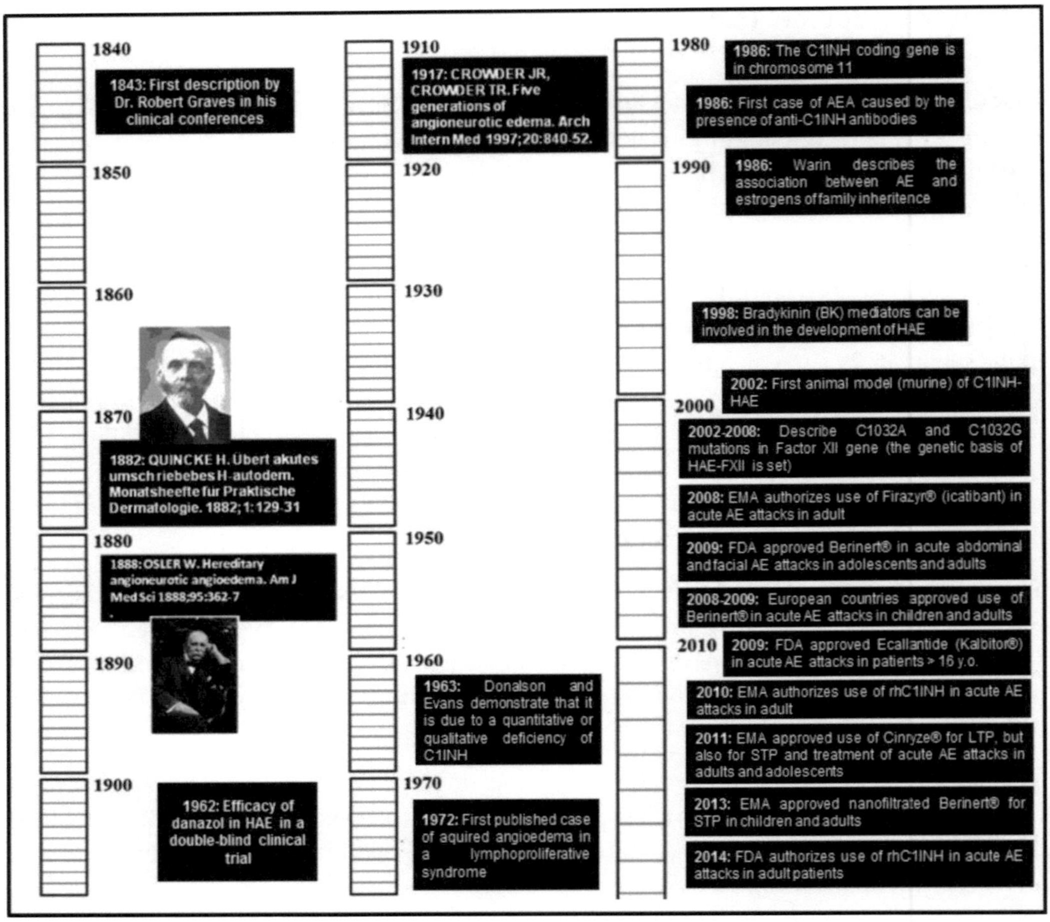

Figure 3. Historical review of angioedema due to C1-inhibitor deficiency.

In 1986, the *C1NH* gene was identified (Gene Bank X54486; Swiss-Prot P05155), which encodes the C1INH protein, also called *SERPING1*, located on chromosome 11 subregion q11-q13.1 [57–59].

Although the possible relationship between AE and estrogens in women was described as early as 1986 [60], it was not until the first decade of the twenty-first century when several series of patients with HAE were described with normal levels of the fractions of the complement system [61, 62]. It was originally called HAE type III [62]. Finally, a mutation was found in *F12* gene in some of the families [63–65].

Initially, C2-kinin, a vasoactive peptide generated by cleavage of the C2b fragment was thought to be involved in angioedema formation in C1-INH-HAE [66].

In 1998, there was growing support for another hypothesis in the generation of AE. It argued that BK was the most important mediator in the development of AE [67] and had been proven through clinical, *in vitro* studies and experiments in an experimental model of C1INH-deficient transgenic mice [68]. In 2002, a transgenic mouse with C1 inhibitor deficiency was developed by Professor Davis [69].

In the last decade, several drugs have been approved and marketed in Europe, in the United States, and in other countries, contributing to improved management of C1-INH-HAE and patient's quality of life.

First, icatibant acetate (Firazyr®, Shire HGT, Zug, Switzerland) [70, 71], a bradykinin B2 receptor blocker, was approved by the European Medicines Agency (EMA) in 2008 for the treatment of acute AE attacks in adult patients with C1-INH-HAE [72] and was marketed in Spain in March 2009.

In 2008, a new C1-esterase inhibitor formulation, Cinryze®, was approved by FDA for the long-term prophylaxis of C1-INH-HAE [73]. This drug incorporated a nanofiltration step as an extra safety procedure to reduce the transmission of enveloped and nonenveloped viruses and possible prions [74, 75] and had been shown to be effective in reducing the number of AE attacks per month [76, 77]. In 2011, the European Medicines Agency (EMA) approved the marketing of Cinryze® for long-term prophylaxis, but also for short-term prophylaxis and treatment of acute AE attacks in adults and adolescents with C1-INH-HAE [78].

Berinert®, which had been marketed in Germany in 1985, was approved in 2008–2009 in different European countries through a mutual recognition agreement for the treatment of acute AE attacks in children and adults with C1-INH-HAE. Later, it also incorporated the nanofiltration step and it was approved by the EMA for short-term prophylaxis in children and adults in 2013 [79]. In 2009, FDA approved Berinert® for the treatment of acute abdominal and facial AE attacks in adolescents and adults with C1-INH-HAE [80].

In December 2009, Ecallantide (DX-88, Kalbitor®, Dyax Corp, currently part of Shire HGT), a kallikrein inhibitor, was approved by the FDA for the treatment of acute AE attacks in patients >16 years with C1-INH-HAE [81]. It was later approved for adolescents (2014).

A recombinant C1 inhibitor (rhC1INH) (Ruconest®, Pharming Technologies BV®, Leiden, The Netherlands) produced in transgenic rabbits [82] was approved by EMA in 2010 for the treatment of acute AE attacks in adult patients with C1-INH-HAE [83]. It was in 2014 when the FDA approved it for the same indication by FDA [84].

Some European centers have developed training programs for self-administration of intravenous and subcutaneous specific drugs for the treatment of C1-INH-HAE [85–90].

The development of new drugs or new uses for old drugs changed the therapeutic approach in C1-INH-HAE in the last decade. However, the development of new drugs will even alter more therapeutic landscape for C1-INH-HAE in the next years.

4. Historical review (from C1 inhibitor to coagulation factor XII)

In hereditary angioedema (HAE) with mutation in *F12* gene (FXII-HAE), symptoms are similar to C1-INH-HAE, there are no abnormalities in the *C1NH* gene and antigenic and functional C1INH, C1q and C4 are usually within the normal range [91]. The final common mediator is thought to be bradykinin (BK). The history of the description of nC1-INH-HAE can be seen in **Figure 4**.

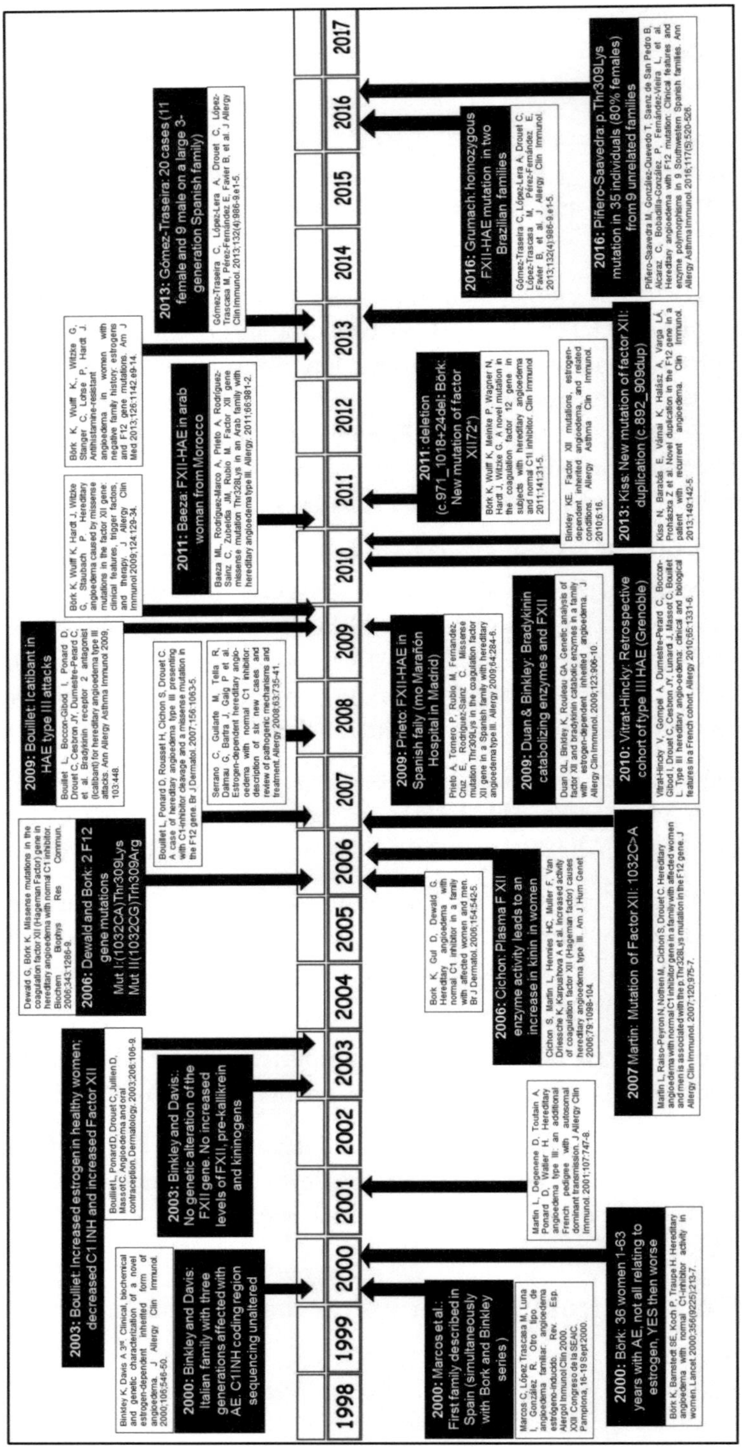

Figure 4. Historical review of angioedema type III.

http://dx.doi.org/10.5772/67714

In 2000, Binkley et al. [92] analyzed the family tree of eight women from three different generations noting that AE episodes were triggered by estrogen treatment (OCPs, hormone replacement therapy in menopause) or by pregnancies, the onset being at 14–21 days after conception, and at 7–14 days after the initiation of hormone replacement therapy. Börk et al. [93] described simultaneously a series of 36 women with angioedema with functionality conserved in the different fractions of the complement system (including C1 inhibitor), and who worsened in relation to situations of increased estrogens. Bork et al. [93] proposed to call this new AE type as HAE type III. Simultaneously, Marcos et al. [94] described in the XXII National SEAIC Congress the first family case in Spain, data that would be extended over the years [95]. One year later, Martin et al. [96] contributed data regarding the transmission of "HAE type III" in France.

Boulliet et al. [97] reported that increased levels of estrogen in healthy women have produced a reduction of C1INH, which entailed an increase in amidolytic FXII activity. Dewald et al. analyzed 20 unrelated women with HAE without C1INH deficiency, finding two mutations in the *F12* gene in the second position of the ACG codon, corresponding to the residual amino acid 309; mutation I (five patients) 1032C>A; Thr309Lys; and mutation II (1 patient) 1032C>G; Thr309Arg (**Figure 4**). This mutation was not found in 145 healthy controls. Later, these authors extended the study to five families with 20 symptomatic patients and 10 asymptomatic family members (eight men and two women), which showed the presence of one of the two mutations [98]. Cichon et al. [99] studied a family proving that the increased amidolytic enzymatic activity of FXII in women produced an increase in the production of kinins. A year later, Martin et al. [100] studied four generations of one family with eight members who were carriers of the *F12* gene 1032C>A mutation (four symptomatic and four asymptomatic), noting that in women symptoms were triggered or exacerbated by estrogens, whereas in men the symptoms were milder.

Börk et al. [101] described 35 symptomatic women from 13 different families with FXII-HAE (with proven mutations p.Thr309Lys/p.Thr309Arg). Triggers were taking OCPs (17 women) and pregnancy (3 women). A symptomatic exacerbation occurred after taking OCPs (8 women), pregnancy (7 women), hormone replacement therapy with estrogen (3 women), taking ACE inhibitors (2 women) and taking type 1 ACE receptor blocker (1 woman). pdC1INH was effective as the treatment of acute AE attacks (6 women) and progestogens (8 women), danazol (2 women), and tranexamic acid (1 woman) were used as prophylactic treatment.

Börk et al. proposed to use FXII-HAE to name those cases of nC1-INH-HAE with a mutation in *F12* gene and unknown-HAE (U-HAE) to those without a known mutation [101].

The series with the largest number of hereditary (related to estrogen) (HAE type III) corresponds to Börk et al., who described 69 patients from 23 unrelated families with HAE-FXII, and 196 patients with U-HAE [102].

An increase in FXII amidolytic activity was initially described as the cause of activation of contact system and the final release of bradykinin with the consequent angioedema in FXII-HAE [99], although other authors could not confirm this. Recently, another study has shown that the different mutations in exon 9 of *F12* gene found in FXII-HAE produce an increase in FXII activability by plasmin [103].

In Spain, several studies have been published focusing on FXIII-HAE: Serrano et al. [104] (six cases; two of them women from the same family) and Prieto et al. [105] (four generations of the same family with mutation 1032C>A; Thr309Lys; three symptomatic women, one male asymptomatic carrier).

Baeza et al. [106] described a nonatopic 27-year-old Arab woman from Morocco with a clinical diagnosis of hereditary angioedema type III and the p.Thr328Lys mutation. Icatibant acetate was prescribed for compassionate use.

Gómez-Traseira et al. [107] describes 20 cases (11 females and 9 males on a large 3-generation Spanish family). The p.Thr309Lys mutation was detected in five female patients who had a phenotypic variant in which AE was exclusively precipitated by high estrogen levels and in six asymptomatic relatives.

Piñero-Saavedra et al. [108] described p.Thr309Lys mutation in 35 individuals (80% females) from 9 unrelated families. In this prospective observational cohort study, 16 females (44% estrogen dependent, 56% estrogen sensitive) were clearly symptomatic. Also, two polymorphisms (XPNPEP2 c-2399A and the ACE insertion/deletion) were detected in 17% of patients.

The University Hospital in Grenoble is a reference center for the study of FXII-HAE in France. As a result of this, Vitrat-Hincky et al. [109] published a retrospective analysis (for the years 2000–2009) with 26 patients, which included four symptomatic men).

Duan et al. [110] not only confirmed the *F12* gene mutation (gene-codifying coagulation factor XII) in women of the same family but also provide certain polymorphisms in the genes encoding aminopeptidase P (APP) and angiotensin-converting enzyme (ACE). It highlights the role of the BK-catabolizing enzymes in the pathogenesis of angioedema.

Börk et al. [111] described a new mutation in the *F12* gene (deletion of 72 base pairs c.971_1018+24del72*). More recently, Kiss et al. [112] described a new mutation consisting in the duplication of 18 base pairs (c.892_909dup) causing the repeated presence of 6 aa (p.298-303) in the same region of FXII to those described above.

Grumach et al. [113] report two Brazilian FXII-HAE families segregating the mutation c.983 C>A (p.Thr328Lys). In each family, one patient with a homozygous mutation was found. The homozygous FXII-HAE mutation status leads to a severe phenotype in females and males, and to an increased risk of manifest symptoms in the latter.

In terms of treatment, there is no approved drug for the treatment of nC1-INH-HAE, either FXII-HAE or U-HAE. The pdhC1INH has been used in the acute attack of AE in some cases of FXII-HAE [102, 114, 115]. More recently, icatibant acetate was effective but also used off-label as this indication is not reflected in the product's prescribing information [115].

Author details

Jesús Jurado-Palomo[1,2*], Irina Diana Bobolea[3,4], Alexandru Daniel Vlagea[5] and Teresa Caballero[2,6,7]

*Address all correspondence to: h72jupaj@yahoo.es

1 Department of Allergology, Nuestra Señora del Prado University General Hospital, Talavera de la Reina, Spain

2 Spanish Study Group on Bradykinin-Induced Angioedema (SGBA), Spanish Society of Allergology and Clinical Immunology (SEAIC), Madrid, Spain

3 Department of Allergology, Hospital Doce de Octubre Institute for Health Research (i+12), Madrid, Spain

4 Highly-specialized Severe Asthma Unit, Hospital Doce de Octubre Institute for Health Research (i+12), Madrid, Spain

5 Department of Immunology, Central Laboratory of Madrid Community—BRSalud, San Sebastián de los Reyes, Madrid, Spain

6 Department of Allergology, Hospital La Paz Institute for Health Research (IdiPAZ), Madrid, Spain

7 Biomedical Research Network on Rare Diseases, CIBERER (U754), Madrid, Spain

References

[1] Koch R. UntersuchungenüberBakterien: V. Die ätiologie der Milzbrand-Krankheit, begründetauddieentwicklungsgeschichte des *Bacillus anthracis*. [Investigations into bacteria: V. The etiology of anthrax, based on the ontogenesis of *Bacillus anthracis*]. CohnsBeitragezurBiologie der Pflanzen. 1876;2:277–310.

[2] Bankston J. Joseph Lister and the Story of Antiseptics (Uncharted, Unexplored, and Unexplained). Bear: Mitchell Lane Publishers. 2004. ISBN: 1-58415-262-1.

[3] Vivanco Martínez F. Hundred years of complement (Cien años de complemento). Immunology (Inmunología). 1990;9:99–107.

[4] Taube M, Gscheidlen. Über faenlniss und den widerstand der lebenden organismen gegen dieselbe. Zweiundfuenfzigster jahres bericht der schlesischen geselischaft für vaterlaendische cultur. 1874:179-95.

[5] Wyssokowitsch W. Über die schicksale der in′s blut injicierten mikro-organismen in Körper der warmblüter. Z Hyg Infektionskr. 1866;1:3–9.

[6] Von Fodor J. Neuere verschue mit infektion von bokterien in die venen. Dtsch Med Wochenschr. 1886;1:321–6.

[7] Von Fodor J. Die faehigkeit des bluts bacterien zu vernichten. Dtsch Med Wochenschr. 1887;13:745–6.

[8] Metschnikoff E. Sur la lutte des cellules de l'organisme contre l'inactivasion des microbes. Ann Ins Pasteur. 1887;1:321–35.

[9] Grohmann W. Über die einwirkung des zellenfrein blutplasma anfeinige pflanzliche miccroorganisme (schimmel, spross, pathogene und nicht pathogene spaltpilze 0.) Dorpat C Maltiesen, 1884;34-45.

[10] Nuttal GHF. Experimente über die bacterien feindlichen. Einfluesse des thierischen körpers. Z Hyg Infektionskr. 1888;4:353–94.

[11] Buchner H. Über die bakterientödtende wirkung des zellfreien blutserums. Zbl Bakt (Naturwiss). 1889;5:817–23.

[12] Buchner H. Über die nähere natur der bakteri-entödtenden substanz I bluteserum. Zbl Bakt (Naturwiss). 1889;6:561–5.

[13] Pfeiffer R, Issaeff R. Über die specifische bedentung der choleraimmunotät. Z Hyg Infektionskr. 1894;17:355–400.

[14] Bordet J. Sur le mode d'action de sérums préventifs. Ann Ins Pasteur. 1896;10:193–219.

[15] Bordet J, Sur l'agglutination et la dissolution des globules rouges par le sérum d'animaux injecties de sang defibriné. Ann Inst Pasteur. 1898;12:688–95.

[16] Bordet J, Gengou O. Sur l'existence de substances sensibilisatrices dans plupart des sérums antimicrobiens. Ann Inst Pasteur. 1901;15:289–95.

[17] Bordet J. Les propriétés des anti sensibilisatrices et les théories chimiques de l´immunité. Ann Ins Pasteur. 1904;18:593–510.

[18] Ferrata A. Die unwirksamkeit der komplexen hämolysine in salzfreies lösungen und ihre unsache. Berlin Klin Wschr. 1907;44:366–75.

[19] Brand E. Über dan verhalten der komplemente bei der dialyse. Berlin Kli Wochsch. 1907;44:1075–84.

[20] Ritz H. Uber die wirkung des cobragiftes auf die komplemente. Z Immunitältsforsch. 1912;13:62–3.

[21] Coca AF. A study of the anticomplementary action of yeast, of certain bacteria and of cobra venom. Z Immunitältsforsch. 1914;21:604–10.

[22] Gordon J, Whitehead KR, Wormall A. The action of ammonia on complement. The fourth component. J Biochem. 1926;20:1028–35.

[23] Ueno S. Studien über die komponenten des komplementes I und II. Jap J Med Sci. VII. Social Med Hyg. 1938;2:201–225.

[24] Pillemer LE, Ecker E, Oncley JL, Cohn EJ. The preparation and physicochemical characterization of the serum protein components of human complement. Exp Med. 1941;74:297–308.

[25] Nelson RA Jr, Jensen J, Gigli I, Tamura N. Methods for the separation, purification and measurements of nine component of hemolytic complement in guinea pig serum. Immunochemistry. 1966;3:11–35.

[26] Inoue K, Nelson RA. The isolation and characterization of a new component of hemolytic complement, C'3e. J Immunol. 1965;96:355–67.

[27] Pillemer L, Blum L, Lepow IH, Ross OA, Todd EW, Wardlaw AC. The properdin system and immunity. I. Demonstration and isolation of a new serum protein, properdin and its role in immune phenomena. Science. 1954;120:279–85.

[28] Green H, Barrow P, Golberg B. Effect of antibody and complement on permeability control in ascites tumor cells and erythrocytes. J Exp Med. 1959;110:699–713.

[29] Borsos T, Dourmashkin RR, Humphrey JH. Lesions in erythrocyte membrane caused by immune hemolysis. Nature. 1964;202:251–2.

[30] Lachman PJ, Bowyer DE, Nicol P, Dawson RM, Munn EA. Studies on the terminal stage of complement lysis. Immunology. 1973;24:135–45.

[31] Haxby JA, Kinsky CB, Kinsky SC. Immune response of a liposomal model membrane. Proc Natl Acad Sci. 1968;61:300–7.

[32] Kinsky SC, Bonsen PP, Kinsky CD, Van Deenen LL, Rosenthal AF. Preparation of immunologically responsive liposomes with phosphoryl and phosphinyl analogs of lecithin. Biochim Biophys Acta. 1971;233:815–19.

[33] Mayer MM. Mechanism of cytolysis by complement. Proc Natl Acad Sci. 1972;69:2954–8.

[34] Tranum-Jensen J, Bhadki S, Bhakdi-Lehnen B, Bjerrum OJ, Speth V. Complement lysis; the ultrastructure and orientation of the C5b-9 complex on target sheep erythrocyte membranes. Scand J Immunol. 1978;7:45–6.

[35] Podack ER, Halverson C, Esser AF et al. SC5b-9 dimer: regeneration of the ability to interact with lipid by the selective removal of S-protein. J Immunol. 1977;120:492–8.

[36] Bieseker G, Podack ER, Halverson CA, Müller-Eberhard HJ. C5b-9 dimer: isolation from complement lysed cells and ultrastructural identification with complement dependent membrane lesions. J Exp Med. 1979;149:448–58.

[37] Bahkdi S, Bhadki-Lehnen B, Tranum-Jensen J. Proteolytic transformation of SC5b-9 into an amphiphilic macromolecule resembling the C5b-9 membrane attack complex of complement. Immunology. 1979;37:901–12.

[38] Podack ER, Tschopp J. Polymerization of the ninth component of complement (C9): formation of poly (C9) with a tubular structure resembling the membrane attack complex of complement. Proc Natl Acad Sci. 1982;79:574–8.

[39] Quincke H. Über akutes umschriebebes Hautodem. Monatsheefte für Praktische Dermatologie, 1882;1:129–31.

[40] Osler W. Hereditary angioneurotic angioedema. Am J Med Sci. 1888;95:362–7.

[41] Crowder JR, Crowder TR. Five generations of angioneurotic edema. Arch Intern Med 1917; 20: 840–852.

[42] Donaldson VH, Evans RR. A biochemical abnormality in hereditary angioneurotic edema: absence of serum inhibitor of C1-esterase. Am J Med. 1963;31:37–44.

[43] Caldwell JR, Ruddy S, Schur PH, Austen KF. Acquired C1 inhibitor deficiency in lymphosarcoma. Clin Immunol Immunopathol. 1972; 1:39.

[44] Landerman NS. Hereditary angioneurotic edema, I: case reports and review of the literature. J Allergy. 1962;33:316–29.

[45] Spaulding WB. Methyltestosterone therapy for hereditary episodic edema (hereditary angioneurotic edema). Ann Intern Med. 1960;53:739–45.

[46] Gelfand JA, Sherins RJ, Alling DW, Frank MM. Treatment of hereditary angioedema with danazol. Reversal of clinical and biochemical abnormalities. New Engl J Med. 1976;295:1444–8.

[47] Agostoni A, Cicardi M, Martignoni GC, Bergamaschini L, Marasini B. Danazol and stanozolol in long-term prophylactic treatment of hereditary angioedema. J Allergy Clin Immunol. 1980;65:75–9.

[48] Lundh B, Laurell AB, Wetterqvist H, White T, Granerus G. A case of hereditary angioneurotic oedema, successfully treated with ε-aminocaproic acid. Studies on C'1 esterase inhibitor, C'1 activation, plasminogen level and histamine metabolism. Clin Exp Immunol. 1968;3:733–45.

[49] Frank MM, Sergent JS, Kane MA, Alling DW. Epsilon aminocaproic acid therapy of hereditary angioneurotic edema: a double-blind study. N Engl J Med. 1972;286:808–12.

[50] Sheffer AL, Austen KF, Rosen FS. Tranexamic acid therapy in hereditary angioneurotic edema. N Engl J Med. 1972;287:452–4.

[51] Brackertz D, Kueppers F. Possible therapy in hereditary angioneurotic edema (HAE). Klin Wschr 1973;51:620–2.

[52] PickeringRJ,GoodRA,KellyJR,GewurzH.Replacementtherapyinhereditaryangioedema. Successful treatment of two patients with fresh frozen plasma. Lancet. 1969;1:326–30.

[53] Hill BJ, Thomas SH, McCabe C. Fresh frozen plasma for acute exacerbations of hereditary angioedema. Am J Emerg Med. 2004;22:633.

[54] Waytes AT, Rosen FS, Frank MM. Treatment of hereditary angioedema with a vapor-heated C1 inhibitor concentrate. N Engl J Med. 1996;20:1630–4.

[55] De Serres J, Gröner A, Lindner J. Safety and efficacy of pasteurised C1 inhibitor concentrate (Berinert® P) in hereditary angioedema: a review. Transfus Apher Sci. 2003; 29:247–54.

[56] Regulation (EC) No 141/2000 of the European Parliament and of the Council of 16 December 1999 on orphan medicinal products of 19 December 1999. Official Journal L 018, 22/01/2000 P. 0001-0005.

[57] Bock SC, Skriver K, Nielsen E, Thogersen HC, Wiman B, Donaldson VH, et al. Human C1 inhibitor: primary structure, cDNA cloning, and chromosomal localization. Biochemistry. 1986;25:4292–301.

[58] Davis AE III, Whitehead AS, Harrison RA, Dauphinais A, Bruns GA, Cicardi M, et al. Human inhibitor of the first component of complement, C1: characterization of cDNA clones and localization of the gene to chromosome 11. Proc Natl Acad Sci USA. 1986;83:3161–5.

[59] Tosi M, Duponchel C, Bourgarel P, Colomb M, Meo T. Molecular cloning of human C1 inhibitor: sequence homologies with alpha 1-antitripsin and other members of the serpins superfamily. Gene. 1986;42:265–72.

[60] Warin RP, Cunliffe WJ, Greaves MW, Wallington TB. Recurrent angioedema: familial and oestrogen-induced. Br J Dermatol. 1986;115:731–4.

[61] Binkley K, Davis A 3rd. Clinical, biochemical and genetic characterization of a novel estrogen-dependent inherited form of angioedema. J Allergy Clin Immunol. 2000; 106;546–50.

[62] Börk K, Barnstedt SE, Koch P, Traupe H. Hereditary angioedema with normal C1-inhibitor activity in women. Lancet. 2000;356:213–7.

[63] Dewald G, Börk K. Missense mutations in the coagulation factor XII (Hageman Factor) gene in hereditary angioedema with normal C1 inhibitor. Biochem Biophys Res Communs. 2006;343:1286–9.

[64] Cichon S, Martin L, Hennies HC, Muller F, Van Driessche K, Karpushova A, et al. Increased activity of coagulation factor XII (Hageman factor) causes hereditary angioedema type III. Am J Hum Genet. 2006;79:1098–104.

[65] Martin L, Raiso-Peyron N, Nothen M, Cichon S, Drouet C. Hereditary angioedema with normal C1 inhibitor gene in a family with affected women and men is associated with the p.Thr328Lys mutation in the F12 gene. J Allergy Clin Immunol. 2007;120;975–7.

[66] Strang CJ, Cholin S, Spragg J, Davis AE 3rd, Schneeberger EE, Donaldson VH, et al. Angioedema induced by a peptide derived from complement component C2. J Exp Med. 1988;168:1685–98.

[67] Nussberger J, Cugno M, Amstutz C, Cicardi M, Pellacani A, Agostoni A. Plasma bradykinin in angioedema. Lancet. 1998;351:1693–7.

[68] Davis AE. The pathogenesis of hereditary angioedema. Transfus Apheresis Sci. 2003; 29:195–203.

[69] Han ED, MacFarlane RC, Mulligan AN, Scafidi J, Davis AE 3rd. Increased vascular permeability in C1 inhibitor-deficient mice mediated by the bradykinin type 2 receptor. J Clin Invest. 2002;109:1057–63.

[70] Bas M, Bier H, Greve J, Kojda G, Hoffmann TK. Novel pharmacotherapy of acute hereditary angioedema with bradykinin B2-receptor antagonist Icatibant. Allergy. 2006; 61:1490–2.

[71] Bork K, Frank J, Grundt B, Schlattmann P, Nussberger J, Kreuz W. Treatment of acute attacks in hereditary angioedema with a bradykinin receptor-2 antagonist (Icatibant). J Allergy Clin Immunol. 2007; 119: 1497–503.

[72] European Medicines Agency. European Public Assessment Report (EPAR) for Firazyr [updated 01.12.11; accessed 11.01.17]. Available from: http://www.ema.europa.eu/

[73] FDA Cinryze® Approval Letter. Accessed 11.01.07. Available from: http://www.fda.gov/

[74] Burnouf T, Radosevich M. Nanofiltration of plasma-derived biopharmaceutical products. Haemophilia. 2003;9:24–37.

[75] World Health Organization. Annex 4 Guidelines on viral inactivation and removal procedures intended to assure the viral safety of human blood plasma products. WHO Technical Report. 2004;924 Series No.

[76] Zuraw BL, Busse PJ, White M, Jacobs J, Lumry W, Baker J, et al. Nanofiltered C1 inhibitor concentrate for treatment of hereditary angioedema. N Engl J Med. 2010;363:513–22.

[77] Zuraw BL, Kalfus I. Safety and efficacy of prophylactic nanofiltered C1-inhibitorin hereditary angioedema. Am J Med. 2012;125:938.e1–7.31.

[78] European Medicines Agency. European Public Assessment Report (EPAR) for Cinryze [updated 23.11.16; accessed 11.01.17]. Available from: http://www.ema.europa.eu/

[79] European Medicines Agency. European Public Assessment Report (EPAR) for Berinert [accessed 11.01.17]. Available from: http://www.ema.europa.eu/

[80] FDA Berinert® Approval Letter. Accessed 11.01.07. Available from: http://www.fda.gov/

[81] FDA Kalbitor® Approval Letter. Accessed 11.01.07. Available from: http://www.fda.gov/

[82] Choi G, Soeters M, Farkas H, Varga L, Obtulowitz K, Bilo B, et al. Recombinant human C1-inhibitor in the treatment of acute angioedema attacks. Transfusion. 2007;47:1028–32.

[83] European Medicines Agency. European Public Assessment Report (EPAR) for Ruconest [updated 24.05.16; accessed 11.01.17]. Available from: http://www.ema.europa.eu/

[84] FDA Ruconest® Approval Letter. Accessed 11.01.07. Available from: http://www.fda.gov/

[85] Agostoni A, Aygören-Pürsün E, Binkley KE, Blanch A, Bork K, Bouillet L et al. Hereditary and acquired angioedema: Problems and progress: Proceedings of the third C1 esterase Inhibitor deficiency workshop and beyond. J Allergy Clin Immunol. 2004;114:S51–131.

[86] Levi M, Choi G, Picavet C, Hack E. Self-administration of C1-inhibitor concentrate in patients with hereditary or acquired angioedema caused by C1-inhibitor deficiency. J Allergy Clin Immunol. 2006;117:904–8.

[87] Longhurst H, Buckland M, O'Grady C. Home therapy for hereditary angioedema: the Barts experience. C1-Esterase Inhibitor Deficiency Workshop. Budapest. 16–18 May 2003. Abstracts Book. 39–40.

[88] Bygum A, Andersen KE, Mikkelsen CS. Self-administration of intravenous C1-inhibitor therapy for hereditary angioedema and associated quality of life benefits. Eur J Dermatol. 2009, 19:147–51.

[89] Cicardi M, Craig TJ, Martinez-Saguer I, Hébert J, Longhurst HJ. Review of recent guidelines and consensus statements on hereditary angioedema therapy with focus on self-administration. Int Arch Allergy Immunol. 2013;161(Suppl 1):3–9.

[90] Caballero T, Sala-Cunill A, Cancian M, Craig TJ, Neri S, Keith PK et al. Current status of implementation of self-administration training in various regions of Europe, Canada and the USA in the management of hereditary angioedema. Int Arch Allergy Immunol. 2013;161(Suppl 1):10–6.

[91] Bork K. Hereditary angioedema with normal C1 inhibitor. Immunol Allergy Clin North Am. 2013;33:457–70.

[92] Binkley K, Davis A 3rd. Clinical, biochemical and genetic characterization of a novel estrogen-dependent inherited form of angioedema. J Allergy Clin Immunol. 2000;106;546–50.

[93] Bork K, Barnstedt SE, Koch P, Traupe H. Hereditary angioedema with normal C1-inhibitor activity in women. Lancet. 2000;356:213–7.

[94] Marcos C, López Trascasa M, Luna I, González R. Another type of angioedema relative: angioedema induced oestrogen. (Otro tipo de angioedema familiar: angioedema estrógeno-inducido). Rev Esp Alergol Inmunol Clin 2000. XXII Congress of the Spanish Society of Allergology and Clinical Immunology (SEAIC). Pamplona, 16–19 Sept 2000.

[95] Marcos C, López-Lera A, Varela S, Liñares T, Álvarez-Eire MG, López-Trascasa M.Clinical, biochemical and genetic characterization of type III hereditary angioedema in 13 Northwest Spanish families. Ann Allergy Asthma Immunol. 2012; 109:195–200.

[96] Martin L, Degenene D, Toutain A, Ponard D, Watier H. Hereditary angioedema type III: an additional French pedigree with autosomal dominant transmission. J Allergy Clin Immunol. 2001;107:747–8.

[97] Boulliet L, Ponard D, Drouet C, Jullien D, Massot C. Angioedema and oral contraception. Dermatology. 2003;206:106–9.

[98] Dewald G, Börk K. Missense mutations in the coagulation factor XII (Hageman Factor) gene in hereditary angioedema with normal C1 inhibitor. Biochem Biophys Res Commun. 2006;343:1286–9.

[99] Cichon S, Martin L, Hennies HC, Muller F, Van Driessche K, Karpushova A, et al. Increased activity of coagulation factor XII (Hageman factor) causes hereditary angioedema type III. Am J Hum Genet. 2006;79:1098–104.

[100] Martin L, Raiso-Peyron N, Nothen M, Cichon S, Drouet C. Hereditary angioedema with normal C1 inhibitor gene in a family with affected women and men is associated with the p.Thr328Lys mutation in the F12 gene. J Allergy Clin Immunol. 2007;120;975–7.

[101] Börk K, Wulff K, Hardt J, Witzke G, Staubach P. Hereditary angioedema caused by missense mutations in the factor XII gene: clinical features, trigger factors, and therapy. J Allergy Clin Immunol. 2009;124:129–34.

[102] Bork K, Wulff K, Witzke G, Hardt J. Hereditary angioedema with normal C1-INH with versus without specific F12 gene mutations. Allergy. 2015;70:1004–12.

[103] de Maat S, Björkqvist J, Suffritti C, Wiesenekker CP, Nagtegaal W, Koekman A, et al. Plasmin is a natural trigger for bradykinin production in patients with hereditary angioedema with factor XII mutations. J Allergy Clin Immunol. 2016;138:1414–23.

[104] Serrano C, Guilarte M, Tella R, Dalmau G, Bartra J, Gaig P, et al. Estrogen-dependent hereditary angio-oedema with normal C1 inhibitor: description of six new cases and review of pathogenic mechanisms and treatment. Allergy. 2008;63:735–41.

[105] Prieto A, Tornero P, Rubio M, Fernandez-Cruz E, Rodriguez-Sainz C. Missense mutation Thr309Lys in the coagulation factor XII gene in a Spanish family with hereditary angioedema type III. Allergy. 2009;64:284–6.

[106] Baeza ML, Rodríguez-Marco A, Prieto A, Rodríguez-Sainz C, Zubeldia JM, Rubio M. Factor XII gene missense mutation Thr328Lys in an Arab family with hereditary angioedema type III. Allergy. 2011;66:981–2.

[107] Gómez-Traseira C, López-Lera A, Drouet C, López-Trascasa M, Pérez-Fernández E, Favier B, et al. Hereditary angioedema caused by the p.Thr309Lys mutation in the F12 gene: a multifactorial disease. J Allergy Clin Immunol. 2013;132:986–9.e1-5.

[108] Piñero-Saavedra M, González-Quevedo T, Saenz de San Pedro B, Alcaraz C, Bobadilla-González P, Fernández-Vieira L, et al. Hereditary angioedema with F12 mutation: Clinical features and enzyme polymorphisms in 9 Southwestern Spanish families. Ann Allergy Asthma Immunol. 2016;117:520–526.

[109] Vitrat-Hincky V, Gompel A, Dumestre-Perard C, Boccon-Gibod I, Drouet C, Cesbron JY, et al. Type III hereditary angio-oedema: clinical and biological features in a French cohort. Allergy 2010;65:1331–6.

[110] Duan QL, Binkley K, Rouleau GA. Genetic analysis of factor XII and bradykinin catabolic enzymes in a family with estrogen-dependent inherited angioedema. J Allergy Clin Immunol. 2009;123:906–10.

[111] Börk K, Wulff K, Meinke P, Wagner N, Hardt J, Witzke G. A novel mutation in the coagulation factor 12 gene in subjects with hereditary angioedema and normal C1I inhibitor. Clin Immunol. 2011;141:31–5.

[112] Kiss N, Barabás E, Várnai K, Halász A, Varga LÁ, Prohászka Z et al. Novel duplication in the F12 gene in a patient with recurrent angioedema. Clin Immunol. 2013;149:142–5.

[113] Grumach AS, Stieber C, Veronez CL, Cagini N, Constantino-Silva RN, Cordeiro E, et al. Homozygosity for a factor XII mutation in one female and one male patient with hereditary angio-oedema. Allergy. 2016;71:119–23.

[114] Börk K. Diagnosis and treatment of hereditary angioedema with normal C1 inhibitor. Allergy Asthma Clin Immunol. 2010;6:15.

[115] Bouillet L, Boccon-Gibod I, Ponard D, Drouet C, Cesbron JY, Dumestre-Perard C, et al. Bradykinin receptor 2 antagonist (Icatibant) for hereditary angioedema type III attacks. Ann Allergy Asthma Immunol. 2009;103:448.

Chapter 15

Pseudoangioedema

Sevgi Akarsu and Ecem Canturk

Additional information is available at the end of the chapter

http://dx.doi.org/10.5772/67850

Abstract

Angioedema is a rapid, localized and temporary subcutaneous edema, which targets the lips, eyelids, gastrointestinal and respiratory mucosa resulting in abdominal pain, asthma and even serious life-threatening conditions like airway obstruction. There are several other disorders such as allergic contact dermatitis, drug rash with eosinophilia and systemic symptoms (DRESS), superior vena cava syndrome (SVCS), orofacial granulomatosis and so on, which manifest with subcutaneous swelling and masquerade as angioedema and are known as 'pseudoangioedema' in the literature. Knowledge of pseudoangioedema for healthcare professionals is crucial to avoid potentially serious results of misdiagnosis such as further investigations, unnecessary applications and delayed diagnosis. We aim to discuss differential diagnosis of angioedema and help physicians recognize the typical features of angioedema and its differential diagnosis in this chapter.

Keywords: angioedema, pseudoangioedema, angioedematous, pseudoangioedematous, angioedema differential diagnosis, angioedema mimickers, swellings mimic angioedema, masquerading as angioedema, angioedema similar disease

1. Introduction

Angioedema is defined as a rapid, localized and temporary swelling of the skin and/or mucous membranes caused by increased endothelial permeability and extravasation of intravascular fluid into the interstitial tissues. It has predilection sites, including the lips, tongue, eyelids, gastrointestinal and respiratory mucosa [1, 2]. Angioedema represents one of the most common airway emergencies, so quick diagnosis and intervention mean the life of a patient. Although coexistence with urticaria is frequent (50%), angioedema without urticaria is defined as a distinct disease. Angioedema without urticaria, called Quincke's edema/angioneurotic edema, is classified into two main categories: hereditary and acquired angioedema [1–3]. Hereditary angioedema is a severe and rare form caused by genetic mutations in the complement C1 inhibitor, factor XII gene or unknown etiology. Four types of acquired angioedema are identified: idiopathic histaminergic angioedema, idiopathic non-histaminergic angioedema, acquired angioedema related to angiotensin-converting enzyme inhibitors and acquired angioedema with C1 inhibitor deficiency [3]. Several disorders can cause subcutaneous swelling and are often misdiagnosed as angioedema. These conditions which mimic angioedema are known as 'pseudoangioedema' in the literature [2, 4]. Misdiagnosis may lead to life-threatening results because of ineffective management of these serious medical conditions. There are some clues help distinguish angioedema from other causes of swelling. Angioedema is characterized by asymetric and transient swelling, typically lasting 24–48 hours. It is essential to be aware of angioedema mimickers for healthcare professionals in both the emergency and outpatient setting [1, 2, 4].

2. Research design

This chapter based on a literature search in Pubmed using the keywords 'angioedema', 'pseudoangioedema', 'angioedematous', 'pseudoangioedematous', 'angioedema differential diagnosis', 'angioedema mimickers', 'swellings mimic angioedema', 'masquerading as angioedema' and 'angioedema similar disease'. Case reports, clinical trials, cohort studies, systematic reviews and meta-analyses associated with these keywords published up until now were evaluated.

3. Differential diagnosis for pseudoangioedematous disorders

The most common and important angioedema mimickers are discussed in this chapter.

3.1. Contact dermatitis

Contact dermatitis is an inflammatory skin disease due to delayed type hypersensitivity response after a direct contact with irritating or allergenic foreign substances. Contact dermatitis of the face frequently causes severe swelling of the facial and periorbital skin similar to angioedema [2, 4, 5], as in our case (**Figure 1**).

The first manifestation of contact dermatitis may be angioedema-like swelling but after a while, superficial erythema, vesicles or blisters and later eczematous dermatitis develop, whereas angioedema does not have these clinical signs [2, 4]. It can also be distinguished from angioedema by a history of exposure to chemical agents, especially cosmetic products. Facial contact dermatitis is becoming a common problem because of the increase in the use of cosmetic products, and the cosmetic market has grown progressively. Unlike angioedema, antihistamines are not effective, and causative agents can be identified by an epidermal patch test [5].

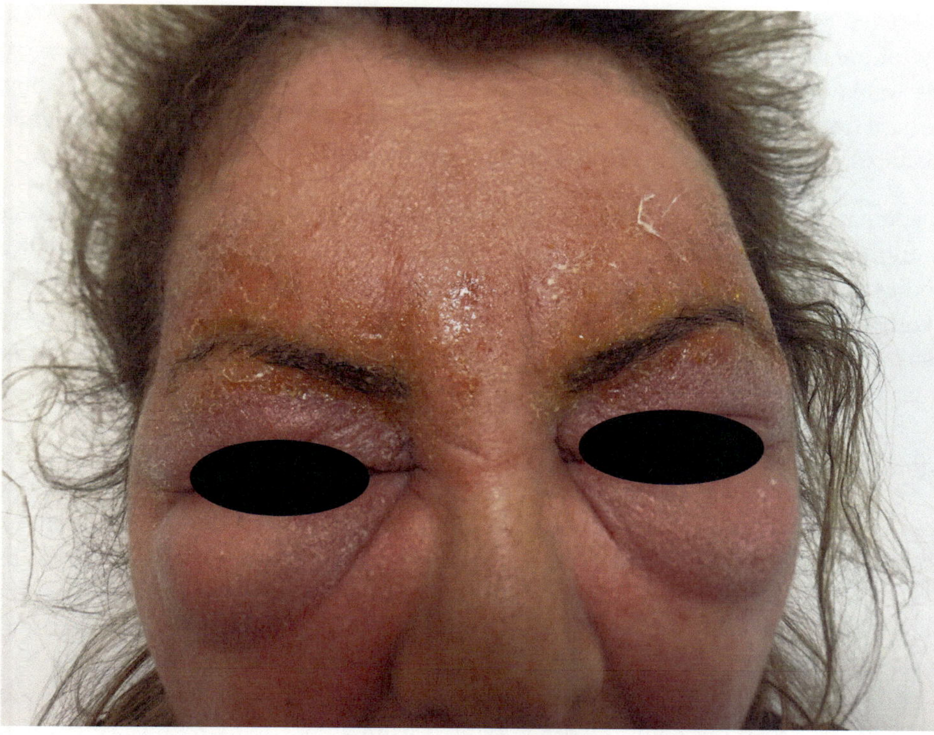

Figure 1. Contact dermatitis with severe facial swelling after hair dyeing.

3.2. Drug rash with eosinophilia and systemic symptoms (DRESS)

DRESS syndrome is a rare life-threatening cutaneous adverse drug-induced reaction associated with 10% mortality. Aromatic anticonvulsants, especially phenytoin, carbamazepine and phenobarbital, are the most common causes of DRESS [6–9]. Although there can be various manifestations, it usually starts as diffuse morbilliform rash later becoming indurated with associated edema. There is often aberrant facial edema, especially in the periorbital and mid-facial region that can sometimes be mistaken for angioedema. 25% of patients have prominent facial swelling [6, 8]. History of medication, lymphadenopathy and other systemic findings and laboratory test results such as eosinophilia help differentiate this medical condition from angioedema. The onset of symptoms occurs 2–6 weeks after drug administration, longer than other drug reactions. There is no reliable standard for the diagnosis of DRESS, and management is the discontinuation of the causative drug [6, 9].

3.3. Dermatomyositis and lupus erythematosus

Dermatomyositis is an autoimmune inflammatory disorder, which affects the skin, muscles and blood vessels. Cutaneous manifestations are intense erythema and edema on the dorsum of the hands and periorbital region [10–13]. Heliotrope rash is a distinctive feature defined as periorbital erythema with symmetrically distributed edema. Gottron papules are erythematous to violaceous plaques often on the extensor joints of hands [10, 12, 13]. Although it may mimic angioedema due to periorbital edema, accompanying symmetrical proximal muscle weakness, fatigue, weight loss and elevated serum creatine kinase levels distinguish the disease from angioedema [14]. Diagnosis is confirmed by typical, clinical electromyography patterns, elevated muscle enzymes and muscle biopsy [12, 13].

Angioedematous appearance of the periorbital area is also a rare presentation of systemic lupus erythematosus. A pathophysiological mechanism of this condition is explained by autoantibodies against C1 inhibitor causing acquired deficiency of C1 esterase inhibitor [15, 16]. Although periorbital edema as the sole presenting manifestation of cutaneous lupus erythematosus is extremely rare, it is very rarely associated with discoid lupus erythematosus and lupus erythematosus profundus [17, 18].

3.4. Morbihan disease

Rosacea is a common cutaneous disease that affects middle-aged individuals present with a variety of clinical manifestations. Morbus Morbihan is a rare complication of rosacea characterized by chronic erythematous edema of the face, exclusively in the forehead and periorbital region which mimics angioedema [19, 20]. There is no specific laboratory and histopathologic findings to verify diagnosis. The patient has no complaint. Furthermore, other clinical features of rosacea like telangiectases, inflammatory papules and pustules may not be present as well [19]. This disorder could be differentiated from angioedema by refractory, aberrant and solid edema without spontaneous involution [4]. Reported therapies include systemic corticosteroids, tetracyclines, isotretinoin, clofazimine and ketotifen. Excision of redundant edematous tissue is a surgical alternative treatment [21].

3.5. Superior vena cava syndrome

Superior vena cava syndrome (SVCS) is an obstruction or severe reduction in blood flow through the superior vena cava. SVCS has been associated with infections and malignancies but more recently, with the increased use of intravascular devices; as in our case (**Figure 2**), more cases have been associated with pacemaker implantations. Despite the increase in thrombus-related SVCS, malignancies remain the most common cause of SVCS. Facial and neck swelling which mimic angioedema is present in 82% of the patients [22, 23].

However, angioedema symptoms are often episodic, whereas SVCS is characteristically persistent and progressive. The other clue to differentiate SVCS from angioedema is increase of signs when the patient is in a supine position [23]. Diagnosis of SVCS is confirmed by a Doppler ultrasound and CT scan of the chest including thoracic inlet. Prognosis and treatment of SVCS depend on the underlying disease [22, 23].

3.6. Subcutaneous emphysema

Subcutaneous emphysema is a rare disease with the sudden onset of swelling as a result of air entrapment under the skin [24–27]. There are various causes including blunt or

http://dx.doi.org/10.5772/67850

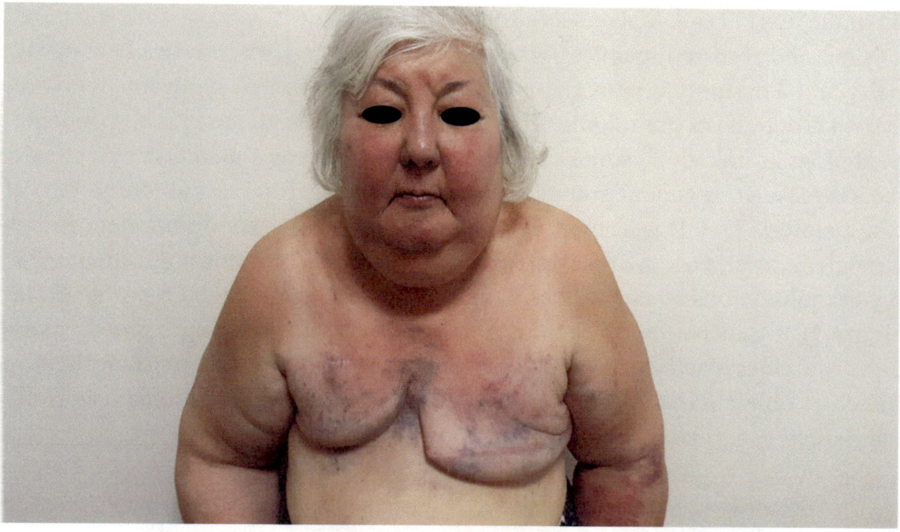

Figure 2. Facial and neck swelling with dilatation of pectoral veins in a patient with superior vena cava syndrome.

penetrating trauma to the chest or neck, following gastrointestinal perforation (corrosive burns of the esophagus, Boerhaave's syndrome, gas gangrene), diving injuries, endoscopy, tracheostomy, cryosurgery, dental surgery or skin biopsy [24]. The majority of the cases which mimic angioedema is reported after a dental surgery [24, 27]. The main clinical clue for differentiation from angioedema is a characteristic crackling sensation created as the gas is pushed through the tissue during palpation which is called crepitus [4, 24, 26]. In doubtful cases, an X-ray or a CT scan could be performed [25]. Severe subcutaneous emphysema can cause compression of the upper airway and jugular venous compression, which can lead to airway and cardiovascular compromise. Trauma-related causes may require emergent surgical intervention [27].

3.7. Hypothyroidism

Low levels of thyroid hormones cause symptoms including weight gain, constipation, dry skin, thinning of hair, hoarse voice, fatigue, lethargy, depression and cold intolerance. Eyelid swelling associated with hypothyroidism is uncommon and can occasionally mimic angioedema [28, 29]. Eyelid swelling is a clinical sign of severe acute hypothyroidism. Other more common dermatologic manifestations of hypothyroidism are thin, dry, rough, hyperkeratotic skin and rough, brittle hair [28]. In the case of sudden-onset, permanent, asymptomatic and bilateral soft swelling, hypothyroidism should be suspected. Diagnosis is confirmed with low levels of thyroid hormones, and treatment is hormone replacement [4, 28, 29].

3.8. Orofacial granulomatosis

Orofacial granulomatosis is a rare disease which presents as a swelling of the oral and maxillofacial region secondary to granulomatous reaction. The most common clinical presentation is swelling of the lips [30–32]. Melkersson-Rosenthal syndrome is an idiopathic disorder involving persistent and recurrent painless swelling of the face and lips, classically associated with facial palsy and a fissured tongue. Cases of Melkersson-Rosenthal syndrome with only labial involvement is defined as granulomatous cheilitis, which masquerades as angioedema [29, 31, 33]. The etiology is unknown, some authors hypothesized it as a manifestation of sarcoidosis or Crohn's disease. Ano-genital granulomatosis may be regarded as the counterpart of orofacial granulomatosis [34]. It is also a rare chronic inflammatory condition that can present as diffuse penile, scrotal, vulvar or ano-perineal swelling which mimic angioedema [34, 35]. In addition, granulomatous reactions after cosmetic dermal filler injection reports, similar to our case (**Figure 3**), are increasing in the last decades due to the growing cosmetic market [36]. Although some clues like the chronic and persistent nature of edema persist, histopathological examination is obligated for differential diagnosis of orofacial granulomatosis from angioedema and other pseudoangioedematous disorders [30–36].

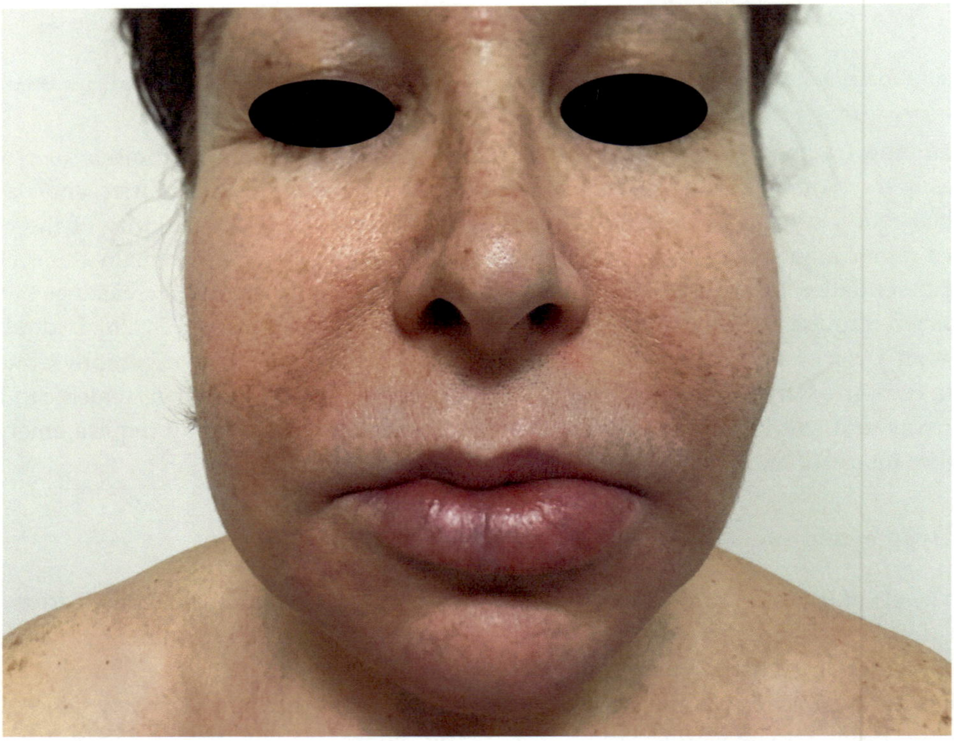

Figure 3. Granulomatous reaction on the lips and mandibular area 7 years after dermal filler injection.

Systemic steroid therapy is widely used for orofacial granulomatosis, Melkersson-Rosenthal syndrome and other granulomatous foreign body reaction such as cosmetic dermal fillers [30–36]. A combination of minocycline, clofazamine, non-steroidal anti-inflammatory drugs and thalidomide is reported as other therapies for Melkersson-Rosenthal syndrome [32, 33]. Surgical excision is another alternative option for Melkersson-Rosenthal syndrome and granulomatous foreign body reaction [32, 36].

3.9. Hypocomplementemic urticarial vasculitis syndrome

Urticarial vasculitis is characterized by recurrent urticarial lesions, angioedema and histologically with necrotizing venulitis. The patients have been categorized into two subgroups: those with hypocomplementemia and those with normal complement levels [37–39]. Hypocomplementemic urticarial vasculitis syndrome is a rare entity associated with urticaria and persistent acquired hypocomplementemia. It was identified as a systemic lupus erythematosus-related syndrome or hypocomplementemic cutaneous vasculitis [37]. Angioedema occurs in up to 50% of patients, frequently involving the lips, tongue, periorbital tissue and hands and can be the first sign of this syndrome. Characteristic cutaneous lesions of hypocomplementemic urticarial vasculitis syndrome are painful and usually resolve with postinflammatory hyperpigmentation. There are also systemic findings such as renal, pulmonary, gastrointestinal, neurologic, rheumatologic and ophthalmic. Treatment is determined by severity and systemic involvement of the disease, including systemic corticosteroids and immunosuppressants [37–39].

3.10. Weber-Christian disease

Weber-Christian disease (relapsing febrile panniculitis) is a very rare lobular panniculitis subtype associated with painful subcutaneous nodules, which are mainly present in the extremities and trunk, and systemic symptoms include fever, malaise, polyarthralgia and so on. [40]. Typically, lesions are distributed symmetrically on the legs and thighs. Furthermore, periorbital lesions which mimic angioedema can be detected in Weber-Christian disease, as well. Diagnosis is based on histological and clinical findings. Treatment of Weber-Christian disease includes systemic corticosteroid, non-steroidal anti-inflammatory drugs, anti-malarial drugs and immunosuppressive drugs in resistant cases [2, 40].

3.11. Infections

Infections localized in the tongue, lips and periorbital area cause swelling and masquerade as angioedema. Such infections persist until treated and thus must be differentiated from acute angioedema [2, 29]. It is important to consider infection as well as angioedema when confronted with lower lip swelling in the emergency department [41, 42]. Few cases of methicillin-resistant *Staphylococcus aureus*-related facial or lip infections mimicking angioedema are present in the literature [42]. Tongue abscess is also a very rare entity, causes enlargement of the tongue, and can be easily misdiagnosed as angioedema. Medical history of injury by foreign body, trauma or piercing of the tongue is helpful for differentiation from angioedema [42, 43].

Parasitic infections may be the reason for pseudoangioedema. Trichinosis and tropical filariasis can present as periorbital edema and be easily misdiagnosed as angioedema as well. Romana's sign is unilateral periorbital swelling detected in Chagas disease (also known as American trypanosomiasis) and mimics angioedema [2, 29].

3.12. Lymphoproliferative disorders

Lymphoproliferative diseases, B-cell lymphomas and monoclonal gammopathy of undetermined significance cause acquired angioedema secondary to C1 inhibitor deficiency.

Previously, a few rare cases of peripheral T-cell lymphoma presenting periorbital, upper and lower lip edema, initially mistaken for angioedema, are reported [44–46]. The clinical findings to differentiate from angioedema are progression and no resolution of these lesions. The final diagnosis is based on histopathologic examination [2, 45, 46].

3.13. Mucinosis and other infiltrating disorders

The most common pseudoangioedematous endocrinopathy is autoimmune thyroid disorder [1, 2]. Thyroid orbitopathy is a gradual swelling of the periorbital tissue related to severe hypothyroidism or Grave's disease. Both facial myxedema due to hypothyroidism and pre-tibial myxedema due to Grave's disease are caused by mucin deposition in the dermis [47, 48].

Scleromyxedema (papular mucinosis) is dermal mucin deposition without thyroid disease. It is frequently detected with paraproteinemia [1, 2, 49, 50]. The clinical features consist of forehead swelling and deep longitudinal furrows cause a lion-like face [49, 50].

The amyloidosis is a group of diseases, which is a result of extracellular deposition of amyloid fibrils. Pathognomonic clinical features of systemic amyloidosis include a combination of macroglossia and periorbital purpura [51]. Macroglossia could masquerade as angioedema which affects the tongue. Other systemic involvements (cardiac, renal and neurologic, etc.) and aberrant persistent edema are helpful to differentiate this clinical entity from angioedema. Diagnosis is confirmed by Congo red staining of amyloid fibrils in the histopathologic examination [2, 51].

3.14. Clarkson's disease (idiopathic systemic capillary leak syndrome)

Idiopathic systemic capillary leak syndrome, called Clarkson's disease, is a rare life-threatening disease manifested by recurrent episodes of sudden hypovolemic shock and massive edema due to the capillary leakage of plasma from the intravascular to the extravascular compartments. Approximately 79–82% of these patients have monoclonal gammopathy of unknown significance [1, 52, 53]. Angioedema should be considered upon the initial presentation of Clarkson's disease. Generalized symmetrical cutaneous swelling and a characteristic triad of hypotension, hemoconcentration and hypoalbuminemia in the absence of secondary causes of shock are helpful clinical features to differentiate from angioedema [1, 4]. Systemic corticosteroids and intravenous immunoglobulin are used in the treatment of this condition [52, 53].

3.15. Gleich's syndrome (episodic angioedema with eosinophilia)

Gleich's syndrome is a rare disorder characterized by episodes of angioedema, eosinophilia and resolves spontaneously without therapy. The etiology is unknown and typical clinical features are angioedema, fever, eosinophilia, elevated serum IgM, increased body weight and benign course without internal organ involvement [1, 4, 54]. The presence of specific laboratory features, together with the other characteristic clinical manifestations, should differentiate this entity from classical angioedema [4]. Systemic corticosteroids and imatinib have been reported beneficial for its treatment [1, 4].

http://dx.doi.org/10.5772/67850

3.16. Idiopathic edema

Idiopathic edema is the persistent self-limited fluid retention in the gravitationally dependent areas, especially on the lower limbs. There is a female predominance and it is prominent in premenstrual periods, which is why the condition is also known as 'cyclical edema' [4, 55]. After a prolonged supine position, the facial and periorbital region may be included as well. It can be differentiated with symmetrical involvement and pitting edema from angioedema. Diagnosis is confirmed by exclusion of cardiac, hepatic, renal or thyroid disease, all well-known causes of edema [4].

3.17. Cluster headache

Cluster headache is a primary headache disorder typically characterized by severe recurrent attacks of unilateral pain with conjunctival injection, nasal congestion or rhinorrhea, ptosis or miosis and periorbital edema. Unilateral edema of the eyelid or the face is reported in 74% of the patients [4, 56]. Pain is intense and unresponsive to antihistamines and topical steroids. The characteristic headache with other clinical signs is helpful in the differential diagnosis of cluster headaches and angioedema [4].

4. Summary

Angioedema manifests with asymmetric, non-pitting and transient edema, which has predilection areas including the lips, tongue and periorbital region. Diagnosis and treatment of angioedema are crucial because it represents one of the most common airway emergencies. As a result, knowledge of typical clinical features and differential diagnosis for healthcare professionals are obligations. It is important to remember that not all swellings are angioedema in the clinical practice. Pseudoangioedematous disorders should be considered in patients presenting with long-lasting and resistant swellings. The most frequent diseases that mimic angioedema are acute contact dermatitis, DRESS syndrome, hypothyroidism, orofacial granulomatosis, idiopathic edema, vasculitis and panniculitis. These conditions do not respond to angioedema treatment and may cause serious life-threatening results. It is possible to recognize pseudoangioedema by detailed medical history and physical examination, but skin biopsy is required for resistant cases.

Author details

Sevgi Akarsu* and Ecem Canturk

*Address all correspondence to: sevgi.akarsu@deu.edu.tr

Department of Dermatology, Faculty of Medicine, Dokuz Eylul University, Izmir, Turkey

References

[1] Gunes A, Akarsu S. Angioedema: diagnosis and treatment approaches. Turkderm-Archives of the Turkish Dermatology and Venereology. 2013; **47**: 7–18. doi:10.4274/turkderm.35651

[2] David W. Differential diagnosis of angioedema. Immunology and Allergy Clinics of North America. 2006; **26**: 603–613. doi:http://dx.doi.org/10.1016/j.iac.2006.09.006

[3] Cicardi M, Aberer W, Banerji A, Bas M, Bernstein JA, Bork K, Caballero T, Farkas H, Grumach A, Kaplan AP, Riedl MA, Triggiani M, Zanichelli A, Zuraw B. Classification, diagnosis, and approach to treatment for angioedema: consensus report from the Hereditary Angioedema International Working Group. European Journal of Allergy and Clinical Immunology. 2014; **69**(5): 602–616. doi:10.1111/all.12380

[4] Andersen M, Hilary J, Longhurst H, Rasmussen E, Bygum A. How not to be misled by disorders mimicking angioedema: a review of pseudoangioedema. International Archives Allergy and Immunology. 2016; **169**: 163–170. doi:10.1159/000445835

[5] Kasemsarn P, Iamphonrat T, Boonchai W. Risk factors and common contact allergens in facial allergic contact dermatitis patients. International Journal of Dermatology. 2016; **55**: 417–424. doi:10.1111/ijd.12880

[6] Walsh SA, Creamer D. Drug reaction with eosinophilia and systemic symptoms (DRESS): a clinical update and review of current thinking. Clinical and Experimental Dermatology. 2011; **36**(1): 6–11. doi:10.1111/j.1365-2230.2010.03967.x

[7] Sharma RK, Tibdewal P, Sharma N, Sikri T, Sikri H, Sharma A, Ankur. DRESS syndrome: (drug, rash, eosinophilia and systemic symptoms) – the hypersensitivity reaction due to antipsychotic drug – quetiapine, the pictorial presentation. Journal of Pioneering Medical Sciences. 2015; **5**(3): 92–93

[8] Husain Z, Reddy BY, Schwartz RA. DRESS syndrome: part I. Clinical perspectives. Journal of American Academy of Dermatology. 2013; **68**(5): 1–14. doi:10.1016/j.jaad.2013.01.033

[9] Jeung YJ, Lee JY, Oh MJ, Choi DC, Lee BJ. Comparison of the causes and clinical features of drug rash with eosinophilia and systemic symptoms and Stevens-Johnson syndrome. Allergy Asthma et Immunology Research. 2010; **2**: 123–126. doi:10.4168/aair.2010.2.2.123

[10] Ramos-E-Silva M, Pinto AP, Pirmez R, Cuzzi T, Carneiro SC. Dermatomyositis – part 1: definition, epidemiology, etiology and pathogenesis, and clinics. Skinmed Journal. 2016; **14**(4): 273–279.

[11] Milisenda JC, Doti PI, Prieto-González S, Grau JM. Dermatomyositis presenting with severe subcutaneous edema: five additional cases and review of the literature. Seminars in Arthritis and Rheumatism. 2014; **44**(2): 228–233. doi:10.1016/j.semarthrit.2014.04.004

[12] Muro Y, Sugiura K, Akiyama M. Cutaneous manifestations in dermatomyositis: key clinical and serological features – a comprehensive review. Clinical Reviews in Allergy & Immunology. 2016; **51**(3): 293–302. doi:10.1007/s12016-015-8496-5

[13] Iaccarino L, Ghirardello A, Bettio S, Zen M, Gatto M, Punzi L, Gatto M. The clinical features, diagnosis and classification of dermatomyositis. Journal of Autoimmunity. 2014; **48–49**: 122–127. doi:10.1016/j.jaut.2013.11.005

[14] Kaplan AP, Greaves MW. Angioedema. Journal of American Academy of Dermatology. 2005; **53**: 373–388.

[15] Bienstock D, Mandel L. Facial angioedema and systemic lupus erythematosus: case report. Journal of Oral and Maxillofacial Surgery. 2015; **73**(5): 928–932.

[16] Habibagahi Z, Ruzbeh J, Yarmohammadi V, Kamali M, Rastegar MH. Refractory angioedema in a patient with systemic lupus erythematosus. Iranian Journal of Medical Sciences. 2015; **40**(4): 372–375.

[17] Makeeva V, Seminario-Vidal L, Beckum K, Sami N. Bilateral periorbital swelling as the initial presentation of cutaneous lupus erythematosus. Journal of American Academy of Dermatology. 2016; **2**(1): 72–76. doi:10.1016/j.jdcr.2015.12.009

[18] Ghaninejad H, Kavusi S, Safar F, Asgari M, Naraghi ZS. Persistent periorbital edema as a sole manifestation of cutaneous lupus erythematosus: report of two cases. Dermatology Online Journal. 2006; **12**(2): 14.

[19] Stephanie W, Robinson M, Meehan SA, Cohen DE. Morbihan disease. Dermatology Online Journal. 2012; **18**(12): 27.

[20] Lamparter J, Kottler U, Cursiefen C, Pfeiffer N, Pitz S. Morbus Morbihan: a rare cause of edematous swelling of the eyelids. Ophthalmologe. 2010; **107**(6): 553–557. doi:10.1007/s00347-009-2083-1

[21] Veraldi S, Persico MC, Francia C. Morbihan syndrome. Indian Dermatology Online Journal. 2013; **4**(2): 122–124. doi:10.4103/2229-5178.110639

[22] Herscovici R, Szyper-Kravitz M, Altman A, Eshet Y, Nevo M, Agmon-Levin N, Shoenfeld Y. Superior vena cava syndrome – changing etiology in the third millennium. Lupus. 2012; **21**: 93–96. doi:10.1177/0961203311412412

[23] Berksoy Hayta S, Güner R, Arslan S, Gümüs C, Akyol M. A case of pseudoangioedema as a superior vena cava syndrome. Cumhuriyet Medical Journal. 2016; **38**(2). doi:10.7197/cmj.v38i2.5000192511

[24] Dhawan AK, Singal A, Bisherwal K, Pandhi D. Subcutaneous emphysema mimicking angioedema. Indian Dermatology Online Journal. 2016; **7**(1): 55–56. doi:10.4103/2229-5178.174304

[25] Jensen P, Johansen UB, Thyssen JP. Cryotherapy caused widespread subcutaneous emphysema mimicking angiooedema. Acta Dermato-Venereologica. 2014; **94**: 241. doi: 10.2340/00015555-1663

[26] Cakmak SK, Gonul M, Gul U, Kilic A, Demirel O. Subcutaneous emphysema mimicking angioedema.JournalofDermatology.2006;**33**:902–903.doi:10.1111/j.1346-8138.2006.00207.x

[27] McKenzie SW, Rosenberg M. Iatrogenic subcutaneous emphysema of dental and surgical origin: a literature review. Journal of Oral and Maxillofacial Surgery. 2009; **67**: 1265–1268. doi:10.1016/j.joms.2008.12.050

[28] Nievasa MS, Santiago SA. Bilateral eyelid swelling associated with acute hypothyroidism. Actas Dermo-Sifiliograficas. 2014; **105**: 427–429. doi:10.1016/j.adengl.2013.05.009

[29] Van Dellen RG, Maddox DE, Dutta EJ. Masqueraders of angioedema and urticaria. Annals of Allergy, Asthma & Immunology. 2002; **88**(1): 10–15. doi:10.1016/S1081-1206(10)63586-7

[30] Tilakaratne WM, Freysdottir J, Fortune F. Orofacial granulomatosis: review on etiology and pathogenesis. Journal Oral Pathology Medicine. 2008; **37**(4): 191–195. doi:10.1111/j.1600-0714.2007.00591.x

[31] Rogers RS. Granulomatous cheilitis, Melkersson-Rosenthal syndrome, and orofacial granulomatosis. Archives of Dermatology. 2000; **136**: 1557–1558

[32] Leâo JC, Hodgson T, Scully C, Porter S. Review article: orofacial granulomatosis. Alimentary Pharmacology and Therapeutics. 2004; **20**: 1019–1027. doi: 10.1111/ j.1365-2036.2004.02205.x

[33] Charlene Kakimoto C, Sparks C, White AA. Melkersson-Rosenthal syndrome: a form of pseudoangioedema. Annals of Allergy, Asthma & Immunology. 2007; **99**: 185–189. doi:10.1016/S1081-1206(10)60643-6

[34] Van de Scheur MR, Van der Waal RIF, Van der Waal I, Stoof TJ, Van Deventer SJH. Anogenital granulomatosis: the counterpart of oro-facial granulomatosis. Journal of the European Academy of Dermatology and Venereology. 2003; **17**: 184–189.

[35] Makatsori M, Manson AL, Gurugama P, Wakelin S, Seneviratne SL. Penile granulomatosis presenting as pseudoangioedema. European Annals of Allergy and Clinical Immunology. 2013; **45**(3): 111–112.

[36] Chen Y, Chen M, Chiu Y. A case of mimicking angioedema: chin silicone granulomatous reaction spreading all over the face after receiving liquid silicone injection forty years previously. Chinese Medical Journal. 2011; **124**(11): 1747–1750.

[37] Saigal K, Valencia IC, Cohen J, Kerdel FA. Hypocomplementemic urticarial vasculitis with angioedema, a rare presentation of systemic lupus erythematosus: rapid response to rituximab. Journal of the American Academy of Dermatology. 2003; **49**(5): 283–285. doi:10.1016/S0190

[38] Jara LJ, Navarro C, Medina G, Lastra OV, Saavedra MA. Hypocomplementemic urticarial vasculitis syndrome. Current Rheumatology Reports. 2009; **11**: 410. doi:10.1007/s11926-009-0060-y

[39] Buck A, Christensen J, McCarty M. Hypocomplementemic urticarial vasculitis syndrome: a case report and literature review. Journal of Clinical and Aesthetic Dermatology. 2012; 5(1): 36–46.

[40] Wang HP, Huang CC, Chen CH. Weber-Christian disease presenting with intractable fever and periorbital swelling mimicking angioedema. Clinical Rheumatology. 2006. doi:10.1007/s10067-006-0235-0

[41] Cohen PR, Kurzrock R. Community-acquired methicillin-resistant *Staphylococcus aureus* skin infection: an emerging clinical problem. Journal of American Academy of Dermatology. 2004; **50**: 277–280. doi:10.1016/j.jaad.2003.06.005

[42] Lucerna AR, Espinosa J, Darlington AM. Methıcıllın-resıstant *Staphylococcus aureus* lip infection mimicking angioedema. The Journal of Emergency Medicine. 2015; **49**(1): 8–11.

[43] Riccardi A, Dignetti P, Tasso F, Caiti M, Lerza R. Tongue abscess: a rare occurrence possibly mimicking angioedema. Emergency Care Journal. 2013; **9**(23): 70–71. doi:10.4081/ecj.2013.e23.e

[44] Fricker M, Dubach P, Helbling A, Diamantis E, Villiger PM, Novak U. Not all facial swellings are angioedemas! Journal of Investigative Allergology and Clinical Immunology. 2015; **25**(2): 133–162.

[45] Patel S, Patel R, Draikiwicz S, Capitle E. Peripheral T-cell lymphoma: a challenging mimicker of angioedema and urticaria. Annals of Allergy Asthma & Immunology. 2015; **115**: 995. doi:10.1016/j.anai.2015.06.013

[46] Harrison NK, Twelves C, Addis BJ, Taylor AJ, Souhami RL, Isaacson PG. Peripheral T-cell lymphoma presenting with angioedema and diffuse pulmonary infiltrates. The American Review of Respiratory Disease. 1988; **138**: 976–980. doi:10.1164/ajrccm/138.4.976

[47] Rebora A, Rongioletti F. Mucinoses. Bolognia JL, Jorizzo JL, Rapini RP. Dermatology, 2012; **8**(46): 687–698.

[48] Heymann WR. Cutaneous manifestations of thyroid disease. Journal of American Academy of Dermatology. 1992; **26**(6): 885–902.

[49] Rongioletti F, Rebora A. Updated classification of papular mucinosis, lichen myxedematosus and scleromyxedema. Journal of American Academy of Dermatology. 2001; **44**: 273–281.

[50] Polat A, Kapicioglu Y, Sahin N, Yilmaz M. A case of angioedema-like atypic scleromyxedema responding to treatment with steroid. Turkderm: Archives of the Turkish Dermatology and Venereology. 2016; **50**(1): 28–30.

[51] Wechalekar AD, Path FRC, Gillmore JD, Hawkins NP. Systemic amyloidosis. The Lancet. 2016; **387**(10038): 2641–2654.

[52] Druey KM, Greipp PR. Narrative review: Clarkson disease – systemic capillary leak syndrome. Annals of Internal Medicine. 2010; **153**: 90–98. doi:10.1059/0003-4819-153-2-201007200-00005

[53] Kapoor P, Greipp PT, Schaefer EW, Mandrekar SJ, Kamal AH, Gonzalez-Paz NC, Kumar S, Greipp P. Idiopathic systemic capillary leak syndrome (Clarkson's disease): the Mayo Clinic experience. Mayo Clinic Proceedings. 2010; **85**(10): 905–912. doi:10.4065/mcp.2010.015

[54] Cho HJ, Yoo HS, Kim M, Shin Y, Ye Y, Kim J, Choi J, Park S, Park H. Clinical characteristics of angioedema with eosinophilia. Allergy & Asthma Immunology Research. 2014; **6**(4): 362–365. doi:10.4168/aair.2014.6.4.362

[55] Grigoriadou S, Longhurst HJ. Clinical immunology review series: an approach to the patient with angioedema. Clinical and Experimental Immunology. 2009; **155**: 367–377. doi:10.1111/j.1365-2249.2008.03845.x

[56] Nesbitt AD, Goadsby PJ. Cluster headache. British Medical Journal. 2012; **344**(2407): 1–9. doi:10.1136/bmj.e2407